Library of
Davidson College

The Language of the Heart,
1600–1750

NEW CULTURAL STUDIES

Series Editors

Joan DeJean
Carroll Smith-Rosenberg
Peter Stallybrass
and Gary A. Tomlinson

A complete list of books in the series
is available from the publisher.

The Language of the Heart, 1600–1750

Robert A. Erickson

PENN

University of Pennsylvania Press

Philadelphia

Copyright © 1997 University of Pennsylvania Press
All rights reserved
Printed in the United States of America on acid-free paper

10 9 8 7 6 5 4 3 2 1

Published by
University of Pennsylvania Press
Philadelphia, Pennsylvania 19104-6097

Library of Congress Cataloging-in-Publication Data

Erickson, Robert A.
    The language of the heart, 1600–1750 / Robert A. Erickson.
      p. cm. —(New cultural studies)
    Includes bibliographical references and index.
    ISBN 0-8122-3394-8 (alk. paper)
    1. English literature—Early modern, 1500–1700—History and criticism. 2. Heart in literature. 3. Literature and science—Great Britain—History—17th century. 4. Literature and science—Great Britain—History—18th century. 5. English literature—18th century—History and criticism. 6. Body, Human, in literature. 7. Emotions in literature. 8. Heart—Terminology. I. Title. II. Series.
PR438.H43E75 1997   96-53150
820.9'36—dc21   CIP

*For Liisa, Martin,
Stephen, and Annaliisa*

Born to no Pride, inheriting no Strife,
Nor marrying Discord in a Noble Wife,
Stranger to Civil and Religious Rage,
The good Man walk'd innoxious thro' his Age.
No Courts he saw, no suits would ever try,
Nor dar'd an Oath, nor hazarded a Lye:
Un-learn'd, he knew no Schoolman's subtle Art,
No Language, but the Language of the Heart.
   —ALEXANDER POPE, "An Epistle . . . to Dr. Arbuthnot"

Contents

Preface · xi

Acknowledgments · xxi

Introduction: Writing the Heart from Plato to Hobbes · 1

1 The Biblical Heart · 25

2 The Phallic Heart: William Harvey's *The Motion of the Heart* and "The Republick of Literature" · 61

3 The Heart of Eve: Satan and Eve in *Paradise Lost* · 89

4 The Generous Heart: Aphra Behn, *Oroonoko*, and the Woman Writer · 147

5 The Written Heart: Clarissa, Lovelace, and Scripture · 185

Notes · 229

Works Cited · 255

Index · 267

Preface

IN THIS BOOK I study the evolving delineation of the human heart in English narrative and culture of the early modern period, from around 1600 to the mid-eighteenth century. The Introduction provides a map of the heart from the Greeks to the early modern period; the five chapters begin with a discussion of the representation of the heart in the Authorized Version of the Bible (the King James Version of 1611) and then trace the development of the rhetoric of the heart in four important English narrative texts, each in itself a unique experiment in narrative form and each having something new and distinctive to say about the human heart, especially with respect to language, gender, and the sexual body. These four works are William Harvey's *The Motion of the Heart and Blood* (originally published in Latin in 1628, with the first English translation appearing in 1653), John Milton's *Paradise Lost* (1667), Aphra Behn's *Oroonoko* (1688), and Samuel Richardson's *Clarissa* (1747–49). My general argument is that these four diverse narratives exemplify a movement from a strongly masculinist heroic version of the heart in Harvey (one that incorporates a projective sense of the heart's power) to a no less powerful but more feminist heroic narrative in Richardson (one that incorporates a more receptive sense of the heart's power). We shall follow two paths to this destination in Richardson, by two roughly contemporary poets, one male and the other female: first, Milton's formulation of Satan's assault upon Eve in *Paradise Lost*, and second, Behn's erotic-heroic figuring of the male and female heart in her fiction and poetry.

Paradoxically, the heart (like the King James Bible) is so taken for granted that it is the quintessentially marginal organ, having received little critical attention until recently. One could even say that the heart is so central to our physiological and symbolic functioning that, for the most part, we hardly pay attention to it. And maybe that's a healthy thing. Jonathan Sawday in *The Body Emblazoned*, a recent study of the "new science" of anatomy and the human body in Renaissance culture, asserts and demonstrates, with a wealth of examples across many disciplines, that "the early modern period sees the emergence of a new image of the human interior, together with new means of studying that interior" (p. viii). We live in a neo-Lucretian age of image bombardment. Never has the power of the sensory image—and "imaging"—in all its forms had such impact on human experience, ranging from medical imaging of the body's interior to cultural "body images" like that of "thinness" for American women caught in its collective grip, or the other fitness hysteria for American men, perhaps lesser in scope but not in intensity, localized in the perfect "abs." Contemporary concerns about the health of the heart and the arteries, about heart, lung, and kidney transplants, about the size of one's breasts or the firmness of one's midsection, contribute to a gradually emerging sense that we are living in a more "cardiocentric" than "neurocentric" world, a world in some respects more like that of the early modern period, when most people thought of the heart as the center of emotion and even of thinking, as I shall try to show. Recent investigations of the behavior and self-image of heart transplant patients suggest that a considerable number of these patients experience marked personality change, not least in their attitude toward sexual orientation and performance.

In this study I attempt a more extensive and intensive kind of "image" criticism, one begun in my earlier book, *Mother Midnight*, and concerned not only with a variety of external images of nature and the human body, but also with *internal* images of the body and the inner organs of the body, with a sense of how the inner body was imagined by people in the early modern world, and with the "worth" of the internal body and the drama of its inner parts, centering on the heart. This approach to talking about images attempts to explain the complex interplay of external, internal, and subliminal images related to the heart—from a range of idioms—in particular dramatic passages from the five major texts I have chosen to discuss in detail. Examples of this kind of analysis are the eroticized movements of the heart and blood in Harvey's version of the drama of the body's interior and Satan's flight over a feminized Paradise imagined under the aspect of an anatomist and his moving probe.

We shall be concerned in this study with "the sexual heart": its links with the male and female genital organs and with "the gendered heart" (the heart constructed according to prevailing notions of "masculine" and "feminine") as well as its relation to the ungendered heart, the important notion that the same heart operates in both women and men. Jeremiah gives voice to this third concept when he quotes the Lord: "And they shall be my people, and I will be their God: And I will give them one heart, and one way . . ." (32.38–39). The sexual heart is the gendered heart. But critics who have discussed the rhetoric of the heart in literary texts have for too long emphasized only the association between the heart and love. As important and complex as that association is, we must recognize that there is much more to the figure of the human heart than that. The early modern era saw the development of new definitions of the nature of men and women and the sexual body. It has even been argued that male and female heterosexuality, as we know it, was invented sometime in the eighteenth century. We need to take a fresh look at how sex and gender are represented in this critical period—and one largely unexplored avenue of this representation is the early modern construction or "writing" of the sexual or gendered heart. That is my subject. The remaking of the sexual body was not so dramatic and abrupt a process as cultural historians like Thomas Laqueur and Randolph Trumbach suggest; this change took place in a multifaceted direction in the early modern period, and the evolving representation of the heart is one telling index to that remarkable process.

The two central depictions of the heart that emerge from this study are a group or cluster of metaphors associating the heart with language, writing, and thought, and another equally important group associating the heart with sex, passion, and gender. The first of these, particularly as seen under the aspect of seventeenth-century anatomical discourse, provides the overarching design of the book and incorporates the second. Observing the dialogue and tension generated between these two metaphorical clusters is a new way of looking at one of the oldest and most important cultural symbols in human history. I wish to suggest that the making of the modern world coincided with reconfigurations of gender, and that the "heart"—in all the variety of its significations—was a central figure which both reflected and helped produce this change. I hope to show as well that an intensive examination of the representation of the heart in these religious, physiological, and literary discursive contexts will help to enlarge our understanding of three important developments in the emergence of the modern world: the interrelationships among gender, science, and literature, the multiform birth of what we now call "the novel," and the changing meanings of "nature" and "human nature." "Cultural studies" in general has continued to raise questions about the usefulness of the very term "human nature." I want to try to determine further whether a close examination of how the human heart was constructed, or "written," in a variety of discourses will yield a deeper sense of how "human nature" in its masculine and feminine embodiments was understood in this transformative period. What *did* it mean to be human? How can a study of the heart help us to answer that question?

Although in the following pages I shall be using terms like "semiotic," "inscription," "gender," "phallic" (and the list could go on), I wish to make clear at the outset that these terms are not meant to invoke a systematic panoply of associations to semiotic, psychoanalytic, Lacanian, feminist, or any other specific theory. From my first published article (in 1965) on the ambiguities of sexual identity in Arbuthnot's and Pope's *The Memoirs of Martinus Scriblerus*, I have engaged the issue of how the sexes are represented in early modern literary, medical, philosophical, and historical discourses, and my work has been influenced, more or less at different times, by the writings of Freud, Jung, Poulet, the Yale New Critics, Frye, Derrida, Foucault, Bakhtin, a variety of feminist theorists, the New Historicists, and others. But my use of these writings is eclectic, intuitive, and "historicist," if a historicist approach to literary and other cultural texts may be defined as one that examines the effects of the mutual impact and interplay of a variety of discourses and texts in a single period, centering on a primary figure or image. Hence my method in this book is one of imaginative reconstruction. I ask my reader to participate with me in re-imagining how these varied early modern texts relating to the heart were understood in their own time, why they mattered then, and why they matter to us now. Such an approach seems to me a viable way of talking about cultural texts in an interpretative period still dominated by competing single or special interest theories and theorists.

I have chosen to cast this material in the form of chapters that are also independent essays, thus encouraging the reader to make connections among these unique works without imposing what I would consider excessive authorial "continuity" among them. I am all too conscious of the limitations of this study, of how many discourses of the heart (such as that relating to the sacred heart in Roman Catholic theology, or to the emblem tradition of the seventeenth century, especially the works of George Wither and Christopher Harvey) are omitted, and of how much more needs to be done to understand even the representation of the sexual heart from the Middle Ages to the modern period in such writers as Chaucer, Shakespeare, or the Romantic poets. As with *Mother Midnight*, which was concerned with what I call "birth studies," I consider this effort to begin to define "heart studies" exploratory, speculative, and ongoing, one that does not argue a narrow, overriding thesis but that attempts to allow each of these diverse narratives to tell its own story of the heart.

Or primary importance to this study, then, are the fundamental notions of the vital *movement*—expressed in literal and figurative narratives—of the heart and blood, the ambivalent scriptural heart and its relation to gender and sexuality, and the enduring connection between the trope of the heart and the activity of language, spoken and written. Our starting place is a consideration, in the Introduction, of the importance of the heart in the vital economy of the body as represented in England in the early modern period; hence the need for "writing" the heart as the Aristotelian/Galenic "humoral body" is redefined in the context of an emerging language of empiricism. Since the Authorized Version of the English Bible was the cultural narrative most influential in expressing the nature of the heart as well as defining the roles of male and female in early modern England, the first chapter is primarily a thematization of how the imaging of the heart evolves from the Old Testament to the New, beginning with the speaking/writing "seminal" relationship between the "Lord God" and humankind, especially God's profound internal communion with the womb and heart of selected women—Eve, Sarah, Rebekah, Rachel, Samson's mother, and Hannah. The analysis then moves to consider the "semiotic" or sign-making and marking activities of God upon the male body, a representation of God's primarily *external* power on man in contrast to his primarily *internal* power in relation to woman. God's signs move from individual to nation and culminate first in the covenant of circumcision with Abraham, a sign of God's claim upon the source of generation in males, and finally in the "circumcision of the heart." In this discussion I emphasize the ancient idea of writing as anatomy (literally, "a cutting up") and that this activity, like circumcision, is done almost exclusively by males in a male context. In the Bible and much of the literature it helped to shape, writing is a male act of power. God's seminal and semiotic "writing" relationship with the deepest essential being of his people, female and male, is explored further in the ungendered "book of life" trope, especially in Psalm 139. This writing relationship separates the chosen people from others but culminates in God's direction to the prophet Jeremiah to announce that the Law or Word of God will be written in *all* his people's hearts, superseding the inscription of the Law on the phallic stone tablets of heroic yet fallible males like Moses and the priests. For the seventeenth-century Puritan reader, God's writing must be reanimated in the heart.

The combined metaphor of God's writing on the heart via the Spirit (which was to have such a resonant effect on Milton's and Richardson's fictive procedures) becomes a figurative bridge to the representation of the heart in the Gospels and St. Paul, as the chapter concludes with a consideration of Mary, Elisabeth, and other New Testament women as rich new versions of divine interaction with the female heart.

The second chapter examines the 1653 English translation of William Harvey's *Exercitatio anatomica de motu cordis et sanguinis in animalibus* (An exercitation on the motion of the heart and blood in animals) (1628)—probably the most important medical treatise of the seventeenth century—in its scientific and biblical cultural context and with special attention to its narrative and rhetorical structure. Harvey the narrator is seen in many roles, as a mischievous wizard, as a new kind of anatomist-priest with a new gospel of Truth, as a cooperative interpreter or minister of Nature, as a diminutive questing hero in an early scientific version of trial at the center of all heroic narrative, and as the inventor of a new English rhetoric of the heart that is still colored by scriptural idiom. The new rhetoric imagines the heart as a powerfully virile figure in a corporeal quest narrative, sending out the warm, live-giving blood to invigorate the colder feminized outer parts of the body, after which it returns home to the heart for restoration in its continuous circular journey of sexual regeneration within the body. The heart is further likened to "a familiar household god" who does his duty to the whole body in a kind of perpetual marriage service. The chapter concludes with a consideration of how the first-person narrative of the "sexuality" of the inner body in *The Motion of the Heart and Blood* has affinities with various aspects of the emerging narratives of the early novel, especially those of Behn, Defoe, Richardson, and Sterne.

The third chapter traces the narrative of the heart in the dramatic action and context of the epic poem *Paradise Lost*, where a phallic and invasive Satan, seen under the aspect of seventeenth-century anatomical discourse and the language of Rochesterian libertinism, seeks to seduce Eve, the Mother of Mankind and the new female embodiment of the human heart, to revolt from God. As Harvey's narrative incorporates elements of heroic romance, so Milton's narrative incorporates elements of the new science of anatomy. After an initial account of the androgynous Spirit and its relationship to "the upright heart and pure" of the imploring male narrator, the chapter surveys the special emphasis in the poem on the heart region in Heaven, Hell, and Paradise; considers Eve as Adam's heart companion and partner; and then moves to a detailed examination of how

Satan, as a perverse anatomist, first subjects the predominantly feminine and generative land of Eden and Paradise to his predatory and fatal gaze, and then begins his carefully calculated attack upon Eve, who is represented not only as a supremely attractive woman in her potent physical beauty and grace, but as one whose emotional life is closely analogous to the seventeenth-century account of the "Corporeal Soul"—a flexible new version of the motion of the heart and blood—found in the physiological writings of Thomas Willis (1621–75). "Satanic sex"—intrusive and possessive, like libertine sex—is contrasted with "blissful," interpenetrative, angelic sex and with unfallen human sex as a prelude to Satan's protracted sexual assault upon Eve's heart, a complex form of rape. This assault is described as an invasion of her body in three progressively internalized and comprehensive stages: first, the violation of her "head," through the dream of disobedience which Satan fashions for her after invading the human pair's most sacred space, their innermost bower; then, in book 9, his penetration of her "hand," the handiwork and artistry of her new *personal* space of creation, her nursery of roses; and, climactically, his subtle and highly complicated entrance into, and seduction of, her "heart" in three increasingly compelling seduction speeches modeled on the classical oration. The chapter continues with an account of Adam as the original man of feeling who senses that he was created by the female Earth, and concludes with an analysis of Adam and Eve's regeneration of the heart (compared again to Willis's psychophysiological account of repentant religious experience), a process in which Eve, despite her inferiority to Adam in intellect and "real dignity," exercises superior adherence to the heroic Christian ethic of "the better fortitude" of active patience and martyrdom.

The fourth chapter continues to explore the act of writing in relation to the heart but now as an ambivalent exercise of female-authored power. The chapter provides a close analysis of, first, Aphra Behn's love poetry in response to her encounter with Thomas Creech's translation of Lucretius (with a look at male poets' praise of her as an androgynous poet), then an examination of the rhetoric of the gendered heart in *The Rover* and of the brilliant playwright-within-the-play, Lady Fulbank, inscribed in Behn's *The Lucky Chance*. In the logic of the developing metaphor of Harvey's masculinist writing of the heart giving way to Behn's more feminist writing of the heart, with *Paradise Lost* as the mediating narrative between these male- and female-authored texts, Behn becomes one of the first important female artists of the *written* word for which Milton's Eve, as oral and visual artist, was a fictive counterpart and prototype. In *Oroonoko*, Behn skillfully fuses oral and written elements into a distinctively fluid textuality as she tells her own scripturally allusive creation myth about a new black Adam and Eve, an implicit gospel narrative of the true and innocent heart of Nature as opposed to conventional and hypocritical Euro-Christian examples of human nature. In the context of Behn's reading of Lucretius, her erotic poetry of the "Generous Heart," and her later "royalist" poems, the chapter considers how Behn expands the Miltonic attribute of Eve's "Softness" (or compassion) into a major virtue of her distinctly masculine hero, Oroonoko, and makes her soft and loving heroine, Imoinda, a potent warrior when the need arises. Oroonoko's capture of the heart of a great She-Tiger—a central moment in the narrative—prefigures his own downfall at the hands of his European colonial masters, and when he severs Imoinda's "Face"—the "Idea" of which he had enclosed in his heart—he severs his own heart and life force as well. This is Behn's unique depiction of a new kind of "heroic martyrdom" far different from the versions in *Paradise Lost*. Imoinda, like Eve, is her husband's heart partner, but Behn gives a turn to the Miltonic Christian dynamic of Eve offering to die for Adam by having Imoinda offer willingly and tenderly to submit to Oroonoko's knife. Oroonoko finally subjects himself—in a scene that echoes the Crucifixion—to a similar sacrificial fate when he is executed in a brutal, quasi-biblical anatomical vivisection of his external members. Behn at the end dedicates *Oroonoko* to the protection of an aristocratic English couple whose tranquil lives are an image of the beautiful pair in Paradise, as at the same time the female author asserts her hope that the reputation of her pen will ensure literary immortality for her own black hero and heroine—and for herself.

The final chapter discusses Samuel Richardson's *Clarissa* in the light of the scriptural and scientific language of the heart explored in the preceding pages. We begin with a comparison of the neo-Platonist John Norris's analogy between the circulation of the blood and the circulation of love in the universe with Richardson's implied doctrine of the epistolary circulation—by way of the receptive and expressive heart—of spoken and written conversation in the social sphere. We then move to a consideration of *Clarissa* as an extraordinarily complex representation of the trial and redemption of the heart through a male-authored reimagining of the female act of writing. In the light of this inquiry, Richardson's novel emerges as a profound and problematic exploration of the major religious issues in the early modern Protestant tradition as his Christian heroine—an eighteenth-century version of Milton's Eve—experiences the meaning of regeneration in a corrupt secular world epitomized by the guile and influence of the obsessive Lovelace and his minions. The chapter reviews the books of the Bible and religious works most important for the kind of reading that went into the writing of this novel, considers Richardson in his role as reader, and discusses Puritan views of the Bible as God's epistolary intercourse with human hearts. Women and men then "write" themselves after the model of Christ, a new form of "imitatio Christi" by way of writing Christ into the heart. We then move to a close examination of Clarissa's struggle with her family and with the "hot" and insistent phallic heart of Lovelace (modeled to some extent on the heart of Milton's Satan), a struggle virtually defined in terms of the experiences of her suffering heart in relation to Scripture and to writing. The chapter includes an assessment of Lovelace and Clarissa as culminating eighteenth-century representations of the long history of the "male" and "female" heart examined in this study. Focusing on Clarissa's two acts of writing after her rape by Lovelace—the self-mutilation of the mad letters, and especially the transcription of Scripture in her *Meditations*—we see how Clarissa "re-collects" and rewrites herself into a powerful new phenomenon: a figure able to vanquish Lovelace, and one whose scriptural activities, according to the advice of Thomas à Kempis, fortify her heart "in the Day of Tryal and Adversity" for Christ's Last Judgment. After considering how both Clarissa and Lovelace are shaped by their "reading" of their own "scriptures"—one modeled on the sacred, the other secular—the chapter concludes with a discussion of Clarissa's calmly reflective "compact" with her future self, her relationship to her future executor, editor, and virtual apostle, John Belford, and her final meaning for the desperate Lovelace, who demands sole possession of her physical heart after her death. All of Clarissa's final "writings"—her will, her last letter read to her assembled family, her eleven posthumous letters, her talismanic coffin on its final journey to her father's house—underscore the quasi-divine influence of the new woman writer as martyr-prophet, a new Christian female Fate who has the power not only to shape the subsequent destinies of everyone who comes into her purview, but to write herself finally into God's own book of the heart—the "book of life"—which will be read by Clarissa's bridegroom and final judge.

Acknowledgments

I WISH TO THANK FIRST the two readers for the University of Pennsylvania Press for their comments and criticism, in particular Terry Castle for her words of encouragement, her grasp of the project, and her suggestions for revision. For help along the way with a design that began as an analysis of the soul and soon became focused on the representation of the heart, I thank Angus Ross and my colleagues Patrick McCarthy for reading an early version of Chapter 4, Michael O'Connell and Porter Abbott for reading an early version of Chapter 5, Anita Guerrini and Charles Bazerman (respectively) for expert advice on the Introduction and Chapter 2, and especially Everett Zimmerman for reading the entire manuscript and making many helpful suggestions for revision.

Portions of Chapters 4 and 5 first appeared in the journal *Eighteenth-Century Fiction* (5[1993]: 201–16; 2[1989]: 17–51), and a portion of Chapter 2 in *Literature and Medicine During the Eighteenth Century*, ed. Marie Mulvey Roberts and Roy Porter (London: Routledge, 1993). I am grateful to the editors for permission to reprint this material, and thank in particular David Blewett and Roy Porter for the benefit of their editorial expertise, knowledge, and acumen. My undergraduate and graduate students have afforded me and their peers a variety of insights into the human heart in seminars I have taught over the past ten years. I wish to thank in particular John Zamarra and Alicia Linquiti for contributions far beyond requirements in surveying the medical literature of the heart. My two graduate research assistants on the project—Fern Kory in the early stages and Michael Austin in the later stages—worked skillfully and with consistent good humor and patience on a variety of sometimes daunting tasks. Special thanks go to David S. Crouch for the two illustrations of the heart. I am grateful to the Committee on Research of the University of California, Santa Barbara, for summer travel research grants for the years 1988, 1990, and 1993 which enabled me to complete the book. Finally I wish to thank, once again, my wife, Liisa Raatikainen Erickson, whose daily conversation, kindness, and wisdom have cherished and sustained me in thirty years of teaching and writing. My chief sources of joy and hope are named in the quadripartite dedication.

Introduction: Writing the Heart from Plato to Hobbes

LITERARY AND CULTURAL INTERPRETATION of recent years has been concerned almost to the point of obsession with the representation of images and figures of the human body in seventeenth- and eighteenth-century texts. But fuller and more careful attention needs to be paid to how various *internal* structures and organs of the body, such as the bones and diaphragm and pericardium, the tongue, the lungs, the liver, the spleen, the gall bladder, the stomach, the "bowels" as the seat of the deepest emotions, the kidneys or "reins" or "loins," the womb, the "seed," and especially the heart as "the Prince of all the Bowels," are made to reflect, in this era, the most complex expressions of human nature moving between life and death.[1]

Because the view of the heart in the ancient world had so deep and pervasive an influence on how the heart was understood and represented in early modern England, we shall begin our inquiry with Plato's *Timaeus* (dating from the early fourth century B.C.E.), one of the earliest and most influential treatises on the nature and function of the human body and soul. Plato notes that the creator, acting through his divine offspring, placed the immortal soul and reason in the head and encased the mortal soul (subject to "terrible and irresistible affections" like pleasure, pain, fear, anger, irrational sense, and all-daring love) in the breast, or thorax, divided the thorax "into two parts, as the women's and men's apartments are divided in houses, and placed the midriff to be a wall or partition between them." The heart, "the knot of the veins and the fountain of the blood which races through all the limbs," was set as a guard to channel "the whole power of feeling in the body" when passion was roused by reason warning of any wrong assailing the body "from without or being perpetrated by the desires within." "But the gods, foreknowing that the palpitation of the heart in the expectation of danger and excitement of passion must cause it to swell and become inflamed, formed and implanted as a supporter to the heart the lung, which was . . . soft and bloodless, and also had hollows like the pores of a sponge." The lungs gave "coolness and the power of respiration," alleviating the heat of the heart, and "when passion was rife within, the heart, beating against a yielding body," was cooled and more ready to join with passion in the service of reason.[2] We see already in this description, and in that of Empedocles (around 450 B.C.E.), as quoted by Aristotle, the all-important linkage in Greek physiology of the two systems of blood flow and respiration, the vital link between the lungs and the heart.[3] We see also the implicit companionate nature of the cool lung offering support to the hot heart in the economy of the Platonic rational body.

From the very beginning of Greek medicine, the heart was thought to be the source of heat in the body, and heat was the source of life and nutrition. There is in the Platonic account of the heart and blood a characteristic Greek emphasis on physical *motion* and *heat*. Galen quotes Aristotle: "the male provides the form and the principle of motion, and the female the body and the matter."[4] Also from very early times, heat was associated with the male gender and with perfection, coldness and wetness with the less perfect female gender. Since the notions of male activity and female passivity, and especially hot maleness and cold femaleness, are pervasive in the early modern construction of the body—and central to our inquiry from Harvey to Richardson—we may at this point look briefly at Galen's classic formulation of the latter doctrine.

For Galen, Nature is the supreme artisan and regulator of all living bodies, a feminized creative force working in concert with a rather obscure male creator. A fundamental paradox in Galen's medical writing is that this wondrous and foresighted maternal fashioner of life creates a female sex inferior in perfection to the male sex. But there is a particular reason for this imperfection, one that ironically posits a view of feminine power uniquely superior to male power: "it was better for the female to be made colder so that she cannot disperse all the nutriment she concocts and elaborates" and thus the fetus gets what it needs for perfect growth. If the female were "perfectly warm" she would disperse too much heat and evaporate it. The innate heat in man may be greater and thus more perfect, but that heat needs to be controlled and moderated or the animal will become disordered and eventually fly apart. Male heat can be too much of a good thing. Woman is thus in the mediating, moderate position between being too cold and too hot, the optimum mode for the preservation of the species. So the female is colder than the male, but not too cold or she would not concoct.[5] The chief implication of this doctrine—surviving variants of which impinge one way or another on all the female characters in this study from Milton's Eve through Behn's heroines through Richardson's Clarissa and Anna Howe—is that Galenic woman, like biblical woman, is the mother and preserver of the human race, thus continuing in finite form the life-maintaining and life-enhancing ministrations of Nature herself.

In Galenic thought, woman or the feminine element is uniquely qualified to control and moderate the innate heat, beginning with a feminized lung and ending with the uterus. Although for Galen the female and the male genitalia are essentially the same organs turned outward in males and inward in females,[6] the structure of the uterus is specially fitted for the nurturing and preservation of life because of its uniquely bipartite form (the uterus is really two uteri), its flexible structure (being "both moderately soft and moderately hard"), and its connection with the nourishing female breasts: "For just as two uteri ending in one neck have been made in woman, so there are also two breasts, each one like a faithful servant of its own uterus."[7] The female heart and breasts also enjoy a special mutual relationship in that the heart supplies the breasts with innate heat and the breasts supply the heart with protection. This mutuality of heat and protection in the female is greater than that in the male, but "the female body as a whole is colder than the male."[8]

We turn next to the short "Hippocratic" treatise *De corde* (probably dating from around 250 B.C.E., later than the major writings in the Hippocratic corpus) because it provides a compact yet detailed picture of the ancient Greek view of the heart. *De corde* notes that the hot, crimson heart is enveloped by a smooth membrane containing fluid in which the heart moves in a kind of protective bladder. The Hippocratic heart was a strong muscle, containing two separate cavities, with the left side of the heart the more important chamber because it was stronger, hotter, and contained "human intelligence, the principle which rules over the rest of the soul."[9] Difficult as it is for neurocentric readers to grasp, the heart, rather than the brain, was the place of mental functioning for the writer of *De corde*; we shall see this idea given different form in Aristotle and Lucretius. The "Hippocratic" heart, fashioned as in the *Timaeus* by an excellent divine craftsman, was wrapped and encushioned by the lung, which helped—along with the massive construction of the heart—to control its tremendous heat.[10] Since breath (*pneuma*) was considered the most necessary and supreme component in human beings, the organs of respiration were the supreme organs, and of these the heart was the chief.[11] Aristotle as an anatomist showed that the brain was lacking in sensation and that its true function was to cool, by means of a secretion called phlegm, the great heat generated by the heart. For Galen, the heart is the central organ of life and ongoing vitality, and since heat is essential to life, the heart is "the hearthstone and source of the innate heat."[12] Aristotle and Galen were agreed that the fundamental element of life was heat, and the notion that the heart was the source of the body's innate heat and life persisted well into the seventeenth century. The Aristotelian heart and even the brain were respiratory organs, and the heart produced the natural pneuma (not to be confused with the breath drawn from the outside in the breathing process) "which is continually created and renewed inside the body so long as there is heat and life. It is the vehicle of the soul, and as such is responsible for reproduction and movement."[13] Since the heart is the central location of the soul as organizing principle of an animal, the heart is the primary "reproductive" organ in the body. And equally important in terms of his later influence, Aristotle placed sensory knowledge, memory, and imagination (but not intelligence) in the heart. For Aristotle, intelligence or *nous* was not located in any physical organ, but this distinction became blurred in early modern discussions of the Aristotelian heart.

Galen parted company from Aristotle and "Hippocrates" by placing the governing part of the soul in the brain, not the heart. He showed that compression of the brain led to loss of movement and sensibility, whereas compression of the heart merely stopped the pulse.[14] The heart was still the central organ of life for Galen, but he complicated the Aristotelian notion of the soul and heart by having nature rule the body in his reinvention of the Platonic doctrine of three souls (or faculties or spirits) simultaneously governing yet serving the body. These are the rational (or "animal," after *anima* meaning "soul"), the irascible (or "vital"), and the concupiscible (or "natural" or "vegetative"), seated in the brain, heart, and liver respectively. The first presides over rational thought and causes sensation and motion; the second governs the emotions and provides the life force; the third controls nutrition.[15] The doctrine will be of special concern in our encounter with Milton's Satan and Eve.[16] Besides the concept of a feminized creative "nature," the other essential feature of Galen's philosophico-medical system is the principle of humoral balance. Galen of course is remembered in connection with the theory of the four humors—blood, phlegm, yellow bile, and black bile—with blood being the most important because it carried nutrients and innate heat to all parts of the body. Health is the harmonious balance, or blending (*eucrasia*), of the four qualities (hot, cold, moist, dry) and humors, and disease is a *dyscrasia* or unbalanced mixture of the humoral body.[17] Galen's view of the heart was essentially a composite of the teachings of "Hippocrates" and Aristotle, with his own version of what he learned from his great predecessor and favorite rhetorical whipping boy, Erasistratus, and his own contributions based on the dissection and vivisection of Barbary apes and other animals. Galen, unlike the Alexandrians Herophilus and Erasistratus, did not practice human dissection (the Alexandrians were even said to practice human vivisection), but in his capacity of surgeon to the gladiatorial arenas in Pergamon and Rome, he must have seen every type of wound to the male body.[18]

Galen devised an elaborate —and not altogether consistent—scheme for how the blood moved in the body.[19] (The reader is referred to the diagram of the Galenic cardiovascular system, Figure 1.) We need to remember first of all that venous and arterial blood are contained in separate and distinct vessels, and that the liver is a primary player in relation to the blood and its movement, almost like a second heart. The venous blood (associated with the liver and the heart) is alimentary, the arterial blood (associated with the heart) is more "spirituous" and the source of the body's vitality, and both kinds of blood flow to all parts of the body. "The theory also depended upon the ability of organs—whether heart or arteries—to dilate and contract with more or less equal activity. They could thereby alternately attract and expel—'draw and drive'—the liquids they contained. Flows in many vessels were therefore reversible, surging first in one direction and then in the other."[20] The blood is formed in the liver under the influence of the innate heat in a process similar to the fermentation of wine, but before the blood can become suitable nutriment for the parts of the body it has to be cleansed of superfluities by three organs, the gall bladder, the kidneys, and the spleen.[21] This purified and nourishing blood is then supplied (via the pulsative motion of the vena cava and the attractive power of the heart and other internal organs) to all parts of the body above and below the liver.[22] Some commentators describe this motion of the nutritious venous blood as an "ebb and flow."[23] A small portion of this blood moves to the right ventricle, where it is acted upon by the intense innate heat of the heart so that it becomes thinner and purer. Part of this thinner blood goes through the artery-like vein (the pulmonary artery) to feed the lung. The rest passes through invisible perforations (or pores) in the interventricular septum into the left ventricle. Here for the first time the blood comes into contact with the pneuma from the outside world and the blood undergoes a profound change. In a rather mysterious

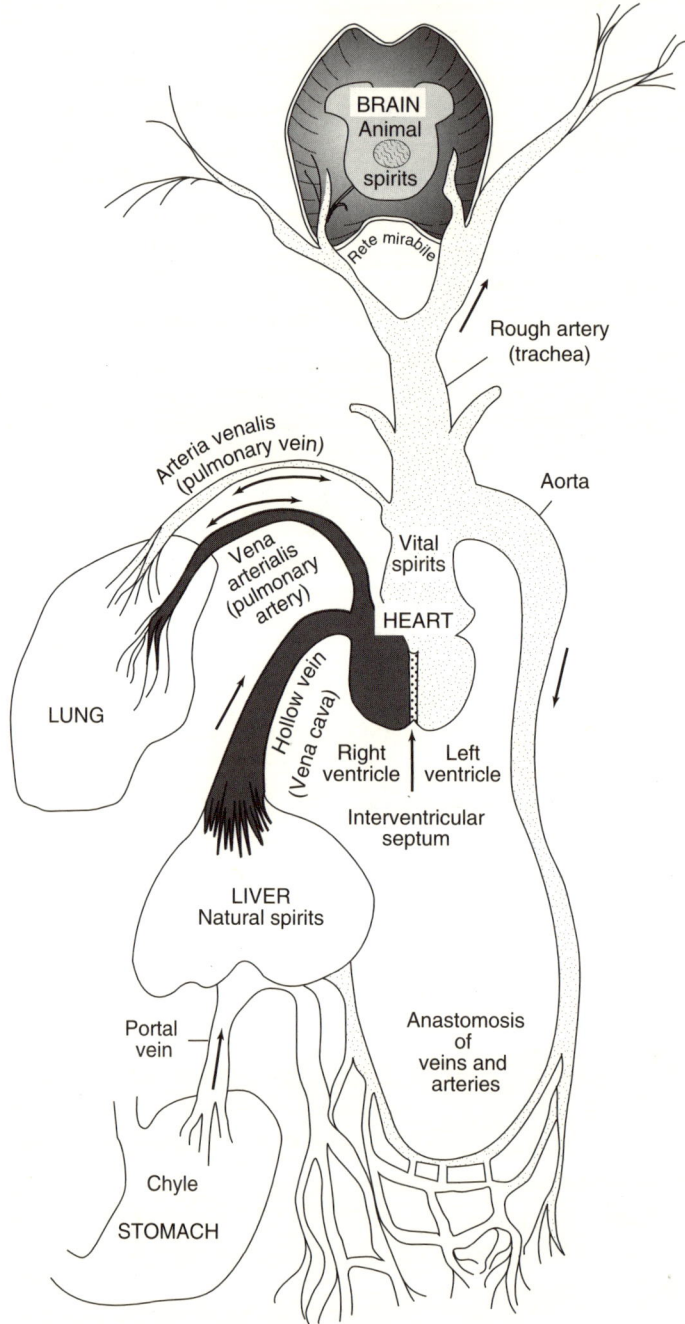

Figure 1. The Galenic cardiovascular system.

process, the pneuma from outside is transformed into a thin, spirituous blood highly charged with life-giving internal pneuma and distributed to all parts of the body.[24] The early modern anatomist Helkiah Crooke (to whose monumental Galenic work the *Mikrokosmographia* we shall make frequent reference) gives the following visionary description of this process in his evocation of the internal "theater of the body":

> This [vital] spirit cherisheth the in-bred heat of euery part, quickens it when it becommeth drowsie, bringeth it forth when it lyes hid, and being spent or wasted restoreth it againe.
> This spirit whilest it shineth in his brightnes and spredeth it selfe through all the Theater of the body as the Sunne ouer the earth, it blesseth all partes with ioy and iolitie and dies them with a Rosie colour; but on the contrary when it is retracted intercepted or extinguished, all things become horred wanne and pale and finally doe vtterly perish. So wonderfull and almost so heauenly are the powers of the heat and spirit, that the diuine *Senior Hippocrates* . . . calleth it the Soule. . . .[25]

Supplemented by a respiratory process through the pores of the skin and the arteries, the complex and at times metaphysical system of blood flow in Galen may be described as carrying nutrition and vital spirit—like a magical internal soup—to the rest of the body. Impurities acquired by the blood from the internal organs were carried off by the pulmonary artery to the lungs and exhaled, so that breathing out was an expulsion of impurities. The ancient art of phlebotomy or bloodletting—again given its classical formulation of Galen—was essentially a method by which residues that have accumulated in the blood because of too much nourishment could be removed in order to restabilize the equilibrium of the humoral body.[26] The doctrine of pure and impure blood was a physiological analogue to the Judeo-Christian notion of the ambivalent heart housing a variety of good and evil impulses, pure and impure thoughts and intentions.

In Galen's scheme, blood is constantly being remade in the liver and moves around the body by means of a complex series of propulsions and attractions. The most remarkable thing about Galen's theory of the movement of the blood is that he considered the heart and arteries primarily organs of *attraction*: "the most powerful action of both heart and arteries was dilation, not contraction. The heart and the arteries were conceived by him as a very powerful form of what we today would call a suction pump."[27] Galen uses the images of the smith's bellows drawing in air, of the flame drawing oil, of the attractive faculties of the lodestone: "the heart, itself, having all imaginable attractive faculties, snatches and, as it were, drinks up the inflowing material, receiving it rapidly."[28] This tremendous attractive power, combined with extremely intense heat, creates an image of the heart with interesting implications for Milton's concept of Hell, as we shall see in Chapter 3, but even more important, the idea of an "attractive," "open" heart came to generate a huge variety of figurative meanings in literary and religious discourse.

Galen saw every organ and tissue in the body attracting from the blood the elements needed for its special function. For Galen, the blood does not circulate but moves primarily in one direction, away from the center of the body; it passes into the heart and the heart sends it out, but the heart does not supply its motive power. It was Harvey's contribution, as we shall see in Chapter 2, to *demonstrate* that the same blood circulates throughout—and nourishes—the entire body, in two virtually simultaneous circulations, *propelled by the heart alone*: the lesser, or pulmonary, circulation, in which blood coming from the veins is pumped (not attracted) from the right ventricle to the lungs through the pulmonary artery and back through the pulmonary veins to the more powerful left ventricle, where in the greater, or systemic circulation the blood is given a stronger push through the aorta to the arteries, organs, and tissues of the body. Even a Galenist like Crooke, however, very much aware of the attractive power of the heart, could anticipate Harvey on the power of systolic action: "The motion of the heart is no trembling but a constant and orderly motion ... the greatest strength of the heart is in the contraction, whereby it hurleth forth (as the lightning passeth through the whole heauen) his spirites into the whole body" (401). Harvey did not know about the actual nature of capillary action but he knew that the blood is somehow transferred from the arteries to the veins in the circulatory process. (The reader is referred to the diagram of the Harveian heart and circulation, Figure 2.)

To sum all this up in rather broad terms, the heart for both Galen and Harvey is a strong, thick, fibrous, sinewy, red, powerful organ controlling (or for Galen, involved in controlling) the flow of the blood. The Galenic heart is essentially *attractive* in its motive power, drawing in the blood in diastole and distributing it to the body in a complex process, originating in the liver, of repeated makings and remakings of the blood. The overall image is of the heart as a four-chambered structure, a receptive vehicle of the blood. Despite its great heat modified by the lung and air, the overall architecture of the Galenic heart is open, attractive, and receptive. The action of the Harveian heart is just the opposite of this. For Harvey the essential action of the heart is *ejaculatory* in systole, driving the blood in

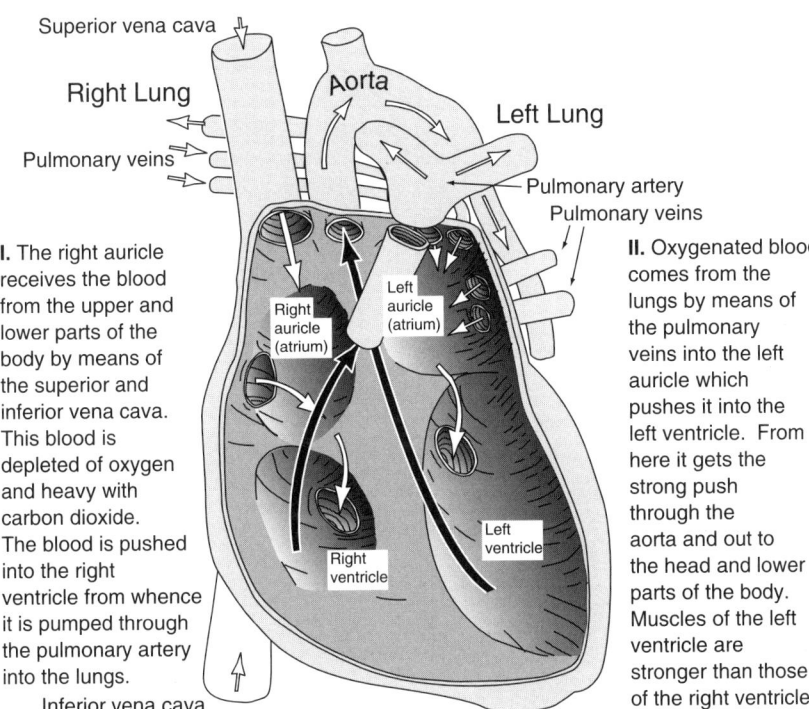

The Two Circulations

Pulmonary – from the right side of the heart to the pulmonary artery and the capillaries of the lungs and then to the left side of the heart by the pulmonary veins.

Systemic – from the left side of the heart by the aorta to the arteries and capillaries of the body tissues and organs, and from there by the veins (and superior and inferior vena cava) back to the right side of the heart.

Veins go to the heart, arteries go away from the heart.

R = right side of heart with carbon dioxide blood
L = left side of heart with oxygenated blood

I. The right auricle receives the blood from the upper and lower parts of the body by means of the superior and inferior vena cava. This blood is depleted of oxygen and heavy with carbon dioxide. The blood is pushed into the right ventricle from whence it is pumped through the pulmonary artery into the lungs.

II. Oxygenated blood comes from the lungs by means of the pulmonary veins into the left auricle which pushes it into the left ventricle. From here it gets the strong push through the aorta and out to the head and lower parts of the body. Muscles of the left ventricle are stronger than those of the right ventricle.

Figure 2. The heart and circulation. (After Harvey)

continuous cycles through the lungs and the outermost parts of the body. The architecture of the Harveian heart is that of a constricting and expanding muscle, analogous to the structure and action of a gun, a comparison Harvey actually makes. Recalling the Galenic notion of the structural identity of the female and male genitalia, it is clear that these two images of the heart—attractive and ejaculatory—have a remarkable similarity to the reproductive organs.

The Galenic heart and the Harveian heart are indexes to two complex images of the human body, the Galenic or classical, and the Harveian or early modern. Since in the Galenic body the blood is constantly being made and then used up, the body is always in a state of remaking itself, concocting or "cooking" itself, with sooty vapors being given off through the skin and the mouth. It is a fragile, unstable, vulnerable body made up of a variety of interconvertible fluids churning around in a constantly precarious state of healthy balance or more often unhealthy imbalance. By the early modern period, as Gail Kern Paster puts it,

[e]very subject grew up with a common understanding of his or her body as a semipermeable, irrigated container in which humors moved sluggishly. People imagined that health consisted of a state of internal solubility to be perilously maintained, often through a variety of evacuations, either self-administered or in consultation with a healer.... [T]his body had a distinct set of internal procedures dependent on a differential caloric economy (most men being hotter than most women) and characterized by corporeal fluidity, openness, and porous boundaries.[29]

In the Harveian body, on the other hand, since the blood is constantly being recycled or renewed, there is a simpler, more stable and consistent internal economy of the body than in the Galenic humoral body. As we shall see in considerable detail in Chapter 2, the Harveian model lends itself to a more regular domestic paradigm of the internal workings of the body, with the kinglike phallic heart ministering via the blood to a feminized outer body. Although it would be far too simple to characterize the Galenic heart, in all its rich accumulations of meaning by the early modern period, as a "female" heart, and the newly emerging Harveian heart as "male," in terms of classical and biblical notions of gender, the Galenic heart has a strongly receptive or "feminine" function, and the Harveian heart a more ejaculatory and "masculine" function. Except for the medical community, which generally accepted Harvey's theory of the circulation by the time of the Restoration, both of these models of the heart and the body were operating together in the minds of people who thought about such matters (and at a subliminal level in others), with the persistent Galenic model predominating through the Restoration and on into the eighteenth century.[30] In considering the interfusion of these two contrasting notions of the action of the heart, one might describe the early modern image of the heart as primarily masculine (as in the image of a king), but having a "bisexual" component.

Examining now in more detail the traditional or Aristotelian/Galenic view of the heart in the early modern period, we need to keep in mind the historicized meaning of "heart" as well as what *we* mean by the word. I have tried in this study to articulate my sense of the various physiological and figurative contours of signification the heart possessed in the early modern period. To help particularize this process, I have drawn occasionally upon the works of several representative seventeenth-century divines, anatomists, and other writers, chiefly the important but neglected "Puritan" divine Thomas Watson and the anatomist Crooke, the older, more conservative contemporary of Harvey's. I emphasize Watson because he has a particularly strong interest in the religious "anatomy of the heart" and because he articulates a theological position close to the "Puritan" concerns of Milton and Richardson.

By the early modern period, the word "heart" had come to mean a variety of things: the center of all vital functions, the source of one's inmost thoughts and secret feelings or one's inmost being, the seat of courage and the emotions generally, the essential, innermost, or central part of anything, the source of desire, volition, truth, understanding, intellect, ethics, spirit. *It was the single most important word referring both to the body and to the mind.* No other word performed what "heart" did, and no other word today quite replaces it. The heart was an organ that both received and projected. In fact, two of the most important words in the language of the heart from Chaucer through the eighteenth century are "impression" and "imagination," the first receptive, the second more active, shaping, outreaching. Chaucer is speaking of the heart when his narrator in "The Miller's Tale" says, "Lo, which a greet thyng is affeccioun! / Men may dyen of ymaginacioun, / So depe may impressioun be take" (lines 3611–13). In "The Blossom," John Donne contrasts the subtle, sedentary heart with the performative penis, and asserts that "A naked thinking heart that makes no show / Is to a woman but a kind of ghost." Let us pause for a moment on that remarkable image of the "naked thinking heart." It cannot be stressed enough that the ancient classical and biblical notion of the heart as the seat of both sensation *and thought* was still strong in the popular and literary mind, though most early modern anatomists considered the brain as superior to the heart. According to Crooke, the so-called "official members" or "principal Parts" of the body—those thought to be absolutely necessary to the preservation of the individual creature—were the heart, the brain, the liver (and sometimes the testicles), with the heart personified as a king, the brain as a judge or governor, and the liver as a prince (31). These organs were the chief actors in the theater of the humoral body, a body whose design was now complicated and enriched by centuries of medical variation upon and redefinition of Galen's original model.

Because the human heart as a physical organ is so fundamental a part of the basic rhythms and forces of life, it has always had a multitude of literal and figurative associations with life processes and with sexuality. Some of the earliest English anatomies describe the heart as virtually a genital organ: "The substaunce of the Hart . . . is spermatike, and an officiall member, and the beginning of lyfe, and he geueth to euery member of the body, both bloud of lyfe: and spirit of breath and heate."[31] Crooke, in characterizing Aristotle's view of the heart, notes that the heart is the first organ to live and the last to die, that it has no notable diseases, that its location in the middle of the body is the most honorable place, and that "by his perpetuall motion, all thinges are exhilerated and doe flourish: and nothing in the whole Creature is fruitfull, vnlesse the powerfull vigour of the Heart do giue foecundity vnto it. . . . [The heart] is the *primum sensorium*," and the seat of the passions, "Joy, Sorrow, and Hope" (39–40).[32]

The basic pattern of the heart's motion of alternate diastole and systole had long been associated with the similar expanding and contracting rhythm of the lungs, reinforcing a sense of the interrelated action of the heart and lungs. As we saw in Plato, the lungs are depicted as a soft, cooling companion to the hot passion of the heart. Again in terms of biblical and classical notions of gender, Crooke gives a feminized portrait of the lungs (cool, soft, and moist), noting that though the lungs are themselves devoid of all motion, "they hang loose and at liberty that they might more freely moove," like internal *mammae*, and conform to the motion of the chest. With their "gibbous and swelling" lobes "they encompass [the heart and pericardium] round about" and "firmly embrace" it. Their substance is fleshy and "covered with a thin Membrane, which varieth in softness" according to age; this "substance also is laxe, spongy and rare, made as it were of the froth of the bloud." They have "a soft motion, which is furthered in that their substance is full of a slimy and viscid moysture," which helps to moderate the great heat of the heart (384–85).

The heart and lungs, as we have seen, were considered "reproductive" and respiratory organs, and the rhythm of expansion and contraction is also seen in the activity of the penis and the womb. In Galen's system the heart, the lung, the arteries, the uterus, and the penis, all operate, in varying sequences, by expansion and contraction, and he goes on to say, "the stomach, uterus, and both bladders, attract, retain, and expel just as the heart does."[33] In fact, his description of the action of the heart—"enlarging when it desires to attract what is useful, clasping its contents when it is time to enjoy what has been attracted, and contracting when it desires to expel residues"—could almost be ascribed to the activity of the uterus.[34] The rhythm of expansion and contraction has more abstract dimensions, such as the motions of Thomas Willis's "Corporeal Soul," to be discussed later in connection with Milton's Eve.

The tactile and physiological nature of the motion of the heart must be supplemented by the aural dimension, the basic two-part rhythm of the iambic heartbeat, as evoked, for example, with memorably uncanny precision in Poe's imaging of a "tell-tale heart." Poe's story is a brilliant compression of constantly recurring discursive links in the long history of the human heart (and evident in the following chapters) between the heart and other important organs of the body, particularly between the heart and the eye and the heart and the ear. The heartbeat would seem to tell a simple story, but the heartbeat is double (as discerned and described at length by seventeenth-century anatomists), and this doubleness was a physiological analogue to the biblical sense of the multiplicity of the heart's deviations (to be discussed more fully in the first chapter) that come under the category of "duplicity." Since one of the core senses of the heart in the seventeenth century was a repository of truth, to have "a heart and a heart" meant to be deceptive or hypocritical. Thomas Watson told his hearers, "Gods eye is principally upon the heart; An humble heart, a broken heart . . . God lookes there most where we look least; some have no heart at all; sin hath stollen away their heart; others have an heart too much, a double heart, Psal. 12.2 . . . an heart & an heart, others have hearts good for nothing, earthly hearts."[35] Watson also said that "the Heart is the greatest Impostor."[36] "The motion . . . of the heart is double," says Helkiah Crooke, "one naturall, the other depraved. The naturall we call the Pulse, the other we call Palpitations: the one preceedeth from a Naturall faculty, the other from an vnnatural distemper; the one is an action of the heart, the other a passion" (501). Crooke echoes the notion that the heart is the hottest of all the "*bowels*" (417), and at the same time imagines the heart as a living machine as he addresses his male reader and inaugurates the theme of male manipulation of the heart, to be seen more vividly in Harvey's experimental descriptions: "Me thinks . . . that every man when he puts his hand into his bosome and feeleth there a continuall pulsation, by which hee knoweth his owne life is gouerned; should also bee desirous to vnderstand what maner of engine this is, which being so small that he may couer it with his hand, hath yet such diuersities of mouing causes therein, especially considering that a little skill to cleere and dresse the wheeles may keep this watch of his life in motion" (401). The doubleness of the heartbeat may be considered as continuous and discontinuous at the same time (continuous over a lifetime, discontinuous in its doubleness), like that all-encompassing image of human fate linked to the womb, the thread of life which must be severed before life in the world can begin. In moments of great poignancy, as in watching a child take its first steps, we still talk about feeling a "catch" in the heart, a momentary cessation. Finally, the continuity of the heartbeat was and is quintessentially vulnerable, subject to instant cessation, like the final cutting of the thread of life.

The other basic rhythm of the heart—that of receiving and discharging the blood—was also open to sexual and other figurative extensions, and here we move from the binary motion of the heart to a consideration of the quadripartite structure of the heart. The four main blood vessels connected to the heart (the incoming vena cava and pulmonary vein, the outgoing pulmonary artery and aorta) were sometimes likened to rivers or fountains and recalled the four rivers of Paradise or of Hades, which we shall revisit in Chapter 3. Helkiah Crooke asks his reader to "Consider and obserue the Heart, his two ventricles, eares as many, foure notable Vessels, which as *Hippocrates* sayth, are as it were . . . the fountaines and well-springes of the humane Nature, and the riuers and sourses whereby the whole body is watered and refreshed: besides eleauen gates or entrances" (15). We see in this passage the irrigational structure of the humoral body, an image analogous to a well-watered garden. As we pause to consider the interior architecture of the heart, let us recall that the ventricles (literally, "small bellies") were a diminutive analogue to the three major "venters" or cavities of the body, the abdomen, the thorax, and the head.[37] The heart itself was sometimes figured as a miniature human body, or a microcosm of the microcosmic body of man, or as a miniature head, with "ears" (auricles) that resembled the organs of hearing in shape and function: "the hert hath two eares . . . yt serue for to let the ayre in and out,"[38] and eyes, as in "having the eyes of your hearts enlightened" (Eph. 1.18 RSV). Also relevant here is St. Peter's cryptic advice to wives to avoid outward adorning of the body: "But let it be the hidden man of the heart, in that which is not corruptible" (1 Pet. 3.4), suggesting primarily that every woman had a hidden, incorruptible version of herself in her heart, but also suggesting the presence of a male element in her inner being. Concluding with the images in Crooke's description, the heart's expulsive power was repeatedly compared to a fountain, maintaining the vital economy of the body. In fact, the comparison of the heart to a fountain is perhaps the primary image of the heart in ancient and early modern discourse.

But the human analogue closest to the Galenic attractive rhythms of the heart was that of the female experience of conception and gestation. And since biblical woman was regarded as the source of evil and the pollution of sin (after Eve), yet at the same time the originator, preserver, and sustainer of life in the family, she exemplified more fully than man the Bible's representation of the ambivalence of the heart. The often noted scriptural binaries of the valiant woman/weak woman, or virgin/harlot, or Bride of Christ/Whore of Babylon, also made the female gender the one more closely associated with the heart, as Bunyan and Milton and Behn—but not Harvey—seem to attest. The rhetoric of the heart in Shakespeare is perhaps strongest in *King Lear*, alternating between the moral extremes of the devoted Cordelia (the name means virgin goddess of the heart), who says, "I cannot heave my heart into my mouth" (1.1.91–92), and her sisters Goneril and Regan: "Then let them anatomize Regan. See what breeds about her heart. Is there any cause in nature that make these hard hearts?" (3.6.76–78). There is a central duality in Shakespeare and the Bible of the soft, open, compassionate heart (usually associated with the "feminine," despite Jezebel, Goneril, Regan, and a few other exceptions) opposed to the closed, hard heart of malice and oppression (usually associated with the "masculine," but again exceptions come to mind), a duality working in varied ways through Milton and Richardson, in particular.

The four-chambered image of the heart gave rise to a multitude of "house" images, often feminized, and ranging from the heart as a storehouse of secrets, memories, or lived experience to the regenerated heart as the dwelling place of Christ. The four "chambers" of the heart may still be imagined, recalling Plato's image of men's and women's separated apartments, as a two-story house, the upper two chambers (the right and left atriums—"rooms," or auricles) connected to the vena cava and pulmonary vein, the lower two chambers (the right and left ventricles—"bellies") connected to the pulmonary artery and aorta. These right and left rooms are divided by a solid wall, which Galen thought had minute holes in it for the passage of blood. The Aristotelian heart as container of the "soul" force, noted above, gave rise in the seventeenth century to the heart as the seat or dwelling place of a femininized soul. The chambers and "strings" or sinews of the heart and its beating suggested images of musical instruments resonating, sounds of the "melody in the heart," as in St. Paul's phrase (Eph. 5.19). Thomas Watson says *"prepare your hearts to the reading of the word*—The heart is an instrument [that] needs putting in tune."[39] The heart was thought of as a multiplex, resonating receptacle for all kinds of impressions from the outside world and from inside the body, leading to images of the sexually receptive heart, as well as to images of the heart being warmed with religious ardor. The fundamental notion of the hot heart had its religious, aspect, as Watson reminded his hearers again and again: "*Leave not off reading in the Bible till you find your hearts warmed....* Let it not only inform you, but inflame you.... Go not from the word till you can say as those disciples, 'Did not our heart burn within us.' "[40]

Going beyond the richly suggestive metaphors of the heart as a house and the sexually generative heart, however, was the multiform figure of the heart as a book. The basic image is the receptive heart as a blank writing surface, a "table" or tablet for recording impressions in the form of words. Since the pulse was taken and counted from earliest recorded history, this activity may have provided the impulse for number systems that led to varieties of inscription.[41] The "people of the book" were numbered from the beginning in a census of the theocratic community (the first version of "the book of life"), and a preoccupation with recording things carried over into the "family theocracy" of Puritanism, with double-ledger books, debt books, account books, "stock" taking, activities intimately related to Puritan rhetorics of the heart.

The bipartite structure of the heart—right side and left side—lent itself to comparisons with the two tablets of the Law in the Old and New Testaments. The "tables of the heart" and the writing on these tables (discussed in more detail in the first chapter) is an important recurring image in Proverbs, the prophetic writings, and the epistles of St. Paul. Even Hobbes, who attempted resolutely to read Scripture unmetaphorically and who stressed God's "Infiniteness, Invisibility, and Incomprehensibility,"[42] saw the heart as the original repository of the written Law of Nature preserved in the language of Natural Reason: "That part of the Scripture, which was first Law, was the Ten Commandments, written in two Tables of Stone, and delivered by God himselfe to Moses; and by Moses made known to the people. Before that time there was no written Law of God, who as yet having not chosen any people to bee his peculiar Kingdome, had given no Law to men, but the Law of Nature, that is to say, the Precepts of Naturall Reason, written in every mans own heart."[43] It was an easy step from the image of the written heart to the image of the heart as an open book, as a treasury of verbal impressions, a storehouse of memories and life impressions, and learning something by heart was like memorizing from a book. The image of the treasure of the heart in the Gospels lent itself to later representations of the book of the heart. One is reminded of Bunyan's response, in his spiritual autobiography, to reading Luther's commentary on Galatians: "I found my condition in his experience, so largely and profoundly handled, as if his Book had been written out of my heart."[44]

Like its empathetic counterpart "my heart goes out to you," "taking something to heart" is one of the oldest figures of speech in English and still has the vivid sense of storing an impression, usually something painful, heavy, or troubling—"something close to one's heart"—as in Hamlet's unforgettable "how ill all's here about my heart" (5.2.212–13). Another important image of receptivity was that of the heart as the ground, earth, or soil. The strength and fertility of the land was often referred to as its "heart" (*OED* 21), an idea that comes down to us in the word "heartland." In "The Flower," George Herbert's "shrivelled heart" goes—like a dormant seed—underground to the "mother root" for later rejuvenation. In Puritan theology the originally hard heart of evil can only be rendered more tender, soft, and malleable for the reception of the divine Word, Christ, through regeneration. The entire conversion process is an ongoing effort to make a new heart, a heart that is holy and receptive to the "seed" of the Word. The Word softens the heart, warms it, makes it better soil, a better medium for the inseparable reception of the Word. "'The heart of a Christian is Christ's garden,' wrote Sibbes, explaining that Christ's spirit, blowing upon his flowers, 'makes them to send forth a sweet savour.'"[45]

The good heart was the good ground, or for the literate Puritan, the paper upon which he or she is writing, imagined as a literal external extension of the tables of the internal heart, or the book of the heart. The process of regeneration is recorded memorably by Bunyan who recounts how he came upon "three or four poor women sitting at a door in the sun, talking about the things of God," and how they were out of his reach, "for their talk was about a new birth, the work of God on their hearts." He thought they were in a special world of grace, and he felt his own heart begin to "shake" at the awareness of his own wickedness and ignorance. After repeated visits to the company of these poor people, he began to experience "a very great softness and tenderness of heart, which caused [him] to fall under the conviction of what by Scripture they asserted," and in a telling tribute to the power of the blood in the humoral body, he concludes his account with a startling image from phlebotomy: "By these things my mind was now so turned, that it lay like a horse leech at the vein, still crying out, *Give, give* (Prov. 30:15)."[46]

Having reviewed the ancient and traditional early modern notions of the nature and movements of the heart and blood, I would like, finally, to consider the newly emerging "empiricist" view of the heart that was to have profound significance as well for the redefinition of gender in early modern England. This new view of the heart was intimately linked with new views of the "self" and the body. I share the conviction—expressed in different terms by writers in this period and by others in our own—that "human being" or "the self" is an ongoing fiction or tissue of narratives constructed from within the body as well as from without. Human beings are governed from within by inner forces and conflicts that early modern writers often saw originating in "the heart." Ancient Greek physiology seems to see human motivation deriving largely from forces *within the body*, as in Galen's classical formulation of the idea that "the powers that govern us" have their source in the brain, heart, and liver.[47] Human beings are governed from without by a newly developing sense in the seventeenth century of the "self" as the human body interacting not only with forces associated with God's will but a sense of "pressure" from powerful external forces in a world characterized or felt more and more as a "machine" and less and less as a living, organic whole of which one believes oneself to be an integral part. In his popular early eighteenth-century dictionary, Nathan Bailey sums up this view by defining "Nature" as "*the machine of the universe.*"[48] Working in conjunction with the traditional sense of a "God force" impinging on human life, this new sense of the impact of the external world might be called a "world force" that can in part be measured and quantified.[49]

In contemplating these varied early narratives of the heart, it is important to remind ourselves as well that "the self" in its philosophical sense of "ego" or that which in a person is really and intrinsically *that person*—the ego as a permanent subject of successive and varying states of consciousness that can be "narrated"—is essentially a seventeenth-century invention, developed first by poets, then by philosophers as English philosophy itself was in the process of being invented in the early seventeenth century by the empiricist thinkers Francis Bacon and Thomas Hobbes. In writing and art from about 1400 to 1650 in Europe—the period still referred to for convenience as "The Renaissance"—there is an ebullient and vivid sense of individual self-shaping given one of its most definitive expressions in Pico della Mirandola's oration on "The Dignity of Man" in 1486. England in the seventeenth century experienced, in a variety of discourses but especially in "natural philosophy," a rediscovery or redefinition of the senses and how they are *acted upon* by and *react* to a variety of powerful stimuli.

The philosophy of imperceptible bodies moving in a stream through a void and interreacting was of course Epicureanism as conveyed primarily through the philosophic poem in six books *De rerum natura* (On the Nature of Things), by Lucretius, the Roman philosopher-poet of the first century B.C.E. Too often in discussions of empiricism, Lucretius, Epicurus, and atomistic theory are invoked and then dismissed.[50] Lucretius's great unfinished narrative poem, in its various impact on seventeenth-century thinkers, had a larger and more pervasive influence on English philosophical and religious thought—and on English culture—than is generally recognized. Lucretius was a key philosophical and poetic text for Hobbes, Harvey, Milton, Behn, and Locke. I will be referring to *De rerum natura* in the brilliant but rarely reprinted translation by Thomas Creech, first published in 1682, and in John Dryden's better known partial translation of 1685.

For introductory purposes, let us look first at Lucretius's discussion of motion and bodies in space. Lucretius inherited the Aristotelian philosophical discourse on the natural world, which, in the *Physics*, is largely a discourse on motion and change. Early in book 1 Lucretius declares,

> This *All* consists of *Body* and of *Space*,
> This *moves*, and that affords the *Motion place*. . . .
> Besides, whatever *is*, a Power must own,
> Or fit to *Act*, or to be acted *on*,
> Or be a *Place* in which such things are *done*.[51]

After this initial assertion of the motion of bodies through space, and the doctrine of action and reaction, he goes on to establish the position that all bodies have stable properties (that is, ones that can be separated from them only by violence), such as weight in stones, heat in fire, liquidity in water, and even the primary sense of *touch* in sentient bodies. Everything else in human experience, such as slavery, poverty, riches, freedom, war, peace, all come and go in the flux of eventuality. He then asserts that time itself is nothing but our thinking about things in motion—our "laboring Fancy" or imagination creates time and "Events" (1.16). We can infer that among the "Sons of Fame," the poets, only Lucretius has seen that the ultimate cause of unstable events is a primary and permanent "Frame" of space—like a great stage—in which indivisible bodies or "Seeds" may act. The poets sing of Helen's rape, or mourn the fall of Troy, without being aware that these events do not exist of themselves but are only contingent accidents produced by the incessant activity of the eternal seeds. "Take heed, nor fancy from such Tales as these / That *Actions* are, that they *subsist* confess" (1.16). The further implication seems to be that all such narrated events are a tissue of fictions which have no essential existence.

After the famous passage on how Nature, the "*all-powerful She*," allows for the "declination" (or swerve) of the streaming seeds so that "perfect Freedom of the Mind" and "Will" may exist in the animal and human worlds, Lucretius, arguing from animal experience, gives the example of the agitated horse who cannot start the race too soon as evidence that "the *Will first* moves" in the "Mind," which further "proves these *Motions* rise within the *Heart* [a corde] / Begun by th' *Will*, thence run thro every part."[52] Let us pause here for a moment to reflect on the genealogy of Donne's trope of the "naked thinking heart." Counterpoised against the Platonic-Galenic tradition of the thinking brain in Greek physiology is the tradition, beginning perhaps with the "Hippocratic" *De corde*, of the heart as the center of intellectual activity, and extending to Aristotle's view of the heart as the source of sensation, memory, and imagination. The trope of the "thinking heart" was an important alternate paradigm to that of the thinking brain from the ancient world through the early modern period. For Lucretius, as for the Stoics, the heart and the breast region is the source of mind, will, and motion. As we shall see in the next chapter, the heart is also the center of understanding and feeling in the Bible. All human action for Lucretius has its source in the heart, and the primary sense which the heart impels is that of touch.

> For *Touch*, that best, that chiefest Sense is made,
> When Strokes from *things without* the Nerves invade,
> Or something from *within* doth *outward* flow,

>And hurts, or tickles, as it passes thro;
>As 'tis in *Venery*.
>(2.47)

The sentient body feels the force of an external impact, like a blow, or the effects of something welling up from within, like sexual desire, and must respond with choices made by the heart. In addition to book 2, book 4 of *De rerum natura* is relevant to seventeenth-century poetics because of its account of how we perceive the external world. We must here imagine ourselves back into a pre-Kantian, pre-Romantic age where the outside world and the inside "forces that govern us" are thought to impinge constantly on human consciousness, and where the imagination is not so much an autonomous originator of the categories of perception as a receiver and shaper of impressions.

Perhaps the best example of the action of two bodies encountering each other in the context of the Lucretian sexual heart is Dryden's vivid translation of the long passage on the "nature of love" from the fourth book of *De rerum natura*. Dryden goes beyond Creech in explicit poetic rendering of the intensity of pleasure and pain in the vigorous conjunction of human female and male bodies in the sexual act. This is the sequence in Dryden's version: the "fiery dart / Of strong desire" emanates from "some beauteous boy's alluring face," or from each part of the body of some "lovelier maid," "transfixing [the] amorous heart" of the male lover, causing him to roam restlessly, "eager to inject the sprightly seed" into the body that has caused a burning distillation of love's "drops" in his heart: here the female projects, the male injects.

>Such is the nature of that pleasing smart,
>Whose burning drops distil upon the heart,
>The fever of the soul shot from the fair,
>And the cold ague of succeeding care.[53]

The woman's entire body projects erotic images that create a boiling fluid in the male heart. The physical dynamic is one of action upon the heart and reaction in the loins. The poet advises the male lover that when these feminine "aerial images of love" molest the mind, "Discharge thy loins on all the leaky kind." The male heart then is the central repository of "cupido" (desire's) invasive darts and the agent that incubates and distills hot erotic fluid, inciting phallic penetration at the same time that it creates the "cold ague" of erotic anxiety. We see how a much more complex erotic discourse stands behind trivialized and inane later representations of the action and effect of Cupid's darts, images and verse that still fuel the multimillion-dollar valentine industry. The poet then proceeds to describe the physical effects and motions of the love combat instigated by these "aerial shapes"—"all the gentle and ungentle pressures of the lover's warfare," as Richardson's Lovelace puts it[54]—culminating in the "vain violence" of the lovers' attempt to interpenetrate each other's hearts:

> When hands in hands they lock, and thighs in thighs they twine,
> Just in the raging foam of full desire,
> When both press on, both murmur, both expire,
> They gripe, they squeeze, their humid tongues they dart,
> As each would force their way to t'other's heart.[55]

Thus the heart in Lucretius is at once the source and the goal of erotic passion.

By the mid-seventeenth century, the notion of an essentially "soft," porous, and permeable human body on the Galenic model, composed primarily of fluids in a state of perilous "solubility" or interconvertibility, was giving way to, or being modified by, a more mechanized view of the human body and a more mechanized view of the heart. The comparatively new sense—inaugurated in part by the rediscovery of Lucretian Epicureanism—of human life as a motive, mechanical process of being acted upon from within and from without is perhaps most forcibly expressed by Thomas Hobbes in the opening of *Leviathan*: ". . . For seeing life is but a motion of Limbs, the begining whereof is in some principall part within; why may we not say, that all *Automata* (Engines that move themselves by springs and wheeles as doth a watch) have an artificiall life? For what is the *Heart*, but a *Spring*; and the *Nerves*, but so many *Strings*; and the *Joynts*, but so many *Wheeles*, giving motion to the whole Body, such as was intended by the Artificer."[56] Echoing and expanding the image of the heart as an "Engine" already used by the traditional Galenic anatomist Crooke, Hobbes transforms the sluggish, fluid internal motion of the "humoral body" and Lucretius's intense physical vitality into the register of mechanical, physical collision as the human body becomes an engine that moves itself, a clockwork automaton.

God is represented as an "Artificer" or artisan, a maker of machines, and the body is a machine in motion. With Hobbes, the soft, permeable humoral body has become hardened into a mechanical, but still vital, body. Whether the cause of the motion is from within or without, however, motion is simply the pressure of one body upon another. In terms of external stimuli on "the Thoughts of Man," Hobbes continues: "The Originall of them all [i.e., ideas, which Hobbes defines with the words *Representation* or *Apparence*], is that which we call SENSE; (For there is no conception in a mans mind, which hath not at first . . . been begotten upon the organs of Sense."[57] He uses a sexual metaphor conceived within the context of mechanism: all mental conceptions are originally "begotten upon" the senses, as if all ideas begin with the sexual body. Hobbes's mechanization of the sexual body and the heart is a more complex articulation of Lucretius on the processes of causation from external stimuli moving inward. Hobbes goes on:

> The cause of Sense, is the Externall body, or Object, which presseth the organ proper to each Sense, either immediatly, as in the Tast and Touch; or mediately, as in Seeing, Hearing, and Smelling: which pressure, by the mediation of Nerves, and other strings, and membranes of the body, continued inwards to the Brain, and Heart, causeth there a resistance, or counter pressure, or endeavour of the Heart, to deliver it self: which endeavour because *Outward*, seemeth to be some matter without. And this *seeming*, or *fancy*, is that which men call *Sense* . . . All which qualities called *Sensible*, are in the object that causeth them, but so many several motions of the matter, by which it presseth our organs diversely.[58]

That is, the pressure from outside on the brain and heart causes a reaction which *seems* to be an external reality but is actually an internal one. I call this "counter pressure" the Hobbesian recoil effect, important for our encounter with Milton's Satan. It is noteworthy that both Lucretius and Hobbes continue the Aristotelian (and biblical) placement of certain mental functions in the heart. The early empiricists still think with the heart. Hobbes's language glides from the brain to focus on the "endeavour of the Heart" (the same phrase Milton will use at the end of *Paradise Lost*) as the central generator of this internal reality. He then reiterates his emphasis on the motion of bodies upon each other as the cause of sensation and uses examples of violent force upon the senses to make his point:

> Neither in us that are pressed, are they any thing else, but divers motions; (for motion, produceth nothing but motions.) But their apparence to us is Fancy, the same waking, that dreaming. And as pressing, rubbing, or striking the Eye, makes us fancy a light; and pressing the Eare, produceth a dinne; so do the bodies also we see, or hear, produce the same by their strong, though unobserved actions . . . Yet

still the object is one thing, the image or fancy is another. So that Sense in all cases, is nothing els but original fancy, caused . . . by the pressure, that is, by the motion, of externall things upon our Eyes, Eares, and other organs [presumably including internal and external ones]. . . .[59]

In other words, for Hobbes, all human images or thoughts are "Fancy" or fiction or imagination generated in a continuous process of material pressures and reactions from within the body and from outside it. Even Locke, eager to distance himself as far as possible from Hobbes and traditional religio-philosophical rhetoric of the heart and "the finger of God," cannot avoid the fountain imagery often associated with the heart in his carefully phrased (and revolutionary) denial of innate principles being stamped or implanted in the human mind: "Our observation employed either, about external sensible objects, or about the internal operations of our minds perceived and reflected by ourselves, is that which supplies our understandings with all the *materials* of thinking. These two are the fountains of knowledge, from whence all the ideas we have, or can naturally have, do spring."[60]

The terms "within" and "without," "external" and "internal," are obviously of great importance to Hobbes and to Locke, and will be to this study. In general, I will be discussing "outward" phenomena as those activities and actions often associated with forces in the external world, with the "visual," with seeing and perceiving as activities of agency, with the "masculine," with the male gaze, with "writing," penetrating, and anatomizing, with the phallic heart and "hardness," with the semiotic Lord God of the King James version of the Old Testament. This Lord God is also represented as presiding over or within the realm of "inward" phenomena, those often associated with the feminized interior world of mind or soul, with the "aural/oral," hearing and listening, with "reading," with the "feminine," with receptivity and the hidden or secret things within the body, with the receptive heart and "softness," with the Christ of the New Testament, who is predominantly a reader, teacher, redeemer, and judge. This schema is far from rigid. As we have seen already in Lucretius, a woman's body may have powerful "external" agency on the receptive male heart, which in turn injects its desires into appropriate bodies. In what follows, terms like "internal" and "feminine" are not to be simply equated but interpreted contextually. We turn now to the most influential narrative of the heart in early modern England.

I

The Biblical Heart

> The counsel of the Lord standeth for ever, the thoughts
> of his heart to all generations.... From the place of his
> habitation he looketh upon all the inhabitants of the
> earth. He fashioneth their hearts alike; he considereth
> all their works.
> —Ps. 33.11–15

> How long wilt thou go about, O thou backsliding
> daughter? for the Lord hath created a new thing in
> the earth, A woman shall compass a man.
> —Jer. 31.22

HOBBES WAS WRITING *Leviathan* (at a safe distance in France) in the midst of the English Civil War, and the social upheaval England experienced in that event and afterward in plague, famine, the Fire of London, and outbreaks of foreign war from 1660 through 1713 certainly contributed to the sense of being acted upon, shaped, and conditioned by largely uncontrollable forces, whether these forces were thought to emanate specifically and retributively from God or from a more generalized mechanical origin of "world" forces in collision, whose cause was still ultimately from God. It is in this Lucretian-Hobbesian context of the dialogue of external and internal forces acting upon the "theatre of the body" that we must situate the languages of the heart in our five principal texts.

The master narrative for this study is that contained in the Authorized Version of the Bible (hereafter referred to simply as the Bible or Scripture). This translation, published in 1611, was the culmination of a long series of English translations. As everyone knows—and takes perhaps too much for granted—this became the most popular and authoritative version of the Bible in English. It is our master narrative in part because the diverse texts examined here are all imbued, to one extent or another, with the ideology and idiom of the Bible. In this first chapter, I discuss the evolution of the representation of the heart in the Old and New Testaments from the point of view of a present-day reader of the Bible concerned with those anatomical, sexual, religious, and literary traditions in the biblical narrative that seem most important to early modern readers and writers, especially the newly emerging woman reader and writer.

With a much wider circulation of the new "Authorized" translation and greater general literacy, more people were reading the Bible aloud, in families, to themselves and to others. So far as we can tell, there was a much wider consciousness of the stories of the Bible gained from this kind of family reading and from sermons. I want to reinvestigate the importance of the Bible from the gendered and heart-centered perspective suggested in the Introduction, looking closely at the "scriptive" or written characteristic of Scripture. (Originally, the word "scripture" applied to all kinds of writing.) By concentrating on the shaping linguistic matrix of the Bible as it relates to God, the word (spoken and written), the earth or land, woman, man (humankind and the masculine gender), sexual generation, the blood, and most of all, the heart, we can understand more fully the evolving process of how the roles of male and female, masculine and feminine, were created in early modern England.

The word "heart" is used (in some form) 858 times in the Authorized Version, far more than the word "spirit" for example (*lev*, or "heart," is used over 1,000 times in the Hebrew Bible).[1] In the Bible, the term "heart" connotes the inner resources of the whole person, especially the mind and will, with somewhat less emphasis on the emotions, and seldom refers simply to the physical organ. "Heart" was and is a mediating word, bringing together mind and emotion, body and soul, human and divine, but the opposition of the head and the heart, of following either the dictates of the mind or the impulses of the feeling heart ("the heart has reasons that reason does not know," said Pascal) was also firmly established by the eighteenth century. The word "heart" is arguably the most significant word in the Bible pertaining to the relationship between deity and humankind. Robert Alter notes that "Samuel the seer . . . mistakes physical for regal stature in the case of both Saul and Eliab, and has to undergo an object lesson in the way God sees, which is not with the eyes but with the heart—the heart in biblical physiology being the seat of understanding rather than feeling."[2] I suggest that the heart in biblical physiology means much more than "understanding," whether applied to God or man. For God too has a heart, but in the Authorized Version at least God's "heart" signifies— besides understanding—inconsistency, reversal, even regret and sorrow, as when God "repents" that he made "man": "And God saw that the wickedness of man was great in the earth, and that every imagination of the thoughts of his heart was only evil continually. And it repented the Lord that he had made man on the earth, and it grieved him at his heart" (Gen. 6.5–6).

The Puritan divine Stephen Charnock gives a particularly informative interpretation (published in 1681) of this passage and of "the biblical heart" as seen by Puritan commentators in the later seventeenth century, one which will serve as the theological counterpart to the Galenic anatomical heart—primarily an organ of attraction—sketched in the Introduction.[3] In preaching about the heart, Charnock started with a respectable anatomical preamble, reminding his hearers that the ribs (the part of the body from which Eve came) are first of all a defensive structure: "How strongly [the heart] is guarded with ribs like a wall, that it might not be easily hurt! It draws blood from the liver through a channel made for that purpose, rarefies it, and makes it fit to pass through the arteries and veins, and to carry heat and life to every part of the body, and by a perpetual motion it sucks in the blood and spouts it out again, which motion depends not upon the command of the soul, but is pure natural."[4]

Charnock may have been aware of Harvey's new theory about the circulation in his allusion to "perpetual motion," but the Galenic model of the heart was still primary for him, and he was far more interested in what the Bible says about the heart. With reference to Gen. 6.5–6, he exclaims, "I know not a more lively description in the whole book of God of the natural corruption derived from our first parents, than these words; wherein you have the ground of that grief, which lay so close to God's heart . . . and the resolve thereupon to destroy man." He goes on to contrast God's pleasure in the goodness of his creation with the utterly inclusive spatial and temporal evil of the human heart, an evil that applies not only to the people before the Flood but also to those coming after: "'Surely all could not be under such a blemish: were there not now and then some pure flashes of the mind?' No, not one."[5] The subsequent burden of his sermon is to explain how this evil heart can only be saved through regeneration. He then gives an etymological analysis of the word "imagination," which, like the opening of *Leviathan*, stresses the internal fictionality of the heart's constructions and the external construction of the imaginative product (his term "figmentum" is related to "fingere," the source of "fiction"): "'Imagination,' properly signifies *figmentum* . . . 'to afflict, press, or form a thing by way of compression.' And thus it is a metaphor taken from a potter's framing a vessel, and extends to 'whatsoever is framed' inwardly in the heart, or outwardly in the work. It is usually taken by the Jews for that fountain of sin within us."[6] As it is in Lucretius, "imagination" (or "fancy") is a physical, material force for him, the kind of power that fashioned Eve. Finally, he explains the four principal features of the biblical heart:

The word "heart" is taken variously in scripture. It signifies properly that inward member which is the seat of the vital spirits: but sometimes it signifies, 1. The *understanding and mind.*—Psalm xii.2: "With a double heart do they speak." . . . 2. For the *will.*—2 Kings x.30: "All that is in my heart," that is, in my will and purpose. 3. For the *affections*—As, Deut. vi.5: "Thou shalt love the Lord thy God with all thine heart"; that is, with all thy affections. 4. For *conscience.*—2 Sam. xxiv.10: "David's heart smote him." . . . But "heart" here [in Gen. 6.5] is used for the whole soul, because . . . the soul is chiefly seated in the heart, especially the will, and the affections, her attendants; because, when my affection stirs, the chief motion of it is felt in the heart. So that, by the "imaginations of the thoughts of the heart" are here meant all the inward operations of the soul, which play their part principally in the heart; whether they be the acts of the understanding, the resolutions of the will, or the blusterings of the affections.[7]

Starting with this reasonably comprehensive Puritan definition for the function and constitution of the biblical "heart" (conceived traditionally as the arena of the soul), I would suggest that the heart appears as the primary symbol of the ambivalence of human existence in Scripture because it is represented at various times as, on the one hand, the fountainhead of all human wickedness, often linked with the "imagination" and duplicity, and on the other hand—particularly with regard to individuals—as the source of truth, understanding, and sincerity.

The Seminal God

God is first imaged in Genesis as a "Spirit" moving over the waters and this Spirit speaks—or as was sometimes thought, sings—light into being. There is no gender reference to God until verse 10 when "he" names the "dry land Earth, and the gathering together of the waters called he Seas." God appears to be a masculine force and the "Earth/dry land" is by implication female. This verse brings into play God as male creator through speech and the Earth as feminine receiver, but hovering over the transaction is the ambiguous "gathering together of the waters," a term that suggests combined male and female agency, as in the great image of the Lord as a female eagle fluttering over her young and bearing them on her wings in Deut. 32.11. So begins the complex relation between "God" (or "the Lord God," or simply "the Lord") and the feminine or "woman" in the Bible.

I will discuss the Fall in more detail in the chapters on Eve and Clarissa, but I wish now to focus on the creation of Eve. Eve has two names, unfallen "Woman" and fallen "Eve." God causes a deep sleep to fall upon Adam, takes a bone out of his midsection or thorax, and fashions it into Woman. Adam then takes over the divine male prerogative of naming the feminine. Adam's first act is naming, and "Adam" is named precisely at the juncture when he will name. He first names his human partner "Woman" because she is taken out of man. She is bone of his bone, flesh of his flesh; they are "one flesh." Woman is his partner in the "flesh" and blood of his body. But Eve is not only Adam's partner in the flesh, she is his heart partner because she was taken from his breast region, from the center of his being. She is central to Adam. (Both the Bible and Galen—not anatomically correct—center the heart exactly in the middle of the thorax.) The two will "cleave" to each other, one of those rare words with two diametrically opposed meanings: to divide with one blow, as with an ax, and to adhere or cling together, to be mutually faithful. Despite Adam's divine prerogative of naming her, in the drama of the Fall that follows, the woman becomes the chief actor.

As with the seed yielding the herb, the creation of Eve comes from the inside out, but now in an anatomical manipulation by the Maker, who carefully closes up the flesh where the rib had been. The Lord God is the original anatomist, and the creation of Eve is an act of vivisection, albeit a painless one. The Lord God creates now in a new way, not through speech "by kind," but by tactile "forming" and reforming (or, as Charnock would say, "framing"), as if man and woman were a form or kind *different* from the other animals because the two are "made" in the image of God. Charnock's definition of man's evil "imagination" has a curious similarity to this divine process of material creation. This is a God working with his hands and fingers, shaping the human material in a process analogous to the act of writing and to the Lucretian emphasis on the primacy of touch and the interaction of bodies. God invades his created bodies to form or inscribe new bodies. But these bodies, made in the image of God, have a special and unique destiny, and the woman's formation out of man's "bone" instead of the "dust of the ground" suggests a more durable and valuable materiality in her being.[8] The Lord works from "deep" inside in the creation of woman, and his working with woman hereafter will be deep in her womb and in her heart. The word "deep" in this context recalls the great blessing of Jacob upon Joseph at the end of Genesis, invoking the creative power of "blessings of the deep that lieth under, blessings of the breasts, and of the womb" (49.25). As external signifiers of the loving, generous heart, the female breasts signify nourishment and nurture at the deepest theological level. We recall also the mutual warmth and protection of the female heart and breasts in Galen. "Blessings," expressions of divine creative love, come out of the depths, out of the cosmic darkness or the darkness of sleep.

God originally creates from the inside out, then he forms and manipulates "man," then after the Fall he makes an ironic adjustment of his creation by changing the terms. He originally anatomized Adam to make Eve, but no pain or sorrow was involved. When his human creatures prove disobedient, he invades both of them in order to create an ironically appropriate form of sorrow and punishment for their crimes. He intrudes, challenges, confronts. He makes them both *feel* sorrow, and he makes the ground or the land a constant reminder of their wrongdoing in the fates of their two sons. In contrast, the male divine force controlling female Galenic "nature" works all things to harmonious perfection. The word "nature" does not appear in the Authorized Version of the Old Testament.

The curse on woman and the ground is virtually coupled, from the beginning, with the theme of women bearing children by God's permission and enabling power, and at his own good pleasure. Childbearing may be painful and sorrowful, but it is Eve's defining role as "mother of all living" and scriptural woman's most important and wished-for function and responsibility. Eve sets the triumphant tone for this theme by saying, "I have gotten a man from the Lord" (Gen. 4.1). Poor Cain, her firstborn, goes on tilling the ground like Adam and gets into new kinds of trouble. Cain is another man of the female ground, but like the "thorns" and "thistles," he is a curse to his parents, to his brother, to himself, and to the other people who have now suddenly appeared on the earth. Abel in his role as presider over "firstlings" is more like the deity: he is a breeder of higher living forms than Cain's "fruits." God has "respect unto Abel" and his offerings but not unto Cain and his. Abel is a "keeper of sheep" but Cain is not his "brother's keeper." Again, ironically, Abel in death becomes a man of the ground and Cain a "fugitive" when Abel's blood "crieth unto [the Lord] from the ground" after the feminized earth "opened her mouth" to receive his blood. The first mention of blood in the Bible (Gen. 4.10) is linked with the voice and signification—with the expression of deep human emotion and loss—as the first use of the word "heart" (Gen. 6.5) is linked, as we have seen, with human imagination and "thoughts" expressing evil. The blood is imagined as a cry rising up to God from the ground; the heart is imagined as the source of multitudes of evil thoughts springing up within God's grieving gaze. Both the blood and the heart, from the first, signify motion, emotion, pain, and evil, whatever other more positive meanings the two terms will come to generate, as Charnock makes clear in his exposition of Gen. 6.5–6.

After Eve's grateful acknowledgment that the Lord has given her the gift of a "man," childless Sarai (Abram's beautiful wife) tells her husband that "the Lord hath restrained me from bearing," and she offers him the sexual gift of her handmaid, Hagar, that "I may obtain children by her" (Gen. 16.2). Sarai has had years to mature this proposal; she has pondered the fact of her childlessness for a long time. So has her husband. When the Lord makes his startling promise of "a son also of her . . . Abraham fell upon his face, and laughed, and said in his heart, Shall a child be born unto him that is an hundred years old? and shall Sarah, that is ninety years old, bear?" (Gen. 17.16–17). For a biblical character, something "said in the heart" is something that is really meant. It is the truest and most sincere of human expressions. When Esau says "in his heart" that he will slay his brother, he means it (Gen. 27.41), though he later relents and makes up with his brother as they kiss and weep (Gen. 33.4), prefiguring Joseph's reconciliation with his brothers.

Despite the consistent subordination of women to men in daily life and ritual, and the purity laws of Leviticus 12 and 15, the richest and deepest experience of the heart seems to be reserved for women in the Bible, and this experience is almost always accompanied by an experience within the womb. The Bible represents woman as the sacred living being—a human temple—in whom God enacts the mystery of the generation of life, propagating his image in humankind. This transaction makes scriptural woman profoundly different from scriptural man. Unlike man, she has two sources of inward communion with God, her womb and her heart, the latter including mind and emotion. There is no suggestion in the Bible of the Galenic paradigm of "one sex."[9]

The ordeal of the scriptural male hero, as he evolves from Abraham to

Moses to David, is expressed primarily through the struggles of transmigration, warfare, and political intrigue in the *external* world. He confronts the will of God at first in person and later via a prophet. The ordeal of the scriptural female hero is expressed primarily through *internal* struggle, in the danger, pain, and triumph of childbirth and child-rearing within the domestic space. Hers is an internalized version of the male hero's ordeal. When Sarah, standing in the tent door just behind Abraham, overhears the Lord's promise, she too laughs "within herself," but she is also struck more by the absurdity of having sexual pleasure with her old husband than by the thought of pain in childbirth (Gen. 18.12). She seems to retain a secret that even the Lord cannot, or will not, fathom: the Lord says, "Wherefore did Sarah laugh?" (Gen. 18.13). Sarah denies having laughed, and she is afraid, but she keeps her feelings hidden. The Lord knows better but lets her alone; he will penetrate her inner feelings only so far, and no farther, but she knows he is working something to fruition within her. Milton and Richardson will reiterate the theme of the male attempting to penetrate to the woman's inmost core and possess her secrets, but their proponents of this theme are the exemplars of phallic evil, Satan and Lovelace.

Rebekah is a darker and more mysterious secret keeper than the cautious Sarah. Rebekah is linked at once with the inner experience of the heart when she appears at the well to Abraham's servant: "And before I had done speaking in mine heart, behold, Rebekah came forth" (Gen. 24.45). When Isaac entreats the Lord on behalf of his barren wife, she has an early epiphany of the Lord's special purpose for her: "the children struggled together within her; and she said, If it be so, why am I thus? And she went to enquire of the Lord. And the Lord said unto her, Two nations are in thy womb, and two manner of people shall be separated from thy bowels: and the one people shall be stronger than the other people; and the elder shall serve the younger" (Gen. 25.22–23). When scriptural woman has a question about what is happening within her womb, she inquires of the Lord about it. The heart or "understanding" of scriptural woman, in contrast to scriptural man, knows what is going on in her womb. Rebekah knows, in a uniquely painful pre-birth experience in her womb and in her heart, that Jacob the younger is favored, and she cannot help loving him more than Esau, "a man of the field," who like Cain will come to have the curse of the female ground on him. Both peoples shall be literally "separated" from her body, but one will be torn from her figurative "bowels," her deepest affections, a dichotomy reflected in the Lord's own affections as declared by the prophet Malachi: "yet I loved Jacob. And I hated Esau, and laid his mountains and his heritage waste for the dragons of the wilderness" (Mal. 1.2–3). Esau's fate is prefigured in a birth simile; he looks like the "hairy garment" (Gen. 25.25) his mother and brother will eventually use to deceive old Isaac. Rebekah seems almost to personify the curse of the female ground when, in reply to Jacob's fear that he "shall bring a curse" upon himself, she says, "Upon me be thy curse, my son: only obey my voice" (27.12–13). The episodes of the birth and the deception are ironically knitted together, steeped in the word-magic of curse and blessing, and issuing, like a blood feud, from the mysterious inner depths—from the heart and womb—of Rebekah the mother.

The third barren woman in the Genesis series, Rachel, implores her husband (in a passage that intrigued John Locke) to give her children, "or else I die," and the final irony is that she will die in bearing her second son, Benoni (her own name for Benjamin), "son of my sorrow" (Gen. 35.18). Jacob knows perhaps better than any patriarchal husband that he is not in possession or control of the power to impregnate her. All Old Testament males seem to know this. The power of fruition is with the seminal God alone, and they are only his instruments. The mystery of human paternity was never so profound or so poignant as in the Bible. And the language of the Authorized Version, charged with the rhythms of generation and violence, gives each story a resonant finality. As the two infants struggled in the womb of Rebekah, so in her adult life Rachel strives with the fecund Leah: "With great wrestlings have I wrestled with my sister, and I have prevailed" (30.8). Their contest is a frantically competitive bout of maternal creativity and symbolic naming as they take advantage—seemingly while the spell lasts—of "God's hearkening" to their procreative efforts.

The story of the birth of Samson and Samson's relationship with Delilah is one of the richest narratives of the womb and heart in the Old Testament. It is a story of secrets. Samson's mother (who is not named, as if her name itself were a secret known only to God) is visited by an angel of God who wears a "terrible" countenance. He tells her that despite her barrenness, she will conceive and bear a son. He will be a Nazarite to God from his womb, and "he shall begin to deliver Israel out of the hand of the Philistines" (Judg. 13.5). The woman tells of her experience with the angel to her husband, Manoah, and he wants to know how they should rear the child. The angel, whom Manoah sees as simply a man in a field, repeats the injunctions concerning what the woman is not to drink but refuses to divulge his own name ("seeing it is secret") or tell Manoah anything about this special child. Manoah's wife and the angel are linked by being unnamed. Only after the man ascends in a flame from the sacrificial altar does Manoah recognize that this is an angel of God and he fears for his life. His wife, however, knows that God will not destroy them, and it is clear that she has a much deeper understanding of the whole experience than does her husband. In several respects, this narrative has strong affinities with the Elisabeth-Zacharias narrative in Luke, to be discussed later. Samson's mother keeps the secret of Samson's deliverance of Israel and does not even tell her husband. She is a strong Israelite woman counterpoised against the valiant and wily Delilah of the Philistines.

Delilah is one of the few women in the Bible to invoke the heart/erotic love association: "How canst thou say, I love thee, when thine heart is not with me?" (Judg. 16.15). She can manipulate language as forcibly as any man, and she "presses [Samson] daily with her words . . . that his soul was vexed unto death" (16.16). It is as if he must tell her "all his heart," the secret God had put into the womb and heart of his mother, just to survive: "I have been a Nazarite unto God from my mother's womb" (16.17)—almost the exact words of the angel. The secret of the womb his mother was so careful not to reveal bursts from the fallible lips of Samson and becomes Delilah's heart secret to reveal to Samson's male rivals and enemies: "Come up this once, for he hath shewed me all his heart" (16.18), or in the words of Milton's Samson, "I yielded, and unlock'd her all my heart" (*Samson Agonistes* line 407). Heart and womb are here virtually equated. If "heart" can also be a metaphor for womb, this image has the shock of a deep feminine secret between women—never meant to be revealed—being suddenly given away by a man. In betraying his heart and his mother's secret, Samson is now vulnerable. It is as if he has just exposed his mother's womb. Samson's revelation is like the shock of seeing a woman's body opened; it has resonance with the first early modern images of a woman's body dissected, and the imagined shock of men seeing something that only God could see before. The two women, Samson's mother and Delilah, are stronger than Manoah or even Samson because of their mastery and control of the innermost secret language imparted by God. They occupy a space somewhere between the vulnerable human utterance of Samson and the terrible angel who refuses to reveal his name.

The most detailed and profound representation in the Old Testament of God's relationship with a barren woman and her desire to bear a son is the story of Hannah in 1 Samuel. Hannah and Sarah are both advanced in years and barren; unlike Sarah and the other barren women, Hannah prays directly to the Lord for a man-child: "she spake in her heart; only her lips moved" (1 Sam. 1:13); she was communing with God in her heart, the deep spiritual domain within all humankind. She, not Eli, is the true priest. No voice is heard in that place, the words are shaped only. God alone hears what she says and only she knows what she has asked for in this realm of the spirit. To outward appearance, to the imperceptive Eli, she is drunk: "No, my lord, I am a woman of a sorrowful spirit . . . I have poured out my soul before the Lord" (1 Sam. 1:15). She opens her heart to God, asking him for a son (the meaning of "Samuel," "asked of God"), and dedicates him as a loan to the Lord, to do the Lord's work. The language of the heart in this story goes beyond words and beyond ordinary verbal intercourse, preserving and enhancing the sense, found also in the previous stories, of divine and human communion in a profoundly secret space. We shall return to the story of Hannah and her son Samuel in connection with Richardson's creation of *Clarissa*, but we must now turn to another crucial aspect of God's relationship with the human heart.

The Semiotic God

Besides being represented as a seminal God of astonishing fertility and creativity (the ultimate fertility god of all such deities in the ancient Near East), the God of the Old Testament is a powerful God of signs or "tokens." I take the term semiotic in its most literal sense of "sign-making," with the emphasis on creating, inflicting, memorializing. I wish first to explore God's marking activity on the human body (especially the male body), and on the earth or land ("the land is mine" [Lev. 25.23]), and why that activity is important to the biblical narrative of the heart. We shall see that the emphasis on written discourse in Exodus (in conjunction with the emphasis on oral discourse in Genesis) is primarily significant for our master narrative because of the eventual metonymic identification of stone tablets and the human heart in Jeremiah and, most importantly for Christians in early modern England, the discourse of the heart in the Gospels and that of the Spirit's writing in the heart in the Epistles of St. Paul. The account which I give here of God's writing, and writing as a male act of power, culminates in the trope of the written heart.[10]

Adam of course is the first man to experience God's invasive anatomical procedures when Eve is formed from his thorax, but Adam's son Cain, who laments being driven "from the face of the earth" (Gen. 4.14) and hidden from God's own "face," is the receiver of a mysterious visible "mark" on his body as a sign to others to spare his life. This mark is a personal "face-to-face" covenant between God and Cain, a life-giving form of inscription. Cain crosses the boundary between individual or generic man and social man. God "signs" Cain and makes him a unique "fugitive," a social being now with a special story to tell others, a man who leaves the tillage of the land to build a city.

In the realm of the earth, God makes another mark, the covenant of the rainbow, to memorialize his promise (first "said in his heart" [Gen. 8.21] and then made visible to all) not to again curse the ground for man's sake, despite his acceptance of the biblical certainty that "the imagination of man's heart is evil from his youth." Because that evil imagination of the heart is ineradicable, however, there are still plenty of local instances of God's cursing the land. A particularly vivid account of the Lord's anger expressed in written characters that have the power literally to descend upon and destroy both man and the land is found in Moses' speech to the multitude in Deuteronomy 29, after the desolating curses contained in chapter 28: "The Lord will not spare him [the disobedient man], but then the anger of the Lord and his jealousy shall smoke against that man, and all the curses written in this book shall lie upon him, and the Lord shall blot out his name from under heaven" (29.20) The curses now have almost physical weight, grinding the man down, obliterating him.

And the Lord shall separate him unto evil out of all the tribes of Israel. . . . So that the generation to come of your children that shall rise up after you, and the stranger that shall come from a far land, shall say, when they see the plagues of that land, and the sicknesses which the Lord hath laid upon it; And that the whole land thereof is brimstone, and salt, and burning, that it is not sown, nor beareth, nor any grass groweth therein, like the overthrow of Sodom and Gomorrah . . . which the Lord overthrew in his anger, and in his wrath: Even all nations shall say, Wherefore hath the Lord done thus unto this land? what meaneth the heat of this great anger? (29.21–24)

As was noted in the Introduction, heat and life are virtually equated in ancient Greek medicine. In the Hebrew Bible, God as the source of life is also the source of destruction, and his great anger is conveyed in heat. The meaning of this heat lies in the memorial, and the significance of the Lord's writing is always as a reminder, lest one forget. It is a permanent record on the land for those who can read it.

The movement of the covenant signs from the individual to the whole of humankind and then to a special nation eventuates in the covenant of circumcision with Abraham. The ritual of circumcision was a widely performed surgical operation in the ancient world. For the Hebrews, it was a sign of God's claim upon the source of generation in males and a sign of God's control of male potency. When the foreskin of the penis is cut off and removed, God has performed a possessive act of surgical marking or inscription on his own male property and has perfect control of the act of generation. He seals the men of the tribe as his own with a sign of special favor and blessing, a further "opening" or enhancement of male fertility and vitality. The thirteenth-century sage Isaac ben Yedaiah even went so far as to praise the circumcised Jewish penis as superior to the uncircumcised penis of the Christian because the Jewish male "will find himself performing his task quickly." He will not become a slave to sexual passion like the Christian male who "devotes his brain entirely to women, an evil thing." The Jewish husband "who says 'I am the Lord's' will not empty his brain because of his wife. . . . He will find grace and good favor; his heart will be strong to seek out God." Here the strong heart supports the full brain in the Jewish male's undistracted fidelity to God. His heart and brain will not be consumed with sexual thoughts, but his wife, who has the fire of passion "burning within her," will rarely experience the pleasure of orgasm.[11]

In circumcision, God subjugates men in a form of "writing" or accounting or numbering, and writing as numbering was almost as important a sign of possession and control as naming. Circumcision is the earliest form of God's "writing" the male body into a book of men chosen, sealed, and confirmed for his exclusive and unique theocratic community, and this phallic sign "shall be in your flesh for an everlasting covenant" (Gen. 17.13). The significance of circumcision as a symbol of phallic domination was continued in the Israelites' practice of forcing their neighbors to undergo circumcision, and in the practice of castrating (or removing "the foreskins") of enemies slain in battle. These foreskins were collected and numbered tokens of military exploitation and superiority—an early form of writing as "body count"—evidenced in the David narratives. As often happens in biblical and early modern narrative, associations arise between the human genitals and the human heart, and we shall see in the prophetic writings and in the New Testament a special emphasis on the "circumcision of the heart."

The Lord of the Pentateuch is not to be worshiped under the aspect of an image or a "similitude" (Deut. 4.12), but as an image-maker, as a *maker of impressions*. He will have no graven images made of anything relating to his power in heaven and earth except the engraved images of the writing on the tables.[12] While being represented as a God of enormous power in the oral and aural realms, he is primarily the "writing" or inscribing God, and for Puritans and Anglicans of the early modern period, the actual author of the Bible, as the Puritan divine Thomas Watson explains:

> Read the Word as a book made by God himself. It is . . . given *by divine inspiration* [2 Tim. 3.16]. It is the Library of the Holy Ghost. The Prophets and Apostles were but Gods amanuenses or notaries to write the Law at his mouth. The word is of divine original, and reveals the *deep things of God* to us. That there is a numen or deity is ingraven in mans heart, and is to be read in the Book of the creatures. . . . But who this God is . . . is infinitely above the light of reason, only God himself could make this known. . . . Other Books may be made by holy men, but this Book is indighted by the Holy Ghost.[13]

In the "Puritan" view, God, besides being the author of the Bible, actively inscribes his divine image and essence in each human heart. Going beyond the activity of literal writing, however, he is the maker of lasting visual impressions and of spectacular events and objects, impressing, inflicting (or "afflicting," in Charnock's word) his power on his creatures, on the land, and on humankind. He is self-defined as "a jealous God, visiting the iniquity of the fathers upon the children unto the third and fourth generation of them that hate me; And shewing mercy unto thousands of them that love me and keep my commandments" (Exod. 20.5). He is the God of visitation, with the etymological stress on "seeing" (*visere*), inspecting, investigating, intervening, avenging, bringing something to bear. He is the God of the curse and the blessing.

The pattern of the Lord intervening in the life of the male writing prophet and commanding him to convey the Lord's will takes many forms, from authorizing the act of writing a wife away in a bill of divorcement (Deut. 24.1) to impregnating a prophetess. In his attempt to reassure the wavering King Ahaz, Isaiah says that the Lord told him to "take a great roll, and write in it with a man's pen concerning Mahershalalhashbaz ['the spoil speeds, the prey hastes']" (Isa. 8.1).[14] Isaiah then says, "I went unto the prophetess [his wife]; and she conceived, and bare a son" (Isa. 8.3). The son is given the prophetic name and becomes a sign for Israel's victory over its enemies. Isaiah produces the prophetic name or sign first by his phallic pen and then through symbolic sexual intercourse; both actions reinforce each other and the truth of the divine revelation. His prophetess wife participates in the revelation, but he is the writer.

It is clear that however powerful and efficacious scriptural woman might be in her traditional roles of helping to provide food, shelter, nurture, and comfort for man, and however close she might be to God in the inner experience of womb and heart, no woman in Scripture is depicted as an important writer. This fact is all the more intriguing in the context of women becoming published writers in England for the first time in the seventeenth century. But many more women were *reading* the Bible after the appearance of the Authorized Version, and they would be reading the stories of Eve, Sarah, Rebekah, Rachel, Deborah and Jael, Manoah's wife, the Levite's concubine (Judges 19), and many other women in the Bible with new eyes. It is not surprising that Aphra Behn seems to have read the Bible as assiduously as she read Shakespeare, especially toward the end of her life when she was writing more furiously and copiously than ever. Chapter 4 discusses Behn (and the seventeenth-century woman writer) in relation to her employment of the rhetoric of the heart in her poetry and drama, and in *Oroonoko*.

One of the most compelling and powerful female characters in the Bible who comes into contact with the male prerogative of writing is Queen Esther. She is represented as in effect "unwriting" Haman's letter to destroy the Jews when King Ahasuerus authorizes her and Mordecai to write new letters (Esther 8 and 9). And the wicked Queen Jezebel's letters written in her husband Ahab's name bring about the stoning of Naboth in 1 Kings 21.8–11. Both of these passages show royal women usurping the traditionally masculine mode of royal correspondence. We shall be returning to the theme of women's expressive artistry and its relation to "the birth of the novel" in the discussion of Milton's Eve, Behn's *Oroonoko*, and Richardson's *Clarissa*.

A final example of biblical writing as a male act of power in relation to women comes from Jeremiah, traditionally regarded as the prophet of the inward realm, of the passions, of the heart. He, Isaiah, and Ezekiel have a great deal to say about women and the womb in relation to Israel and its God. After excoriating the reckless and unheeding King Jehoiakim as, in the Lord's words, one who will be ashamed and confounded for all his wickedness, the prophet levels the full force of the Lord's displeasure against him with these words directed against his son: "Write ye this man childless, a man that shall not prosper in his days: for no man of his seed shall prosper, sitting upon the throne of David, and ruling any more in Judah" (22.30). Far more even than "writing" a woman away with a bill of divorcement or rendering a woman barren for life, this writing has the impact of a death blow. God and Jeremiah are writing the king and his offspring into impotence and oblivion.

It is with the Moses narratives, however, that we move into the most complex representation of God's literal "writing" relationship with his people and its significance for the biblical narrative of the heart. When God delegates Moses as his spokesman to the people, and Moses wonders how he is going to tell God's "name" to them, God defines himself orally as "I AM THAT I AM" and as "the Lord God of your fathers . . . this is my name for ever, and this is my memorial unto all generations" (Exod. 3.14–15). As God exercises his power of creating spectacular signs with the plagues visited on the bodies of the Egyptian people, and particularly with the "hardening of Pharaoh's heart," he explains to Moses how and why these signs have been performed: "I have hardened his heart, and the heart of his servants, that I might shew these my signs before him: And that thou mayest tell in the ears of thy son, and of thy son's son, what things I have wrought in Egypt, and my signs which I have done among them; that ye may know how that I am the Lord" (Exod. 10.1–2). When Elaine Scarry talks about God intervening in the human "interior," she could also be talking about God's anatomizing of the heart. Scarry emphasizes how human resistance to God as "the withholding of the body—the stiffening of the neck, the turning of the shoulder, the closing of the ears, the hardening of the heart, the making of the face like stone—necessitates God's forceful shattering of the reluctant human surface and repossession of the interior," a process that culminates in God's taking of the Egyptians' firstborn.[15] God's total power over Pharaoh is manifested in the control of Pharaoh's heart, the center of his being and purpose. God's treatment of the male heart of Pharaoh stands in striking contrast to God's working with the womb and heart of women in the Bible. Instead of communing with the receptive heart and opening the barren womb, God hardens and closes off the oppressor's heart. This process also stands in contrast to the ritual of male circumcision, and to the figurative motif of the circumcision, or opening, of the heart. The hardening of Pharaoh's heart is a form of divine inscription whereby God makes the vital core of the Israelites' oppressor an external, visible, fixed sign that the chosen people will then internalize in their communal historical memory. This dynamic of making the internal heart external and then internalizing it in new ways is one we shall see played out variously in the subsequent chapters, culminating in the rhetoric of the written heart, chiefly in the letters of Clarissa and Lovelace in *Clarissa*.

Moses is the first important human "writer" in the Bible. As long as his hands are held up during the battle with the Amalekites, Israel prevails.

When Moses can finally put down his hands he is able to write the memorial. The divine power through the hand moves from military conquest to written memorial. Paradoxically, but all the more powerfully for that, God tells Moses to memorialize a defeat that will forever banish Amalek from remembrance, as if the *very act* of writing will utterly blot him out. After the Amalekites have been discomfited with the edge of the sword, God directs Moses to "write this for a memorial in a book, and rehearse it in the ears of Joshua: for I will utterly put out the remembrance of Amalek from under heaven" (Exod. 17.14). We recall that the heart was thought to have "two ears." A seventeenth-century reader might hear God's injunction going directly to Joshua's heart. The first mention of literal "writing" in the Bible is juxtaposed with destruction by the sword, and God's first command to Moses to write is to memorialize, for the mind and heart of the great warrior-to-be Joshua (the type name of Jesus), the utter extermination in holy war of a powerful enemy.

Some of the earliest forms of writing record military accounting, exploits, and the enumeration of the dead. One thinks of a stick notched to record the number of fallen enemies. The original writing instrument may not have been a stylus but a knife. The word "write" is akin to German *reissen*, to tear, rip open, pull apart, divide. Writing has always been closely associated with the predominantly male-centered activities of war and conquest, with judicial and legal processes, particularly those involved with criminal proceedings and criminal apprehension, and with priestly rites of separation, exclusion, and purification. I want to emphasize at this point the ancient idea of writing as cutting, as anatomy, and that this activity, like circumcision, is done almost exclusively by males in a male context. Moses as God's male priest is represented as a man who has mastered the special art of writing down God's word and the art of cutting up animals for sacrifice. In his role as dissector of animals, he is the biblical precursor of the early modern anatomist, as Democritus was the ancient Greek precursor.[16] And he is a master swordsman when the time comes for him personally to execute wrongdoers.

The idea of the male priest as anatomist, and the priest's activities as a metaphor for God's anatomy of man's heart, is graphically expressed by the Puritan divine Thomas Watson in *Gods Anatomy upon Mans Heart. Or, A Sermon Preached by Order of the Honorable House of COMMONS, At Margarets Westminster, Decemb. 27. [1649] Being a Day of Publique Humiliation. . . . For we must all appear before the Judgment-seat of CHRIST, that every one may receive the things done in his body, according to that he hath done, whether it be good or bad. 2 Cor. 5. 10.* . . . Watson was speaking at the end of the terrible year that saw the execution of Charles I as the culminating act of bloodshed in the Civil War:

> We are met this day to humble our soules, and to bring our Censer, as once *Aaron* did, and step in, that the wrath of the great GOD may be appeased. And was there ever more need to lie in *sackcloth*, then when the Kingdome almost lies in *ashes*? Or to shed *teares*, then when this Nation hath shed so much *blood*? . . . Our condition is low, but our hearts are high. God sees with what hearts we now come, what is our spring, what is our center; his eye is upon us. . . . *Brethren*, did our hearts stand where our faces do, this would be a day of blushing, we would be ashamed to look one upon another; remember God hath a key for the heart. . . . This Nation is sick of a Spirituall Plurisy . . . no wonder if we begin to say who is this *Moses*? . . . Every sinne after we are in Christ, is a sinne of unkindnesse, it is a sinne against bowels.[17]

In expounding or "opening" his text from Hebrews ("But all things are naked, and open'd unto the eyes of Him with whom we have to do," 4.13), Watson speaks in the idiom of the seventeenth-century anatomist (as we shall see more fully in Chapter 2), when he begins with the "map" of the skin, and then moves inward:

> We have here a *Map of Gods Knowledge*. . . . All things are [*naked.*] Some expositors render it *Excoriate*. . . . It is a Metaphor from the taking off the skin of any beast, which doth then appeare naked. Thus our hearts are said to be naked; they lye open to the eye of God, they have no covering; there is no vail over the heart of a sinner, but the vail of unbelief; and this covering makes him naked. . . . They are naked and [*open*]. The word . . . alludes to the cutting up of the Sacrifices under the Law, where the Priest did divide the Beast in peeces and so the *intestina*, the inward parts were made visible. Or it may allude to an Anotomie, where there is a dissection and cutting up of every part, the Mesentery, the Liver, the Arteries.[18] (Square brackets in original.)

He then explicitly reconstructs the role of God as a master anatomist who cuts up the heart, distinguishing the material from the immaterial, and genuine spirituality from hypocrisy:

> Such a kind of Anatomy doth God make in the soul; an Heart-Anatomy: He doth cut up the inward parts, and makes a difference; This is Flesh, that is Spirit; this is Faith, that is Fancie: this is Grace, that seemes to be so. He makes a dissection, as the knife that divides between the flesh and the bones, the bones and the marrow, the sinews and the veins. . . . *They are cut up before him*.[19]

Throughout this commentary, I am reminded of Donne's trope of "the naked thinking heart," as if the divine anatomist were cutting and probing to find a core of genuine faith or grace in the evil "Fancie" or imagination of the heart. Watson talks about lifting the veil from the sinful heart, but he may be creating at the same time a vivid yet indirect memorial of the "anatomy" or execution of Charles as a sacrifice for his sinful nation.

Let us now conclude our examination of the Moses narratives and their relevance to *writing* the biblical heart. By the time Moses receives the "two tables of the testimony" engraved with the "finger" of God himself (Exod. 31.18), Pharaoh's heart has been repeatedly hardened to the accompaniment of God's spectacular signs, interpreted even by the Egyptian magicians as "the finger of God," or the writing of God as expressed through indelible natural calamities and plagues (Exod. 7.3). Hence biblical characters themselves enlarge the meaning of God's "writing" from the literal to the figurative. With respect to his human creatures, God's "writing" comes first, then interpretation of that writing. When Moses descends with the tables and sees the people worshiping the golden calf in an orgiastic dance, he angrily "cast the tables out of his hands and brake them" (Exod. 32.19). Later God commands him to make new tables and directs him, as his scribe, to write out a second version of the Commandments. What is the significance of the interplay of God and Moses as writers, and why should Moses be allowed to break the tables of God's own writing? When Moses' task of forty days and nights is finished, he has made his second complete transcription of the Word of God. But God wrote the first version and he empowers Moses as his scribe to write the second.[20] God is the original speaker and writer of himself, and the creator of all subsequent prophets. If the act of writing may be described as the transformation of thought or speech into body—visible, tangible, material being—writing is the medium of exchange between God and Moses. But this reduction of spirit into body lives only if reanimated by the physical and mental activity of a reader who may in turn become another writer. It would seem as if God's purpose with his mediator is to make him as familiar as possible with his written words, even to the point of destroying them and making him feel their loss. Even *God's own writing* on stone is just another fragile victim of human passion and error unless the words are learned, remembered, and passed on through oral/aural performance from the teacher to the student and finally stored in the heart as the ultimate biblical repository of mental, spiritual, and emotional understanding. In other words, the living heart endures longer and thus prevails over the book or the stone tablet.

For the Puritan preacher of the Word, writing also came first in the form of a meticulously constructed learned commentary on Scripture, but this labor was all in the service of the sermon performed before a congregation, when the preacher would occasionally abandon his prepared text and "speak from the heart." For the Puritan hearer of the Word, the figurative "caul of the heart" must be broken before true regeneration can occur, as in the case of Christian's wife Christiana in the second part of *The Pilgrim's Progress*. Christiana's recollection of her need to "harden her heart" against the entreaties of her husband to go with him on his spiritual journey "returned upon her like a flash of lightning, and rent the caul of her heart in sunder."[21] The "caul of the heart" was a rich metaphor. The "caul" was literally the pericardium, the thin membranous sac surrounding the heart, but it was also the term for the amnion or inner membrane enclosing the fetus before birth, and it could even mean a woman's hair net. The caul of the heart was then a birth metaphor and a woman's word. It enclosed a pun on God's "call" of the heart to regeneration. But the "caul of the heart" was often interpreted as a symbol of the hard, unregenerate heart and was thus analogous to the foreskin that had to be removed for acceptance into the male theocratic community. Hence the image of the caul of the heart was found in everyone and not confined to one gender.

In the context of our reading of the Moses narratives, shattering this caul could also be seen as analogous to Moses breaking the tablets before all the people. In the story of the broken tablets, God will make his words more meaningful and memorable to the children of Israel by requiring Moses first to destroy and lose them, then to rewrite them with his own hand and to teach them with his own mouth.[22] There is a movement in the Moses story of the law going further and further into the sensory, tactile, internal bodily experience of all of God's chosen people, culminating in the understanding of the heart. God writes his covenant for humankind by having *them* write it and learn it in their own hearts and bodies. But sometime during Moses' sojourn with God on the mountain, he becomes aware that God is writing his own book. For the early modern Christian, this was a book different from the Bible, and in a very personal sense, even more important.

The "Book of Life"

In what I have called "the literature of generation," those works in English from about 1550 through 1750 that discuss the conception and birth of humankind (mostly midwife manuals and treatises on human reproduction), one encounters frequent allusions to Psalm 139,[23] the most richly and deeply "interior" of all the psalms:

For thou hast possessed my reins: thou hast covered me in my mother's womb.
 I will praise thee; for I am fearfully and wonderfully made: marvelous are thy works; and that my soul knoweth right well.
 My substance was not hid from thee, when I was made in secret, and curiously wrought in the lowest parts of the earth.
 Thine eyes did see my substance, yet being unperfect: and in thy book all my members were written, which in continuance were fashioned, when as yet there was none of them.
 (Ps. 139.13–16)

This passage might be taken as the paradigm for how our ancestors, at least up to the nineteenth century, viewed the postlapsarian creation of human life. In trying to read the passage in something like the way an early modern Protestant might have read it, all persons are originally "written," member by member, in God's book (at other points in the Old and New Testaments called the "book of life") even before they come into being. The Psalmist was imagined as David, or even as Christ, one who has been given a supernatural view into the working of God's creation at its source, a biblical prefiguring of the vision into the divine world that Milton will implore of the Spirit in the opening of *Paradise Lost*. To "possess" the "reins" means to have control over the source of one's life, or one's generative power. "Reins" could mean the kidneys or "the loins." "Covered in the womb" means to be protected and cherished there. God "writes" man "to the moment" (the members "in continuance were fashioned"), before, during, and after his conception. The image is of God writing people into his book as if it were an unfolding divine narrative—different from the Bible—populated by everyday people. The first novel, as it were. In Psalm 139, God presides over a manufactory operation that results in a human artifact, the body "wrought" in the secret workshop of the womb; God then continues to think about and care for his human creature: "How precious also are thy thoughts unto me, O God!" (v. 17), protecting the person from deadly enemies ("Surely thou wilt slay the wicked, O God" [v. 19]). That all this is an ongoing process within an encompassing narrative, a continuing spiritual dialogue between the caring, guiding God and the inmost being of the praying person is asserted at the end of the psalm: "Search me, O God, and know my heart: try me, and know my thoughts: And see if there be any wicked way in me, and lead me in the way everlasting" (vv. 23–24). For the seventeenth-century reader, the Psalmist David, whose sins were naked and public, asks for God to probe and know him, challenge him, so that there will be no secret or wicked thought left unexamined or unknown. All of this, especially the motif of searching the heart, is profoundly relevant to the representation of the heart in *Clarissa*.

Thomas Watson, in his commentary on Psalm 139, seems to fuse Christ with the Lord God of the Old Testament, and equates man's thoughts with the heart:

First, here is the Judge that sits upon the bench, that is God. . . . The persons to be adjudged either for life or death, [*We*] saith the Apostle, that is, every individuall person: There is none exempted from this Generall Assize. . . . *The most secret Cabinet-designes of mans heart are all unlocked and clearly anatomized before the Lord.* . . . in the originall it is . . . *the hidden things of the heart*, those which are most veiled and masked, and *Psal.* 139 2. *Thou knowest my thoughts afarre off.*[24] (Square brackets in original.)

Watson is struck by the extraordinary "subtility" of God's workings: "Man is a Microcosme or little world" and God sees the "first *embryo and forming of the thought*, that is, a thing very subtle, and scarce discernable." Furthermore, God knows the thoughts of our hearts before we know them, and better than we know them. Finally, he keeps a book in which he records those thoughts for all time, and there will be a heavy reckoning if the writing of sin is not "crossed" with the writing of Christ's blood. This is one of the clearest expressions of the idea that Christ, who, like scriptural woman, does virtually no writing in the Bible, overrides or cancels the sins of the human heart with the redemptive, resurrective power of his blood:

our thoughts are *twisted* and *tangled* one within another, they have no dependance, they may be *inter anomala*: yet even these thoughts are knowne to God, and set in their proper Sphere: what David saith of his members, may be said of our thoughts, *Are they not all written in thy Book?* . . . God knows our thoughts before we our selves know them. He knows what designes are in the heart, and men would certainly pursue, did not he turne the wheele another way. . . . [God] sees what blood and venome is in the heart of a sinner, though it never comes to have vent. . . . God knows our thoughts when we have forgotten them: they are *afarre off* to us, but they are present with him. *Psal.* 50.21. . . . Millions of years are but as a short Parenthesis between: and that we may not thinke God forgets, he keeps a Book of Records, *Rev.* 20.12. *I saw the dead, small and great stand before the Lord, and the Books were opened.* God writes down, *Item* such a sinne: and if the Book be not crossed, there will be an heavy reckoning; to every beleever, the debt book is crossed, the black lines of sin are crossed out in the red lines of Christs blood . . . we cannot write our sinnes in so small or strange a character, but God can read them, he hath a key for them . . . we cannot read his hand-writing: but He understands our Hearts without a commentary. . . . He hath an eye in your heart, He is *kardiognostes*.[25]

The Lord's dynamic of creation-by-writing appears in figurative contexts other than that of the "book of life," particularly in Isaiah, where the Lord says, "Behold I have graven thee upon the palms of my hands" (49.16), as if to suggest that God's hand is always upon humankind. Then there are the instances of God represented as assigning or inscribing a new name for some of the most important characters in his Old Testament narrative, like Abram-Abraham, Sarai-Sarah, Jacob-Israel, a new name that in ancient Hebrew culture (as early modern writers steeped in the Bible would have known) becomes virtually a new identity, and a biblical name, even in the seventeenth and eighteenth centuries, was thought to help shape a person's character. God writes the Old Testament through his chosen scribes, but in a deeper sense, he writes all of human history. There are finally the examples of God making people themselves a "sign" of his works, from the people in Deuteronomy 28 becoming a sign of God's displeasure when they embody God's curses, to the prophets who are individually, in the shape of their very lives and in action parables like Isaiah, being required to walk naked for three years "for a sign and wonder upon Egypt" (20.3), signs of the divine will. Body is transformed into words and signs; alternatively, it is the experience of prophets like Ezekiel to turn words into body by eating the Lord's scroll, internalizing and virtually digesting the Word within his "bowels" (3.3): "Moreover . . . Son of man, all my words that I shall speak unto thee receive in thine heart, and hear with thine ears" (v. 10). This is a suggestive instance of the recurring scriptural "ear" within the "heart" figure, and the passage plays upon a primitive sequence of nutrition, the food passing through the bowels to fortify the heart. When the Word is properly received, heard, and known internally, the prophet can then go and "speak unto [the children of thy people] . . . and tell them, Thus saith the Lord God" (v. 11). In the Gospels, this complex process is miraculously replayed in the dynamic of the Word becoming flesh, and in subvariants like John eating the little book in Revelation 10.

In all these examples, as we saw in the Moses narrative, there is the sense of a deep physical communion between the inward, secret, aural domain of God and the visible world of humankind through the medium of "writing." Since words are the Lord's only acceptable graven images, they remain the visible translation from God's language into humankind's. Writing is something that can be seen and read and reiterated, a permanent engraving upon a surface, but like any language passing through fallible human hands, God's Word can be lost, destroyed, corrupted, or misread in the mortal realm, as the blood of God's "Word," the crucified Christ, was shed to become the redemptive element in the kind of "writing of the blood" Watson describes as operating in the Last Judgment.

We noted that the word "scripture" only gradually evolved into signifying the holy and sacred medium of God's communication with humankind. But some radical Protestant thinkers, Milton in particular, called attention to "a double scripture," external and internal, especially in relation to the Gospels. "There is the external scripture of the written word and the internal scripture of the Holy Spirit which he, according to God's promise, has engraved upon the hearts of believers. . . . Nowadays the external authority for our faith, in other words, the scriptures, is of very considerable importance and generally speaking, it is the authority of which we first have experience. The pre-eminent and supreme authority, however, is the authority of the Spirit, which is internal, and the individual possession of each man."[26] It is as if for Milton there are two scriptures for man as there are two scriptures for God. God's two scriptures are the Bible, the external Word of God mediated by his male scribes, and his own private book of life. The two scriptures for human beings are the Bible, now in part corrupted by human tradition and error, and the perfect internal scripture of the Spirit, written in the hearts of every believer. For Milton, and I would suggest for Richardson also, it is only by the power of this internal scripture that any Christian has hope of being written into God's book of life.

Coinciding with the motif of humankind "being written" in God's book of life is the corresponding anxiety or fear, recorded many places in the Bible, of being "blotted out" or erased from this book. After the golden calf of the Israelites is destroyed, Moses implores God, "Yet now, if thou wilt forgive their sin—; and if not, blot me, I pray thee, out of thy book which thou hast written" (Exod. 32.32). This book is the register of the members of the theocratic community, the one referred to by the Psalmist when he says of his enemies, "Let them be blotted out of the book of the living, and not be written with the righteous" (69.28). There are several allusions to God's "book of life" in the Old Testament, but this passage is the only explicit reference to "the book of the living."

In the New Testament, the trope of the "book of life" is given even more explicit verbal detail. St. Paul singles out "those women which laboured with me in the gospel . . . and with other my fellow labourers, whose names are recorded in the book of life" (Phil. 4.3), and the writer of Revelation, invoking the authority of Jesus in Luke 12.8, has the Lamb say, "He that overcometh, the same shall be clothed in white raiment; and I will not blot out his name out of the book of life, but I will confess his name before my Father, and before his angels" (3.5). The writing of Christ's redemptive blood has its oral parallel in Christ's public "confession" or identification of the saved.

The writing process in the Bible is an act of translation, either a cutting away into a state of separation, or a memorializing into a world of new life. According to Jeremiah, those that separate from the Lord "shall be written in the earth" (17.13), or cast into the underworld, while "he that is left in Zion," according to Isaiah, "shall be called holy, even every one that is written among the living in Jerusalem" (4.3). When Jesus appears to write on the ground in John's account of the woman taken in adultery (the only instance of Jesus apparently writing something in the New Testament and a reversal of the typical prophetic denunciation of the harlot Israel/Jerusalem), he is literally marking the earth, and many commentators thought he was recording the names of her accusers. This is another way of blotting out the names, writing them in the dust to which they will all go in the obliteration of the mortal body.

Written in the Heart

We have seen how the semiotic Lord of the Old Testament inscribes his will in a variety of ways. He leaves his mark on the land (after first laying his curse on it) by such means as drought, fire, or flood (calamities very much in the anxious collective mind of English people in the 1660s), and on humankind by way of the curse on woman's childbirth in pain and on man's toil, the mark upon Cain, the signing of male circumcision, the inscribing of his commandments in stone, the hardening of Pharaoh's heart, the recording of the names of his elect in his book. As the chosen people's most revered military commander and king, and the reputed author of the Psalms, the man God chose "after his own heart" (1 Sam. 13.14) and the man with "a perfect heart" (Ps. 107.2), David was the royal patriarch best fitted to articulate the Old Testament writers' idea of God's will and the wisdom of the heart:

I know also, my God, that thou triest the heart, and hast pleasure in uprightness. As for me, in the uprightness of mine heart I have willingly offered all these things. ... O Lord God of Abraham, Isaac, and of Israel, our fathers, keep this forever in the imagination of the thoughts of the heart of thy people, and prepare their heart unto thee: And give unto Solomon my son a perfect heart, to keep thy commandments, thy testimonies, and thy statutes. (1 Chron. 29.17–19)

The Lord fashions all human hearts in his creation, but each individual heart must also be tried, sifted, tested: "Examine me, O Lord, and prove me; try my reins and my heart" (Ps. 26.2). We see in these biblical allusions to the heart how all the organs of the body from top to bottom, from outside to inside—the eye, the ear, the bowels, the kidneys, the genitals—connect significantly with the heart at the vital center of bodily life and thought. The upright heart survives the trials inflicted by God from without and from within and will be saved (Ps. 7.10). Milton in the opening of *Paradise Lost* knows that the Spirit prefers before all temples and scriptures "the upright heart and pure," and he implores the Spirit to instruct his tried and purified heart and thus help him begin his epic poem. David's heart was also imagined as being tried and purified. In its reversal of the old formula of "every imagination of the thoughts of [man's] heart" as irredeemably evil (Gen. 6.5–6), and in its movement ever inward, the above passage is certainly one of the most remarkable expressions in the Old Testament of the deep interiority of God's domain in humankind (woman and man) and of the plea to God to prepare the heart for his reception. But the culminating expression of this inwardness is the Psalmist's succinct fusion of the motifs of the "book of life" and the writing in the heart: "in the volume of the book it is written of me, I delight to do thy will, O my God: Yea, thy law is within my heart" (40.7–8). This formulation suggests that the writing in the heart may be translated into the book of life, or even that one's final "writing in the heart" may be one's place or passage in the book of life itself.

David as the undisputed author of Psalms and Solomon as the reputed author of Proverbs (for the early modern reader) continually reiterate the vital relation between speaking, writing, and the heart. The heart is both the source and the instrument of language: "My heart is inditing a good matter ... my tongue is the pen of a ready writer" (Ps. 45.1), and God's words are like sharp arrows "in the heart of the king's enemies" (45.5). We notice how the proverbial darts of the god Cupid, given such terrible wounding urgency in Lucretius's erotics of physical desire, are counterpointed by these divine verbal darts in the Old Testament, and how these biblical and classical images of divine or erotic power over the heart coexisted in the minds of early modern readers. (This may also be the time to recall that neither Lucretius nor Galen were Jewish or Christian.) The proverbial father's advice to the son applies also to the daughter: "keep thy father's commandment and forsake not the law of thy mother. Bind them continually upon thine heart" (Prov. 6.20–21); "Bind them upon thy fingers, write them upon the table of thine heart" (7.3). Again we note the image of the tablets or book of the heart and that this binding is an ongoing activity of memory.

The Psalms may contain the richest and most varied language of the heart in the Bible, but the most powerful and concentrated rhetoric of the heart is found in the Book of Jeremiah, beginning with the injunction to "Circumcise yourselves to the Lord, and take away the foreskins of your heart, ye men of Judah" (4.4) and recognizing that "all the house of Israel are uncircumcised in the heart" (9.26).[27] The injunction is directed against Jewish males, telling them to remove—by their own volition—the foreskins of the stubborn heart they all have in common. Again, as in traditional early modern medical discourse, the heart is linked with the organs of reproduction and Jeremiah more than once pairs the heart and the reins (17.10 and 20.12). Jeremiah here transforms the phallus claimed by God as his special male instrument of procreation into the rigid, disobedient inward heart in need of softening. The inward heart, usually associated with the experience of Old Testament women but also with the hardened heart of Pharaoh, as we have seen, is now associated with men of Judah, and the male heart must be circumcised, opened, revitalized, made receptive to a new truth. The fierce anger of the Lord is coming from the north in destruction so appalling that "the heart of the king shall perish, and the heart of the princes; and the priests shall be astonished, and the prophets shall wonder" (Jer. 4.9)—the entire male structure of authority will be rendered impotent. The prophet exhorts polluted Mother Jerusalem to "wash thine heart from wickedness, that thou mayest be saved" (4.14). All of these admonitions culminate in the anguished scream that fuses Jeremiah's voice with the Lord's: "My bowels, my bowels! I am pained at my very heart; my heart maketh a noise in me; I cannot hold my peace" because the vision of impending destruction is so terrifyingly inevitable (4.19). In Jeremiah 4 we see again the heart under its two most characteristic discursive aspects, sexual and verbal. After entreating the Jewish men to circumcise their collective stubborn phallic heart, Jeremiah represents his own heart as a voice, an uncontainable expressive instrument. His heart is in pain and makes a noise of warning that also seems to reverberate the impending sounds of destruction. Jeremiah then represents himself as the passive dupe or the one who, like a woman, is "deceived" and violated by the Lord: "thou art stronger than I, and hast prevailed: I am in derision daily" (20.7). Even when Jeremiah feels that the Lord has deceived him, and he makes up his mind not to speak any more in his name, still "his word was in mine heart as a burning fire shut up in my bones, and I was weary with forbearing, and I could not stay" (20.9). The hot heart that signified life in ancient Greek medicine is here a mortal extension of the ferocious destructive heat of the Lord's anger.

The Christian version of the "circumcision" of the heart, for seventeenth-century Anglicans and Puritans, is summed up graphically in Richard Sibbes's "An Exposition of the Third Chapter of the Epistle of St. Paul to the Philippians, verse 3. *For we are the circumcision*":

> I say a Christian must circumcise himself, his heart, and those parts that are uncircumcised, before he can ever think to go to heaven, whither nothing that is corrupt or unclean entereth. Religion therefore is no easy thing, circumcision is painful and bloody. Mortification is very hard. Corruption it must be cut off though the blood follow, else it will kill thee at length. Wherefore we are also to labour for circumcised hearts to understand God's truth, his will, and commandments. Cut off all extravagant desires.[28]

How did women of the seventeenth century hear this—read this—injunction? How were they to "labour" for circumcised hearts? What Sibbes is describing sounds remarkably like the business of childbirth. Women who had given birth knew something about this kind of cutting off being "painful and bloody," about mortality in childbirth, about the blood flowing till it kills thee at length. They know more about "circumcision" than men do; *they* are the circumcision. Sibbes of course has in mind all hearts, but women are subsumed under the masculine gender. The profound emphasis on God communing with the female heart and womb that we have explored in this chapter was only beginning to be recognized by early modern readers. The prevailing notion (as we shall see further in the next chapter) was still that women's hearts were colder and less powerful than men's, and women were the marginal and subsidiary gender.[29]

Jesus, Heart, Woman

Jeremiah, after Moses, is the prophet who has the most compelling relationship to the act of writing in the Old Testament. In the supreme utterance and vision of this prophet of the inward realm, there is a constant tension between two kinds of writing on the heart, the writing of sin and the writing of renewal and forgiveness. The "iniquity of the fathers" is now summed up in the "sin of Judah . . . written with a pen of iron, and with the point of a diamond: it is graven upon the table of their heart" (17.1), for Jeremiah knows the potential power of the heart for good actions or more likely for wicked ones ("The heart is deceitful above all things, and desperately wicked: who can know it?" [17.9]). In opposition to the sin engraved upon the heart, Jeremiah announces the "new covenant" by introducing "a new thing in the earth, a woman shall compass a man" (31.22). To Christian women readers of Scripture in the early modern period, this claim of the importance of women to the new covenant was unmistakable. A preacher like Watson, however, puts the covenant in the customary seventeenth-century androcentric context:

The *Covenant* is *Nodus Connubialis* a marriage knot; for a woman to go away from her husband after solemne Contract, is of an high nature. The Covenant is *zona virginea* a girdle, or golden claspe that bindes us to God and God to us. The girdle in ancient times was an Embleme of chastity. When the *Covenant* is broken, the Church looseth her virginity. This was Israels Arraignement; after she had been espoused to God, she defiles her Virgin-breasts 1 Jer. 2.3 . . . when she had stained this federall relation by idolatry . . . God gives her a Bill of divorce. *Plead with her*, saith he; *she is not my wife* . . . and remember God sees, hee writes it downe.[30]

For Jeremiah, God will make a new marriage with his bride Israel, not like the old covenant with "their fathers" (31.32) when the law was written only on stone tablets and the onyx stones of the fallible male priests. The new covenant says, "I will put my law in their inward parts," with the suggestion also of a new generation in the womb and loins, "and write it in their hearts," the deepest of all inward parts, the seat of spiritual regeneration, "and will be their God, and they shall be my people" (31.33). Ezekiel's version of this transaction, presented in the context of Israel's rebellious behavior "as the uncleanness of a removed woman" (36.17) and coming just before the vision of the resurrection of the dry bones, is characteristically more anatomical: "A new heart also will I give you, and a new spirit will I put within you: and I will take away the stony heart out of your flesh, and I will give you an heart of flesh. And I will put my spirit within you, and cause you to walk in my statutes" (36.26–27). The "stony heart" is associated with the hard heart of Pharaoh, the "stiffnecked" momentum of the chosen people against the will of the Lord, the covenant-breaking of their fathers who refused the Lord as their "husband" (Jer. 31.32). The new covenant is a new spirit (invoking overtones of the voice and orality), something fluent and invigorating, a kind of vital "writing" that permeates and fructifies and leaves an impression upon the "inward parts" of every hearer—man, woman, child—creating in them a new understanding of God ("they shall all know me, from the least of them unto the greatest of them," Jer. 31.34) and new life in God's communal covenant of the heart.

Since Christian readers of the seventeenth and eighteenth centuries already read the presence of Christ into the Old Testament, the metaphoric leap from this "new covenant" to the "new testament" of the Gospels and St. Paul was not a large one. In the words of Jesus, the heart is still the origin of language and ultimately of evil or good; "out of the abundance of the heart the mouth speaketh . . . for by thy words thou shalt be justified, and by thy words thou shalt be condemned" (Matt. 12.34, 37). In the Judeo-Christian tradition as it had evolved by the seventeenth century, humankind was a collective creature of words or signifiers, "words" taken in the largest sense to include actions also, but words nonetheless, and for the Christian every person was created by the Word who became flesh—the ultimate Signifier, as it were. These human "words" are "characters," like the letters in a book, and they would all be assembled or re-collected at the Day of Judgment to receive their final definition. But it would be a mistake to conceive of Christ as he was read in the early modern era as a "writing God" in the same way that the Lord of the Old Testament is a writing God. Christ is imagined as the instrument that carries out the will of the Father, but the power of the Father God inscribing his people was not easily reconciled with the activities of Christ as the Word. The Lord of the Old Testament writes human beings into existence, inscribes the law for them on stone tablets, impresses the heat of his anger on the land, inscribes his possession of male bodies (and by extension all human bodies) in the covenant of circumcision, tests and proves and searches the human heart, and, in Jeremiah and Ezekiel, ultimately puts his law in everyone's heart. Christ on the other hand is presented in the four gospels as one who fulfills the will of the Father, who reads and understands the human heart, who knows its inmost desires, who will ultimately judge the words and deeds of all humankind at the last day, and who saves the righteous with the redemptive power of the "writing of his blood." Christ becomes the ultimate representation of the prophetic emphasis on putting the law in the inward parts. It is the author of Revelation who finally fuses in one image the Christ of the Gospels with the God of war and judgment of the Old Testament.

In the Gospels, the "iniquity of the fathers" continues to be embodied in Pharisaic "hardness of heart" (Mark 16.14), but in the parable of the sower there is also the good ground of those who are of "honest and good heart," hearing the word, keeping it, and bringing forth fruit with patience (Luke 8.15). In John, Jesus tells the disciples that the Father will send the Holy Ghost in the Son's name, and "he shall teach you all things. . . . Peace I leave with you, my peace I give unto you. . . . Let not your heart be troubled, neither let it be afraid" (14.26–27). When Jesus appears to the disciples after the Resurrection, he twice says, "Peace be unto you," shows them his hands and his side, and then breathes on them saying, "Receive ye the Holy Ghost" (20.19–22). His breathing on the disciples is a reiteration of the divine breath that animated Adam, and a regenerating of the hearts of the disciples to do the new work of the Lord. In the Hellenized world of the New Testament, Jesus' breath is the Holy Spirit, the supreme *pneuma* going out from him into their hearts, working on their hearts and giving them new life. Ancient Greek notions of the vital link between respiration and vitality, the lungs and the heart, are at work in this passage, and the notion of the Spirit cleansing, purifying, and regenerating the heart is given varied new expressions in Paul's epistles and in Acts.

Speaking of the Gentiles, Peter says, "And God, which knoweth the hearts, bare them witness, giving them the Holy Ghost, even as he did unto us" (Acts 15.8). Paul says to the Galatians, "And because ye are sons, God hath sent forth the Spirit of his Son into your hearts, crying Abba, Father" (Gal. 4.6), and in his second epistle to the Corinthians, perhaps the most significant "book of the heart" in the New Testament, he tells them, "Ye are our epistle written in our hearts, known and read of all men: Forasmuch as ye are manifestly declared to be the epistle of Christ ministered by us, written not with ink, but with the Spirit of the living God; not in tables of stone, but in fleshy tables of the heart" (2 Cor. 3.2–3). He later exclaims, "O ye Corinthians, our mouth is open unto you, our heart is enlarged . . . be ye also enlarged" (2 Cor. 6.11–13), in preparation for receiving Paul's message. The Spirit in Paul is a purifying fluid or moving ethereal agent that cleanses and "writes" at the same time. For Paul, following the logic of Jeremiah 31, the good Jew is not good because he is circumcised, but because he has the "circumcision . . . of the heart, in the spirit, and not in the letter" (Rom. 2.28–29). Hence Paul makes explicit the deep association of the "heart" and inward human experience emphasized throughout this discussion of the biblical rhetoric of the heart. He asserts that God does not respect persons. The "work" of the law is "written in [the] hearts" even of the good Gentiles since they are performers of the Law, not just hearers. Their "work" will be shown "when God shall judge the secrets of men by Jesus Christ according to my gospel" (2.15–16).

The image of the Spirit reinscribing the heart is Paul's version of the circumcision of the heart, the culmination of the link between inscription and circumcision we have traced from Genesis to the New Testament. Paul talks about a kind of writing that is beyond even the fixed impressions of the God of Moses who commanded that his words be preserved in stone tablets. The ultimate form of the writing in the heart, though still contained in the fleshy body, is vital and meaningful in a way that can be perceived only by the Spirit, the final medium of expression (bequeathed by Christ) between deity and humankind, but the heart is the place where this communication occurs and is "read." The final form of the writing in the heart is beyond writing, as Milton and Richardson attempt to demonstrate.

To conclude our exploration of the narrative of the heart in the Bible, let us return to the trope of God working through the hearts and wombs of women by looking closely at the opening of the Gospel of Luke. The story of Jesus begins with three birth narratives, one from the Logos's creation of the world in John, one told from the viewpoint of male Judaism in Matthew, and the richest, longest, and most suggestive in Luke, told from the point of view of the two women—Mary and Elisabeth—most deeply involved in the story of the birth of Jesus. Luke is the only gospel writer to establish something like a historically verifiable narrative context for his account of the ministry of Jesus, an account that had a significant (and incalculable) effect on the beginnings of modern historiographic methodology in the early modern world. He attempts to create the illusion at least that the story of Jesus happened in a way that could be verified by those who had been there and could testify to his deeds.

We begin with the now traditional story of the older barren woman and her husband, Elisabeth and the priest Zacharias. The priest repeats the ancient Aaronic ritual of entering the temple to burn incense when an angel appears to him to tell him that his prayer has been heard and that his wife will bear him a son, and his name shall be called John. He "shall be great in the sight of the Lord," and like Samson, "shall drink neither wine nor strong drink" according to the Nazarite law of those specially chosen by God for his purposes. He "shall be filled with the Holy Ghost, even from his mother's womb." He shall go forth in the spirit of Elijah to "turn the hearts of the fathers to the children" (echoing the last words of the Old

Testament in Mal. 4.6), and "make ready a people prepared for the Lord" (Luke 1.13–17). Zacharias then errs by asking in what manner he shall know this to be true; for his unbelief he is stricken dumb when he emerges from the temple. Entrusted with the priestly power of sacred utterance, he is, ironically, rendered speechless. Unlike the Samson birth narrative, however, the angel here appears first to the male, but Elisabeth's state of mind may be discerned by her pleased acknowledgment that the Lord has "dealt with" her favorably and taken away the reproach of childlessness. The angel then goes to Mary, "espoused" to Joseph, and she, like Zacharias, is apprehensive about the announcement that she will bear the "Son of the Highest": "How shall this be, seeing I know not a man?" (1.34). Concealed under the angel's explanation is the unspoken sense that "a man" has nothing to do with it. The "Holy Ghost shall come upon" her, with no reference to the Spirit's gender, and "a holy thing" shall be born of her called "the Son of God" (1.35). As in the Old Testament formula, all the proper names must be stated at once, as if to ensure the truth of the ensuing narrative. But Mary is not punished for her skepticism as Zacharias is, and this account differs from the earlier birth narratives in that here two women are approached by the angel and both are foregrounded over their male counterparts. Manoah's wife is presented as knowing more than her husband about the divine transaction, but here, while the male priest is still speechless, Elisabeth blesses her kinswoman in "a loud voice" and says, "as soon as the voice of thy salutation sounded in mine ears, the babe leaped in my womb for joy. And blessed is she that believed: for there shall be a performance of those things which were told her from the Lord" (1.42–45).

Though Zacharias did not believe, both women affirmed the promise, and John becomes the active hero from the beginning, leaping in the womb for joy and heralding the rewards of the poor in heaven who will "rejoice . . . and leap for joy" in the words of Jesus' Sermon on the Plain (Luke 6.23). The women are the active ones in this account; Zacharias is dumb and Joseph is only mentioned. And Elisabeth, "filled with the Holy Ghost" and its authority (1.41), is given the divine mandate of "blessing" her younger counterpart. Mary is a younger and more favored version of Hannah, who also knew more and saw more deeply into her special experience than did the old priest Eli, and she is given her own version of Hannah's song of praise, a "Magnificat" that exalts not only the lowly but that stresses the power of the Lord to elevate lowly women above mighty men. It is still very much the Lord *doing* things to women, but women are more favored than men in the story, and Jesus, who will define himself as being "meek and lowly in heart" (Matt. 11.29) is identified from the beginning with the lowly estate of women.

The climax of this exaltation of women motif occurs when Elisabeth intervenes in the circumcision ritual on the eighth day; the men have called the child "Zacharias" after his father, and she directly contradicts them: "Not so; but he shall be called John" (Luke 1.60). By this time old Zacharias has seen the light, calls for a writing table, and writes, "His name is John." No wonder they all marvel. Not only has a woman disrupted a sacred male ritual by giving the authentic name, but her husband, a priest, has endorsed her claim. Only after the act of writing the name is "his tongue loosed" and he speaks, praising God. Everyone throughout Judea who heard these things "laid them up in their hearts," wondering what kind of child this should be, and old Zacharias too is finally "filled with the Holy Ghost" (1.66–67), uttering an Old Testament blessing that parallels Mary's song of praise. Hence both female and male figures play constructive roles in the prologue to Jesus' advent.

Only after Mary has given birth to the child, and the reader of the Gospels is aware that the wise men have visited the child with their gifts and that an angel has announced to the shepherds that a Savior, Christ the Lord, has been born to them, do we learn that "Mary kept all these things, and pondered them in her heart" (2.19). It is *her* heart that is the climactic focal point of the birth narrative in Luke. "Mary" means "bitter," a recollection of the curse of sorrow upon Eve in childbirth. For the early modern Christian, Mary is the second Eve, and the virgin birth is the Christian miracle that answers the culminating miracle of the redemptive Mother Jerusalem in Isaiah: "Before she travailed, she brought forth; before her pain came, she was delivered of a man child. Who hath heard such a thing? who hath seen such things? . . . Shall I bring to the birth, and not cause to bring forth? saith the Lord. . . . Rejoice ye with Jerusalem. . . . That ye may suck, and be satisfied with the breasts of her consolations. . . . As one whom his mother comforteth, so will I comfort you. . . . And when ye see this, your heart shall rejoice, and your bones shall flourish like an herb" (66.7–14). The final redemptive image of "heart" and "bone" flourishing like a verdant plant recalls Eve being formed from the bone around Adam's heart. Mother Jerusalem and Mary as the second Eve both redeem Mother Eve.

Mary is represented as feeling both exaltation and sorrow, exaltation prevailing at the birth of Christ, sorrow at his death. In the enigmatic prophecy of old Simeon to Mary, Christ will be a "sign which shall be spoken against; (Yea, a sword shall pierce through my own soul also,) that the thoughts of many hearts may be revealed" (Luke 2.34–35). She is characterized as one who keeps things inside and ponders them, she is thoughtful and questioning, and her heart is a storehouse of memory that continues to grow as her son grows, reaching a new but impenetrable phase when at twelve years of age he preferred to remain in his Father's house but went home with his parents nonetheless and was subject unto them: "but his mother kept all these sayings in her heart" (2.51). Since the early modern reader would form in her or his mind a composite narrative of the events from all four gospels, the reader would "read" this narrative into the pondering, questioning, and perhaps now sorrowful "heart" of Mary. And the reader might recall that the prophet Daniel, after seeing night visions of "one like the Son of man" coming with the clouds of heaven to be given everlasting dominion, glory, and a kingdom over all the people, nations, and languages of the earth, says, "'I . . . was grieved in my spirit in the midst of my body, and the visions of my head troubled me . . . my cogitations much troubled me, and my countenance changed in me: but I kept the matter in my heart'" (Dan. 7.13–15, 28). This passage and the ones in Luke are the only places in the Bible where someone "keeps matters" and "ponders" them in his or her heart.

In Matthew, Jesus endures the agony in Gethsemane ("My soul is exceeding sorrowful, even unto death," 26.38), and then, before the high priest, he answers, "I say unto you, Hereafter shall ye see the Son of man sitting on the right hand of power, and coming in the clouds of heaven" (26.64), a specific restatement of the vision of Daniel applied to himself as the Son of man. At this critical moment in his career, Jesus replicates, in a more extreme form, the ambivalent heart experience of his mother and of the troubled prophet Daniel. In this context, Mary (situated temporally in this narrative of the heart between Daniel and her own prophetic son) takes on the characteristics of a prophet herself. She gives birth to a "holy thing" whose name has already been given him before he is conceived, she is present as he begins his ministry in the wedding at Cana, and she is present at his death on the Cross. The importance of Mary and the feminine is punctuated in John by Jesus' five crucial invocations of the word "Woman," to his mother at Cana (2.4), to the Samaritan woman at the well (4.21), to the woman taken in adultery (8.10), to his mother while he is on the Cross (19.26), and finally to Mary Magdalene after the Resurrection (20.15). The narrative progresses from Mary to Mary. Mary the mother of Jesus, who is present at the beginning and at the end of his ministry in John, is the principal Mary among several others who accompany Jesus throughout his ministry, including Mary Magdalene, the Mary who listens to Jesus' words and who anoints his feet with costly ointment (John 12.3), Mary the mother of James and Joses (Matt. 27.56), and Mary the wife of Cleophas, one of the three Marys at the Cross (John 19.25). The climactic reference to the heart in John is Jesus' reminder to the disciples that they will experience sorrow and then joy, like that of "a woman when she is in travail . . . because her hour has come." When she is delivered she has no more "anguish" because "a man is born into the world." Jesus compares the disciples to the woman in travail: "ye now therefore have sorrow: but I will see you again, and your heart shall rejoice, and your joy no man taketh from you" (16.20–22).

The "heart" of Mary, in the various manifestations of "Mary," is a brooding presence that encompasses the entire career of Jesus, from before his birth to his death and after his resurrection. The word "heart" is used only six times in John, the most inward and mystical of the four gospels, yet the refrain "let not your heart be troubled" seems to be directed as much toward the women disciples of Jesus as it is toward the male disciples, a haunting suggestion of ultimate peace for the woman who seems always in the four gospels to be standing in the divine presence and preserving it.

2

The Phallic Heart
William Harvey's *The Motion of the Heart* and "The Republick of Literature"

> Sweet is the lore which Nature brings;
> Our meddling intellect
> Misshapes the beauteous forms of things—
> We murder to dissect.
>
> Enough of Science and of Art;
> Close up those barren leaves;
> Come forth, and bring with you a heart
> That watches and receives.
> —WILLIAM WORDSWORTH, "The Tables Turned"

> There are as it were at one time two motions.
> —WILLIAM HARVEY, *De motu cordis*

> The following history is given in a series of letters written principally in a double yet separate correspondence.
> —SAMUEL RICHARDSON, preface to *Clarissa*

A STORY IS TOLD by an anonymous contemporary of William Harvey's that when asked what his opinion was concerning witchcraft, "the Good Doctor" gave him the following account. When he was at Newmarket with King Charles I, Harvey heard that there was a woman who dwelt in a lone house on the borders of the heath who was reputed to be a witch. Harvey, being curious about her, went alone to her house and found her home alone. She was at first very distrustful of him, but "when hee told her he was a vizard, and came purposely to converse with her in their common trade, then shee easily believed him; for, say'd hee to mee, you know I have a very magicall face, and looking upon mee, and gathering up his face, I indeed thought hee had." Harvey asked the woman where her familiar was and desired to see it. She immediately fetched a saucer of milk and, making sounds "as toades do when they call one another," went to a chest with the milk. A toad soon emerged from under the chest and drank some of the milk. Harvey then asked if she had any ale to sell, "for they being Brother and Sister must drink together." While she was away fetching the ale, Harvey took some milk, went to the chest, called the toad, and when he came out caught him with his tongs, opened the toad's belly with his dissecting knife, and out came the milk. "Hee examined the toades entrayles, heart, and lungs, and it no ways differed from other toades." The old woman, who was "melancholy and poore," had found the toad one evening eating spiders and insects and had brought it home, making it tame by feeding it, "and so it became a spirit, and that spirit a familiar."

Harvey's "argument in effect" was "A Woman had a tame toade, which she believed to bee a spirit and her familiar, the toad upon disection proved an arrant naturall toad, and had really eaten milk, and not in appearance onely, therefore there are no witches." When the woman returned she found the good doctor busy with the toad "in the Pickle hee had put him in, and was in danger to have a more magical face than hee had before." The woman threw down her pitcher of ale and flew "like a Tigris at his face; twas well hee had nothing but bare bones and tough tanned skin, neyther hair nor bearde, and twas well his eyes were out of reach, well guarded with prominent bones, otherways it had gone ill with him." Harvey was saved by his "very short old black coat ... that pay'd for killing the poor Woman's Divell." Harvey entreated her fairly, offered her money, and tried to persuade her it was not a devil but a mere toad. "That way not prevayling, hee turned his tale, sayd hee was the King's Phisitian, sent by the King to discover whether indeed shee was a witch." The name of the king brought her into better temper, and after giving the doctor a thousand bad names, she let him go. Harvey regaled the king with the story at dinner.

In 1645, a few years after the time of this purported story, a "witch" was hanged at Cambridge for keeping a frog, and, as everyone knows, belief in witchcraft was widespread in the seventeenth century.[1] I rehearse this anecdote to place the legendary Harvey in the narrative context of his age; whatever the authenticity of the story, it tells us something important about the Harvey I see writing the most influential medical narrative of the heart in the modern world. It serves to remind us that Harvey was perceived as a storyteller who went out of his way in the search for truth and enjoyed sharing his discoveries, and in that guise he presents himself as "a vizard" (the word can mean "wizard" and "mask") with a magical face who is in possession of a truth known only to a few adepts. It is also a seventeenth-century gender story about how the learned Doctor Harvey deceived an ignorant but feisty old woman, and how she got back at him. We shall recall the story when considering Satan and Eve's dream in the next chapter. In the context of seventeenth-century storytelling, Harvey is an amphibious creature and creator, both an inquisitive, self-dramatizing wizard and a careful, deliberate, rational early modern scientist.

The English have always been keen explorers, especially in the later Renaissance, of St. Augustine's two books of God, Scripture, and Nature. Not many years after Drake's circumnavigation of the globe came the new English Bible authorized by King James I (who was Harvey's first royal patient). At almost the same time two great English explorers of the human heart were making their own discoveries: William Shakespeare, figuratively, in his last plays, and the thirty-seven-year-old Harvey, physician, wizard, and anatomist, more literally than anyone had before, including his great master at Padua, the "venerable old man," Fabricius ab Aquapendente.[2] Harvey probably made his discovery of the circulation of the blood sometime between 1619 and 1625.[3] He published his findings in *Exercitatio anatomica de motv cordis et sangvinis in animalibvs* (An anatomical dissertation on the motion of the heart and blood in animals), which appeared in Frankfurt-am-Main in 1628. At this time Harvey was at the commencement of an enduring friendship with the new king, Charles I, as his "physician extra-ordinary" (later promoted to the more important "physician in ordinary"), and it was to Charles that he dedicated *De motu cordis*.[4]

Twenty-five years later, in 1653, less than four years after the execution of Charles and the same year that Cromwell became Lord Protector, *The Anatomical Exercises of Dr. William Harvey Professor of Physick, and Physician to the Kings Majesty, on the Motion of the Heart and Blood in Animals*, containing translations of *De motu cordis* and *De circulatione sanguinis* (the two letters to the French anatomist Jean Riolan *fils*, written in 1649 after the King's execution), first appeared in English.[5] *De motu cordis* was now a new book for a more troubled generation; I will refer to this edition as *The Motion of the Heart*. Harvey had waited until he was fifty to publish his treatise; he was now seventy-five, fatigued and ailing, at the end of a career in which he was privileged to see his opponents vanquished and his discovery hailed by an international audience. As his friend Thomas Hobbes said, perhaps with a bit of envy, "*he is the only man, perhaps, that ever lived to see his owne Doctrine established in his life-time.*"[6]

Previous commentators on Harvey have, in general, found small literary merit in *The Motion of the Heart*. Marjorie Hope Nicolson, basing her remarks on the Latin text and Robert Willis's nineteenth-century translation, says Harvey's treatise "is very different from most scientific works of the earlier seventeenth-century, consisting largely of careful reports of experiments with a minimum of theory, with almost no 'philosophizing' of the kind usually found in 'natural histories' of this period. There is no poetry here, and almost no overtones of any sort."[7] Charles Singer gives an even more sweeping estimate of Harvey's mind and art: "Harvey is extremely conservative, a philosopher by temper, cautious, slow, devoid of literary or oratorical charm or gift."[8] Very little attention has been paid to the first English translation of *De motu cordis* as an independent expository text. One of the few to comment on this translation is Sir Geoffrey Keynes:

> The writer of the translation remained anonymous. It is unlikely that Harvey himself had any hand in making it, but there is no reason for supposing that he disapproved of the undertaking. The first Latin edition of 1628 had been very inaccurately printed, and later editions repeated many of its mistakes. The translator of 1653 also allowed himself to take liberties in doing his work, and either he or his printer allowed words and even whole sentences to drop right out of the text. . . . The vigour of the seventeenth century is found there with a sufficient sprinkling of expressive, if now unusual, terms to produce the feeling that Harvey himself is speaking. No such illusion is fostered by the dull excellence of the Victorian text [of Robert Willis], which on a closer inspection, is even found to be not always more accurate than its despised predecessor.[9]

This chapter, largely exploratory in nature, examines the narrative and rhetorical dimensions of the English *De motu cordis* of 1653, focusing on the narrator and his attitudes toward his audience, "Nature," the act of writing, his book, his precursors, his subject (the motion of the heart and blood), and on some of the possible narrative implications this seminal text might have had for the gestating eighteenth-century novel. In so doing, I hope to show that there is more "poetry"—and more literary significance—in the English Harvey than earlier commentators have allowed.[10]

The Anatomist as Author

To begin to appreciate what the first English readers of *The Motion of the Heart* felt and thought when they encountered this text, we must start with the dedication "*To the Most illustrious and Invincible Monarch* Charls [*sic*] King of Great Britain, France, and Ireland, Defender of the Faith."

Harvey begins, "Most Gratious King, The Heart *of creatures is the foundation of life, the Prince of all, the Sun of their Microcosm, on which all vegetation does depend, from whence all vigor & strength does flow. Likewise the King is the foundation of his Kingdoms, and the Sun of his Microcosm, the Heart of his Commonwealth, from whence all power and mercy proceeds* (vii). The language here recalls not only the opening of Genesis concerning God, the land, and the creatures, but also that of Harvey's contemporary, Robert Burton, in *The Anatomy of Melancholy* (1621): "The second region [of the body] is the chest, or middle belly, in which the heart as king keeps his court, and by his arteries communicates life to the whole body."[11]

A dedication is a consecration; the king is in some respect godlike; Harvey chooses the king as the royal champion of his new doctrine of the heart and blood. Charles I, who was the heart of his commonwealth for Harvey and Burton and their generation of the 1620s, is now dead and gone—an executed criminal, like the anatomist's raw material—and this new England has no king at all. From a royalist perspective, the great heart of England has been destroyed, but Harvey allows his original dedication to Charles to stand unchanged in the English version. The English reader begins with what is already a historical narrative whose original royal and in some sense ideal reader can now only be evoked by the historical imagination. Harvey in the persona of "Gulielmus Harveius" wrote the original dedication in part to show the king that the workings of the heart are a model for the proper relationship of king and commonwealth, a relationship that has since gone tragically awry. For the first English readers, the death of the royal heart imbues their experience of Harvey's text in something like the way Thomas Watson's audience experienced his sermon, *Gods Anatomy Upon Mans Heart*, discussed in the previous chapter.

But in another sense, this new English text of an older Latin treatise has an independent language character all its own, one that allows the seventeenth-century English reader (and later readers) to recuperate the executed king in a new light. The reader also recreates the "Author" of the text, "William Harvey," professor, physician, and anatomist, now translated (by a skillful but anonymous hand) from his professional and scholarly Latin persona and refashioned into an English physician speaking plainly in his mother tongue. (I will henceforth distinguish between the historical Harvey and "Harvey" as the narrative voice, or self-styled "Author," of the English text.) The actual William Harvey, now at the end of his natural life, begins a new life as the Author of this work. The first

English readers, and we subsequent readers, must recreate the relationship between this "William Harvey" and this "King Charls." "Harvey" presents the historicized king who now exists in the limbo of the reader's imagination with a model heart serving as a kind of ideal mirror in which the royal person is implored to read, contemplate, and understand his own heart and the divine creative wisdom that shaped heart, man, and king. For us the effect of reading *The Motion of the Heart* is a bit vertiginous, something like standing in one of the rows of the steeply sloped Paduan anatomical theater and looking down past the heads of all those previous readers at the text of the heart that lies exposed on the table in the operating pit below ground level.[12]

"Harvey" styles himself in the dedication as the "*bold*" presenter of things so far written concerning the heart. In the male homosocial world of the epistle to Dr. Argent, president of the Royal College of Physicians in London, now addressing a learned audience of his peers and colleagues, he takes a more modest and conventional tone. The king may have ceased to exist, but the Royal College of Physicians continued to function in the 1650s. "Harvey" reminds Dr. Argent that he has "opened" his new opinion about the motion of the heart and the circulation of the blood many times already in his lectures. Harvey was an oral and visual performer in his own anatomical theater. This was the public Harvey, the master of "performative" anatomy. He had a vivid sense of theater, of himself as a performer in a public theater, and of the "theater of the body" (in Helkiah Crooke's resonant phrase), which he opened to perform upon. His specific performative role was as a professor working from his lecture notes in the *Prelectiones* (written in Latin with occasional English phrases, a style almost the reverse of Burton's), long before he committed his "*opinion*" to permanent Latin form in an anatomical treatise. As a classical scholar with a genuine affection for the Roman poets, he has observed Horace's advice and kept his piece for "*nine years and more.*" In thinking about how Harvey reinscribed the heart and circulation, we would do well to remember Harvey in the role of classicist as well as Harvey the public physician and anatomist.

The Author adopts the prefatorial convention, popular in much seventeenth-century expository and fictional writing, of the "*little Book*," the vulnerable child of an anxious author who hopes his intellectual offspring will "*come abroad entire and safe.*" Since the book affirms a new and unheard of doctrine, that the blood passes and returns "*through unwonted tracts, contrary to the received way,*" the Author "*was greatly afraid to suffer this little Book, otherways perfect some years ago, either to come abroad, or go beyond Sea,*" lest it might seem too arrogant. Harvey elaborated on the metaphor of the book as an infant in the second letter to Riolan, where the printing press serves as implicit midwife: "Most learned *Riolan*, by the help of the Presse, many years ago, I published a part of my labour: But since the birth-day of the Circulation of the Blood, almost no day has past . . . in which I have not heard both good and evil of the Circulation of the Blood which I found out: Others rail at it, as a tender babie unworthy to come to light; Others say, that its worthy to be foster'd, and favour my writings, and defend them; Some with great disdain oppose them; Some with mighty applause protect them" (145). We hear the rhetoric of the ambivalence of the heart in new accents. At the age of fifty, Harvey, though married, was childless. Like the narrator of *Don Quixote* (part 1, 1612 in English), who refers disparagingly to his work as "a child of understanding," "Harvey" is modest about his book and refuses "to ostentate his memory" with profuse quotations from famous authors and philosophers.[13] The little book containing its vital and subversive message is the author's "babie," a male-generated intellectual offspring that will provoke a new circulation of ideas in the masculine "republick of Literature" (18).

The Author's written ambivalence about his undertaking, "*bold*" to the King, "*greatly afraid*" with his peers, is reflected throughout the work. Like anyone with a new story to tell, he is influenced by previous conventions, and he attempts to invent new ones to enhance and enable his enterprise. Harvey knows he has discovered a startling new truth about the human body, but how can he convey that truth convincingly to his peers? How "William Harvey" inscribes his new anatomical gospel in a new English text, in a new English rhetoric of the heart, to a new set of readers that now numbers those he would consider the "vulgar," including the unlearned and women, is one of our chief concerns in this chapter.

In the epistle to Argent, "Harvey" appeals to "*Philosophers*" who are so perfectly in love with truth and wisdom that they will be willing to put aside received notions and accept a new opinion, acknowledging "*that the greatest part of those things which we do know, is the least of the things which we know not*" (xi). The language echoes the "least . . . greatest" formulas of the Gospels (e.g., Matt. 23.11; Luke 9.46–48) and the rhetoric of St. Paul.[14] The Anglican Harvey is a new kind of "opener" of texts. To us, looking back at the pastoral cultures of England and ancient Israel, aware of the central economic and mythic importance of sheep to those cultures, Harvey seems not unlike an Old Testament priest reincarnated, cutting up sheep, goats, female deer, and a variety of other animals as sacrifices to a new goddess, philosophical Truth. Robert Frank says that "the very essence of [*De motu cordis*] was vivisection." Harvey, rather like Moses or Elijah with their swords, was a master of vivisection, the performing of surgical operations or other experiments on living animals, such as prawns, lobsters, snails, small fish, eels, frogs, toads, snakes, lizards, doves, pigs, and dogs.[15] Lest we take too comfortable a view of Harvey the wizard and storyteller, let us try to imagine him tying down a living pig and performing surgical operations upon it. These animals were the external subjects of Harvey's exploration of the internal "subjects" in his anatomical narrative. Such musings present with startling clarity the fine line between Harvey the anatomist as dissector and death-dealer and Harvey the physician, healer, life-giver, writer of "Truth."

At about the same time that Harvey was composing *The Motion of the Heart*, his acquaintance and erstwhile patient Francis Bacon was writing his *New Atlantis* (published in 1627, the year after his death), in which he imagines the scientists who preside over "Salomon's House" (a kind of early organized research unit or institute) as a new kind of Levitical priesthood, clothed in the majesty of priestly robes and riding in rich chariots decorated with images of Old Testament cherubim.[16] Bacon deliberately clothes his new scientists in the garb and authority of the Old Testament priesthood. Harvey, according to John Aubrey, made some rather contemptuous remarks about Bacon, noting that he had "the eie of a viper" and that "he writes philosophy like a Lord Chancellor."[17]

Harvey, I am sure, had a more modest idea of his role as a priest of science than the patriarchal scientists of Salomon's House, and he seldom betrays anxiety about probing into God's hidden and mysterious knowledge, in large part because he has fashioned an intimate and friendly rhetorical relationship with God's handmaid, Galenic Nature, who is always her own best interpreter. He presents himself not as a rival to Nature's God (or God's Nature) but as one who listens to and observes her own interpretations of God's animal world. He is attempting to discover the original Truth of God's Nature, a Truth that has been obscured by generations of error. Hence Harvey is a minister not of the divine Word of Scripture, but of God's chief artisan, and "Nature being perfect and divine, and making nothing in vain" (113), allows him to open and publish the secrets of her book. It is significant in this regard that when Harvey was designing the Latin title page to his *Prelectiones* (1616), he proudly called his manuscript "Lectures on the Whole of Anatomy by me William Harvey, Doctor of

London, Professor of Anatomy and Surgery, anno Domini 1616, aged 37, delivered on April 16 17 18 on the male and female body." At the top he wrote a line from Virgil's *Eclogues* (3.60), *Stat Jove principium, Musae, Jovis omnia plena* (From Jove is the beginning of all things, Muses, with him all things are filled), and he used this line twice more in *De generatione animalium*. Harvey's primary image of God is that of a potent, impregnating, masculine Maker, a scientist's version of the seminal God discussed in Chapter 1, but in mortal language this God appears in many forms. Harvey even went so far as to give an androgynous depiction of this God, as seen under the aspect of human naming: "Nor can these Attributes appertain to any, but to the Omnipotent Maker of all things, under what name soever we cloud and veil him: whether it be *Mens divina*, the divine Mind, with Aristotle, or *Anima mundi*, the soul of the Universe, with Plato; or with others, *Natura Naturans*, Nature of Nature herself."[18] This depiction of God has intriguing affinities with Milton's evolving seminal and sexual God discussed in the next chapter.

If Harvey and his peers saw themselves as new interpreters of the divine wisdom that authored the Book of Nature, they must, in some respects, have considered that their teachings went far beyond those of their brethren in the pulpit. Harvey, clearheaded, analytic, rational as he was, had an almost visionary sense of the beauty and power of his momentous discovery. Part of his feeling of achievement lay in his awareness of the difficulty of the task and the difficulty and challenge of explaining how he found out the truth and returned to tell about it. Harvey as a scientific explorer made two discoveries about the heart and blood. The first occurred in the process of his activities as an anatomist, as a dissector of dead and living tissue, the "fabric" or *textus* of the bodies of all kinds of "animals," creatures possessing the pneuma of life. The second discovery was how to tell about the first one in writing, in appropriate scientific language. It was not simply a matter of choosing the *exercitatio* form. Harvey himself was very much aware of the difficulty of this task. At the end of his provocative preface to *De generatione animalium*, presumably written long after his discovery of the circulation of the blood, he equates the operation of divine "Nature" with her "generation or Fabrick," and notes that

Whoever entereth this new, and unfrequented path, and inquires for truth in the vast volume of *Nature*, by Anatomical dissections, and experiments, he meets with such a croud of observations, and those too in such exotick shapes, that to unfould to others the mysteries himself hath discovered, will bee more toyl, then the finding of them out: for many things occurr which have yet no name; such is *the plenty of things, and the dearth of words*.¹⁹

Using his notes in Latin and English, he had to retrace or recapitulate (in the original Latin sense of "to draw up in heads" or chapters) the steps of the original journey of discovery in a consecutive written exposition. From all indications, this may have been even more arduous a task, but perhaps equally challenging. As an anatomist-author, Harvey was recreating in his finite capacity the divine role of the original anatomist-author of humankind in Genesis 2 who dissected Adam in order to create a new human being, Eve. It is significant that the rise of the printed book coincided with the rise of Renaissance anatomy. The Renaissance anatomist literally deconstructed the human body in order to reconstitute or rewrite it according to Nature's own "true" image in the discourse of "natural history," a genre that Harvey included in his idea of "the republic of letters."²⁰ Without perhaps their being quite aware of it, the anatomists were new creator gods or authors, and the human body was never the same after Harvey had finished remapping and "re-creating" it.

A large part of the difficulty of the enterprise of interpreting the goddess Nature also lay in the fact that Nature herself had an almost equally powerful rival in "*Mistris Antiquity*" (xi), an emblem of "Habit" as the artificial Second Nature who in Harvey's view of scientific investigation all too often supplants her divine original. "Mistress Antiquity" was an extension of the original Mother Night, the elemental figure of darkness, error, superstition, and the ally of Chaos, always at war with light and order, an abstract version of lowly "Mother Midnight," the cant name for a bawd or witch who (as I have argued) figures significantly in the early English novel. "Mistress Antiquity" is Harvey's Mother Midnight, a counterpart to the woman with her toad familiar. Out of strategic necessity in his rhetorical scientific project, Harvey had to pay homage to ancient and modern authorities, especially to Aristotle, to "that divine Man Galen," "the Father of Physick," and to his own teacher and mentor, Fabricius, and he quotes abundantly from their works when their teachings are reasonably "firm." He knows, however, that genuine "*Philosophers*" do not "*suffer themselves to be addicted to the slavery of any mans precepts, but that they give credit to their own eys*" (xi). Harvey, masculinist-Aristotelian scholar though he was in many respects, yet preaches the "eyewitness" gospel of ocular proof in the service of the scientific philosopher's "*Friend Truth*," and the metaphor of "seeing" recurs throughout his text. "*I do not profess to learn and teach Anatomy from the axioms of Philosophers, but from Dissections, and from the fabrick of Nature*" (xiii). The "fabric" of Nature is his text, as it was for Vesalius in his famous *Fabrica*. And he can ultimately disclose his opinion—his refashioning or rewriting of the body—only within the world of letters. His is a literary endeavor. He claims to *"follow the truth only,"* and he bestows his pains *"to bring forth something which might be both acceptable to good men, agreeable to learned men, and profitable to literature"* (xiii).

By following only the truth of Nature, Harvey brings forth his perfected *"little Book,"* his literary offspring. In 1657, after Harvey's death, his friend and fellow M.D. the poet Abraham Cowley portrayed the heroic Harvey with a somewhat different metaphor. In his "Ode: *Upon Dr. Harvey*," Cowley creates a little pre-Restoration comedy by fusing the roles of Truth and Nature into the unconventional image of Nature as an aged but "Coy" and "beauteous" virgin whom Harvey, as "our *Apollo*," pursues with a "violent passion."[21] But instead of stopping to touch the leaves of this new Daphne transformed into a tree, Harvey the anatomist penetrates right on through the bark and fibers into the root of the plant, forcing Nature, like "the Deer long-hunted" taking to a river, to leap for refuge "into the winding streams of blood" and then the confines of the heart where she thinks she shall be safe—"the heart of Man, what Art can e'er reveal?" Harvey himself, in *De generatione*, recounted how, through the kind generosity and protection of King Charles, he was allowed to dissect live does from the king's deer park.[22] Cowley's Harvey/Apollo surprises Nature in her retreat and, holding "this slippery *Proteus* in a chain," forces her to reveal all her "mighty Mysteries." Her former attempt to hide her secrets was, with typical Cowleyan wit, "the first Thing that Nature did in vain." In effect, Cowley's Harvey rapes Nature in the most hidden recesses of the heart's chambers. Though in this poem Cowley perverts what appears to be Harvey's own deepest sense of trusting—never forcing—Nature to divulge her mysteries, the poet here presents us with an often rehearsed paradigm of the seventeenth-century masculine scientist's domination of Nature, which has its analogues in Milton's Satan's stalking and violation of Eve and in the Restoration libertine rake's domination of women. This motif culminates, as I show in the final chapter, in Richardson's *Clarissa* with Lovelace, the naturalist-libertine authority on women and the most complex re-creation of the phenomenon of "the phallic heart" in eighteenth-century fiction, violating Clarissa and ultimately demanding possession of her actual heart.[23]

The Anatomist as Fate

"Harvey" begins his treatise proper (in the "Proeme") with an exposure of previous obscure and false hypotheses about the activity of the heart, but amidst the conventional expository rhetoric one hears the voice of the exasperated and ambivalent son confronting the ignorance of venerable but blind forefathers: he "beseeches" his opponents in a series of quasi-rhetorical questions. He exclaims at their folly: "Good God," how can they miss the evidence in front of their eyes? He scorns the "hidden pore" hypothesis (postulated by Galen) for getting the blood from the right to the left ventricle: "But by my troth there are no such pores, nor can they be demonstrated" (13). In the first chapter, he continues this autobiographical mode, explaining "*the Causes which mov'd the Author to Write*." Thus the motion of the heart has a corresponding movement in the writer; he is like the blood that the heart causes to move and act. Again he points out difficulties, but now he goes back to the original problem. He acknowledges that Fabricius had learnedly and accurately described almost all the parts of living creatures, but "left the *heart* only untouched" (18). He does not mention that Fabricius was his master teacher at Padua, but he may have thought that his mentor left the heart for him.

"Harvey" is confronted and apparently intrigued at first by the near impossibility of accurately describing the movement of the heart and blood: "with *Fracastorius*, I did almost beleeve, that the motion of the Heart was known to God alone" (16), but he cannot leave it there. What was especially difficult was distinguishing the systole and diastole because of "the quickness of the motion," appearing often like "the twinckling of an eye, like the passing of Lightning" (16). The uncertainty of his observations caused him to be "much troubled in mind," an anxiety similar to the kind he expresses in the epistle to Argent, but far more severe. The reader soon discerns that "Harvey" is writing about a quest, a kind of travel narrative of what happens inside the body. His goal, as he puts it, was to gain "both the motion and use of the *heart*" (17). He worked away at the problem, "using daily more search and diligence," examining a variety of creatures, until at some point "he hit the nail on the head." The sense of manual discovery and the capital force of nailing the problem suggest reaching a goal or destination, with a workmanlike nuance of inevitability, of destiny and "destinare," to fasten down or secure.

This suggestive phrase immediately gives way to a richer poetic figure of fate: with the discovery "I . . . unwinded and freed my self from this

Labyrinth" (17). Aubrey tells us that Harvey had a house in Surrey with "a good aire and prospect, where he had Caves made in the Earth, in which in Summer time he delighted to meditate." Aubrey also notes that Harvey was "very Cholerique; and in his young days wore a dagger," which he would draw out upon every slight occasion.[24] Contemplative and quite possibly irritable in real life, the narrator of *The Motion of the Heart* emerges as a modern Theseus—fearless and bold, but also meditative. He works himself into an anatomical labyrinth, then conquers his own Minotaur in his own way when he "unwinds" himself from this figurative cave by means of a cautious and careful mapping and unravelment of the course of the blood. We might extend the metaphor to say that Nature herself was his Ariadne, offering him the threadlike course of the blood vessels to follow. But he had to trust to Nature, not Mistress Antiquity, and to his own powers of perception and dissection in order to tease the secret of the circulation (his "tender babie," as we recall from the letter to Riolan [145]) out of her mysterious womblike "Labyrinth" in the body. We see in this language a new and much more cautious empiricist version of the workings of the seminal God within the womb of his chosen women.

The image of thread is especially appropriate for Harvey. As an anatomical surgeon and physician, he worked skillfully with surgical thread to make a "handsome" ligature, recalling the dexterous midwife who ties off the umbilical cord. In the new English literary persona that now emerges from this text, "little Harvey" incorporates the feminine roles of weaver and seamstress with those of knight errant and the brave little tailor in English folktale.[25] As sewer, surgeon, anatomist, and *writer*, he is an androgynous but predominantly male fate figure, rerouting and remapping the course of the blood, reinscribing the very bloodlines of life, reconstituting and redelivering the human body in an irreversible process. Augmenting the maleness of his enterprise is the strong phallic impulse in his love of handling and manipulating daggers, needles, and "lances" (or lancets, p. 81), surgical knives, probes, and pincers, and he is expert with his fine tools. Indirectly then, Harvey and his translator give us a complex picture of the anatomist as hero, setting himself a quest, searching for the answer to a problem, finding the solution, vanquishing his Thesean monster and his opponents, overcoming his anxiety: "Since which time I have not been afraid, both privately to my friends, and publickly in my Anatomy Lectures to deliver my opinion" (17). And Walter Pagel, one of the foremost Harvey scholars, asserts that "the nearest approach to a circular movement of the blood is found in the speculations of Giordano Bruno whose spectacular death at the stake in 1600 [in Rome] was an event that could hardly have escaped the knowledge of any academic citizen of Padua, including Harvey."[26]

"Harvey" concludes the first chapter with an even more specific claim to a place in the "republick of Literature" (18) than he made in the epistle to Argent, and Harvey the classicist reinforces his claim with a quote from Terence's *Adelphi* (The Brothers). This comedy is built upon the complications that arise because of diametrically opposed theories of child rearing adhered to by two Grecian brothers, men in their sixties. Micio, "A Rich Citizen of Athens, a mild, sweet-natur'd old Gentleman . . . extream loving and kind to his Nephews," has never married, but he had adopted one of the two sons of Demea, "His Brother . . . a Country Gentleman, and a violent, angry, fretful, busie, medling Fellow; strict and severe to his Sones, and a great Pretender to Education."[27] Micio's unusual system or theory is that the son who is reared by kindness instead of severity will turn out better in the long run, and his doctrine is partially validated at the end of the play by the sardonic Demea, who, claiming to see the error of his harsh parental ways, says (in the passage translated in the *The Motion of the Heart*):

> *No man so well e'r laid his count to live,*
> *But that things, age, and use some new thing give,*
> *That what you thought you knew, you shall not know,*
> *And what you once thought best, you shall forgoe.*[28]

"Harvey" the narrator responds, "This may perchance fall out now in the motion of the heart, that from hence the way being thus pervious, others . . . may take occasion to doe better, and search further" (18). "Harvey" indirectly (and hopefully) casts his opponents in the role of the brother who comes to accept a gentler, more open ("pervious"), and correct theory. Since Demea finally suggests the merging of the two brother's households, the play has an even more striking aptness to the characterization of the heart and blood in this text, as we shall see.

This Familiar Household God

The Motion of the Heart is an early scientific version of the metaphor of trial at the center of all heroic narrative in the dynamic of quest, ordeal, travel and travail, transcendence. Before we undertake this search with "Harvey," it may be well to supplement the traditional seventeenth-century English context of the natural history of the heart sketched in the Introduction with the following comprehensive account given by Robert Burton in *The Anatomy of Melancholy*. I would like to stress Burton's characterization of the heart as a predominantly masculine organ, his conventional sense of the heart as the seat of the passions, his geographical metaphor for describing the contours of the heart, and his traditional Galenic linking of the left side of the heart with the seat of life and attractive power. It is interesting that the spatiality of the "left," so often associated with the wayward or marginal "feminine," is in the Aristotelian Lucretian model of physiological discourse of the heart (from the time of the Hippocratic *De corde*) firmly bound to the source of life and intelligence. We should recall Burton's description of the heart when we come to Milton's Paradise and Eve as Adam's "heart" partner. Burton says, of the middle region or chest,

the principal part is the heart, which is the seat and fountain of life, of heat, of spirits, of pulse and respiration, the sun of our body, the king and sole commander of it, the seat and organ of all passions and affections. *Primum vivens, ultimum moriens*, it lives first and dies last in all creatures. Of a pyramidical form . . . a part worthy of admiration, that can yield such variety of affections, by whose motion it is dilated or contracted, to stir and command the humours in the body: as in sorrow, melancholy; in anger, choler; in joy, to send the blood outwardly; in sorrow, to call it in; moving the humours as horses do a chariot. This heart, though it be one sole member, yet it may be divided into two creeks right and left. The right is like the moon increasing, bigger than the other part, and receives blood from *vena cava*, distributing some of it to the lungs to nourish them; the rest to the left side, to engender spirits. The left creek hath the form of a cone, and is the seat of life, which, as a torch doth oil, draws blood unto it, begetting of it spirits and fire; and as fire in a torch, so are spirits in the blood; and by that great artery called aorta it sends vital spirits over the body, and takes air from the lungs by that artery which is called venosa; so that both creeks have their vessels, the right two veins, the left two arteries, besides those two common anfractuous ears, which serve them both; the one to hold blood, the other air, for several uses.[29]

"Harvey" the narrator's language to describe his search for the true understanding of the motion and use of the heart becomes even more particularized than the concrete discourse of Burton's natural philosophy, with the narrator's "labyrinth" becoming the delusive "contexture" of the heart and lungs, a pitfall for earlier explorers of the function of the heart. The narrator as preeminent reader of the "contexture" or textus of the "*fabrick* of the *heart* and *arteries*" (101), the pioneering "first" man—recalling Adam—who "hitherto has said anything aright concerning the

Anastomosis," or network of interconnections among the heart, arteries, and veins (67), will explore the darkest recesses of the microcosmic body of the heart—the ventricles (literally, "little bellies"), the "bosom" (10), the "cellars" and "cisterns" of the cave of the heart (30, 35), the secret "fountain" (95), the source of "treasure" or a "treasury" of blood (95, 30, 118), then record what he has seen. The explorer must find the hidden region but he cannot get lost in it—he must also come back home.

In the second chapter, the minute anatomist as surgical knight with his lance cuts through the capsule environing the heart of a living creature to show that "the *heart* moves sometimes, sometimes rests" (19). The traditional anatomical view of the heart, as we saw in the Introduction, called attention to its density, durability, intense heat, and continuous motive power: "The substance of the heart is a thicke . . . and red flesh, being made of the thicker part of the bloud; it is lesse redd then the flesh of muscles but harder, more solide and dense, that the spirits and inbred heate which are contayned in the heart and from thence powred into al parts of the body should not exhale; and that it might not bee broken or rent in his strong motions and continuall dilatation and constriction."[30] "Harvey"'s first description stresses the heart's erectile-contractile nature: while it is moving, the virtually phallic "*heart* is erected, and . . . it raises it self upwards into a point" (19), beating against the breast; "the *heart* being grasp'd in ones hand whilst it is in motion, feels harder" (20). These are certainly the most vivid early descriptions in English of the tactile manipulation of a living heart. To the narrator it seems that "the motion of the *heart* was [*sic*] a kind of *tention* in every part of it" as the fibers constrict; "in all its motions, it was erected, received vigour, grew lesser, and harder," like the motion of "muscles," and "having thrust out the blood contained within it," its white color gives way to "purple and crimson" in its relaxation (20–21).[31] We recall that as early as 1616 Harvey had concluded that the heart acted as a muscle in systole with the ventricles contracting and forcibly ejecting blood outward, rather than drawing it in during diastole as traditional Galenic doctrine taught. The unmistakably phallic—even masturbatory—characteristics of "Harvey"'s depiction of the heart recall the phallic, life-giving power of the seminal God discussed in the previous chapter and will be contrasted with the destructive phallic and phallocratic power of Milton's Satan, Rochester's libertine poetic persona, and Richardson's Lovelace in later chapters.

"Harvey"'s remarkable account of the ejaculatory power of the heart is punctuated by noting that if a "wound" is inflicted by the lance in the ventricle the blood contained within will leap out. In the new rhetoric of the natural philosophy of the heart, this intensely literal "wound in the heart" supplants the worn-out convention familiar in more traditional quest-romance narratives. We are also told that the sides of the ventricle are girded together like a "noose" for greater expulsive force. The reader who recalls the equation between the king and the heart at the opening of the treatise and in Burton's rhetoric of the heart may feel somewhat uneasy at these operations, and even more so a few pages later when the narrator gives a detailed and poignant account (based on Aristotle but with his own variations) of how the heart dies. We hear again (as in Burton's account) that the heart has "ears" (auricles) and "four motions distinct in place, but not in time" (28). The heart now begins to take on, rather eerily, the aspect of the head: "drawing towards death, it ceases to answer by its motion, and only by nodding its head seems as it were to give consent" (29). One recalls the poise and grace of Charles proceeding to his death in a highly controlled dramatic performance, giving the final signal to the executioner.[32] But this heart dies a lingering death, adumbrating the protracted dying of a heroine like Richardson's Clarissa a century later. The narration continues: "And whilst by little and little the *heart* is dying, you may see after two or three beatings of the *ear*, the *heart* will, being as it were rowsed, answer, and very slowly and hardly endeavour and frame a motion" (29), as if the heart were trying to speak. The narrator presents himself as someone in touch with, and virtually in control of, the very source of life itself: "putting your finger upon the ventricle of the heart, every pulsation is perceived" (29), as later, in the description of ligatures, the physician, like a new Heraclitus, "shall feel the blood as it were passing by under his finger" (75).

This sense of the anatomist as a godlike or magical figure, a semidivine wizard having control over life functions, is intensified in his description of an experiment on the immobile heart of a "*dove.*" Recalling the language for Christ's curing of the blind and the deaf, the narrator says: "I wetted my finger with spittle, and being warmed kept it a while upon the *heart* . . . as if it had received strength and life afresh, the *heart*, and its ears began to move, to contract, and open, and did seem as it were recall'd back again from death" (31).[33] Here also the narrator gives a personal eyewitness account of his experience, deeply implicated in his own story, and ends with a climactic meditation on the circular nature of the life processes,

Nature in death returning to her beginnings, a blurred interpenetration of being and not being:

Nay its doubtfull too . . . whether we may say that with this beating [of the heart in death] the life begins, seeing the Sperm and prolifique Spirit, of all living creatures, goes from them with a kind of leaping, as if it self were a living creature. So Nature in death making as it were a recapitulation, returns upon her self with a retrograde motion, from the end of her race to the beginning of it, from whence she first issues thither she returns, seeing the generation of living creatures . . . is . . . as from a non entitie to be an entitie, so by the same steps, corruption passes from an entitie, to a non entitie; whence it is, that that which in living creatures is last made, fails first, and that which is first made, fails last. (32)

Here "Harvey" specifically identifies the ejaculative nature of the heart with "the Sperm, and prolifique Spirit of all living creatures," a metaphysical evocation of the generative power of the heart and blood.[34] Nature's "recapitulation" suggests her bond with Harvey the anatomical writer, Nature as divine allotter, original Fate, and forward-moving inscriber of all her living "Phaenomena's" (118), the Author participating with her in this enterprise to reinscribe or rewrite and restore the course of the blood according to Nature's true, original plan. *Natura Naturans*, Shakespeare's "great creating Nature," is another name for God, as we have seen, and Harvey is thus her prophet, and his book is her Revelation. Hence Nature, in Harvey's own definition, becomes a "veil" of the semiotic God of the Old Testament.

As he moves closer to his revelation of the circular motion of the blood, the Author explores the subtheme of the apparent duplicity of the heart, whose real motion can only be perceived by the skilled anatomist. Contrary to the common Galenic opinion, the heart is contracted when it is emptied (21), and one continuous motion of the heart appears, "as it were keeping a certain harmony, and number" (35) when two motions ("one of the *ears*, the other of the *ventricles*") are actually at work. Here it becomes even more apparent that "Harvey" sees the heart, lungs, and blood vessels as an interconnective "contexture," or "fabrick of the *heart*" (37), a text that has been misread by his precursors who (again recalling the image of the cave or labyrinth) "stumbling as it were in a dark place . . . seem to be dim-sighted, and clamper up [jumble together] divers things" in a confused way (37). But though Galen misunderstood the function of the aorta and arteries, he gave an accurate indication of Nature's writing in "the orifice of the *vena arteriosa* [pulmonary artery]," where three "doors, made like a Σ or half-Moon" (the three semi-lunar valves) (51), keep the blood from flowing back into the heart. Galen describes the valvular action of the heart as a kind of invisible and minute "kissing," and the passage is quoted approvingly in full. Such internal kissing is another example of divine Nature's ever-active artifice in the interior of man, expressed as a kind of gentle and harmonious lovemaking taking place continually within and between even the smallest of the internal bodily parts. This action too is an allegorical model, now a nostalgic one, for the king and his relation to his queen and commonwealth, and the interrelationship between the parts of the body politic.

Chapter 8 of *The Motion of the Heart*, almost midway in the narrative, might be considered the heart and center of the work conceived as a literary offspring. The Author has wound his way through the "contexture of the heart and lungs" to establish the outline of what came to be called the pulmonary or lesser circulation. He now prepares to show the new way through the second, larger, and more complex labyrinth, "the Anastomosis" or interconnective system of the arteries and veins, that which came to be called the systemic circulation. By this point in the narrative, the Author has unobtrusively established himself as a godlike narrator with his finger on the very pulse of life-and-death as an ongoing process. Yet here his anxiety and fear, first seen in the epistle to Argent, are at their height, as his anatomic gospel is "so new and unheard of" that he not only fears the mischief of the envious but that "every man almost will be my enemy," so strong is the power of Mistress Antiquity and "custome and doctrine once received and deeply rooted as it were another Nature" (57). This other Nature is a malign and perverse man-made Nature, an unnatural Nature. So far as we can tell, Harvey, despite an occasionally testy spirit, was a quiet, contemplative, gracious man of well-regulated habits, an Anglican royalist, jealous of his prerogatives as a Fellow of the College of Physicians in London who genuinely abhorred the conventional scholarly controversy and rancor of the time, a man not given to revolutionary pronouncements. What he was about to do was as heroic in his personal life as it is in his narrative life in this text. Aubrey testifies that "I have heard him say, that after his Booke of the Circulation of the Blood came-out, that he fell mightily in his Practize, and that 'twas beleeved by the vulgar that he was crack-brained; and all the Physitians were against his Opinion, and envyed him; many wrote against him."[35]

From his examination of the valves in the veins, he postulated that the blood must "pass back again by some way out of the *veins* into the *arteries*" and this might be "a *circular* motion" (58). "Harvey" then describes this circular motion in one succinct paragraph, likening it to Aristotle's cycle of air and rain in evaporation. The story he now tells is memorable and vibrant not so much because of its disinterested "objectivity" as because of the rich metonymic possibilities derived from its highly concrete language and multilayered cultural "contexture." It is this context we must now unfold in somewhat more detail.

In almost the same words he used to begin his dedication to Charles, and as he had affirmed in the great passage on Nature's "recapitulation" of life and death, the Author reminds us that "the *heart* is the beginning of life, the *Sun* of the *Microcosm*" of man's body (59). As we saw in the Introduction and then echoed in Burton's traditional account of the heart, it was believed that heat was the defining principle of all life and (after Galen) that in the left ventrical of the heart the blood was "perfected" into "vital spirit" in its interaction with air from the outside world. Let us also recall from the Introduction the traditional association of heat with maleness and cold with femaleness. The French physician Nicholas Venette gives a convenient version of this conventional medical view at the end of the seventeenth century:

Every body agrees that generally speaking, the Temperaments of Men and Women are very different; that Men are hotter and drier, that their Flesh is more firm, their Skin more rugged, their Limbs stronger, and their Wit more penetrating; that they live upon hotter, harder, and drier Food, and that their Exercise for the most part is more violent. Women to the contrary are colder and moister, less hot, and less dry; their Flesh is softer, tenderer, and smoother; their Mind easier; they use colder and moister Food: And lastly, live almost always in Idleness.[36]

Harvey, at least in his writings, did not share this simplistic and antifeminist view of the constitution of the sexes, but in general he would have agreed with the basic association of vital heat with the male and coldness and softness with the female. Especially interesting is the language used to bring the inner and outer parts of the body together. "Harvey" calls the outer parts of the body the "habit," the dress or outer physical apparel of the body, as it were, and cold in proportion to their distance from the heart.[37] The blood leaving the heart "is warm, perfect, vapourous, full of spirit . . . and . . . alimentative" (59). One might characterize this fresh blood, from the point of view of an early modern reader, as a host of "vital spirits" moving eagerly and affectionately to the feminized outer parts of the body where "all the parts are nourished, cherished, and quickned with blood" (59). "Harvey" has already associated the external "Habit" of age-old custom with the feminine, with Mistress Antiquity, and we see here a movement away from the biblical fusion of woman, the heart, and interiority to an association of the feminine, the marginal, the dependent. "Cherish" has its full seventeenth-century resonance of showing love to (related to "charity"), taking good care of, fostering. The active power of the blood is characterized elsewhere in *The Motion of the Heart* as moving "largely, impetuously, by impulsion, as it were out of a spout." It is "wonderful to see, with how great force, how great protrusion, how quickly" (65–66) the blood moves in its "in-thrusting, and straight-in driving" force (78), impelled by the heart, "so forcibly, so abundantly, so easily, so suddenly" when viewed in the experiments with ligatures (82).

In "the parts," however, this warm, fructifying blood becomes "refrigerated, coagulated, and made as it were barren" (59). If the blood were to stay in the cold outward parts it would "congeal and be immovable" (92); in effect, it would die (93). There is a hint here of the ancient idea that the life-giving masculine life force is depleted by the insatiable female body. The action of the blood thus correlates with the seventeenth-century notion of the male "dying" in intercourse, and with the little death of detumescence. It is necessary therefore for the blood to "resume and redintegrate" (93) itself again by a return to its source, a passage effected "through the little *veins* into the *vena cava*, and to the right ear of the heart" (58). The blood "returns to the *heart*, as to the fountain or dwelling-house of the body" (59). This is "Harvey"'s revolutionary assertion: the blood is powerfully impelled from the heart on a long circuitous mission and then returns to its original dwelling place or home in the heart where it is restored for its next journey. Hence the blood does not simply circulate: it continually makes a heroic circuit of quest, mission, and homecoming, a journey of sexual regeneration within the body.[38] Once returned to the heart, the blood is "melted" by a powerful natural heat (the text retains the ancient notion of the heart as a kind of internal oven) and then recovers its perfection by again "being fraught with spirits, as with balsam" (59). "Balsam" is a gummy aromatic medicinal resin, sometimes associated with sperm. It also has heroic connotations; balsam soothes and cures the knight's wounds when he returns to his home court or other refuge,[39] and we recall Burton's image of the heart as a king keeping his court. *The Motion of the Heart* consistently fuses new contexts with older images.

But we need to make one final link with the old anatomy. Galen thought that the testicles were an "official" member of the body. According to Crooke's *Mikrokosmographia*, "*Galen* in his first book *de semine*, preferreth the testicles to the heart.... The Testicles are another Fountaine or well-spring of in-bred heate; the Feu-place or Fire-hearth, where the *Lares* of household-Gods of the body, do solace and disport themselues . . . their power is very great, and almost incredible" (45). Crooke reiterates this image, even indulging in wordplay: "Surely the power and vertue of the Testicles is very great & incredible, not onely to make the body fruitefull, but also in the alteration of the temperament. . . . In these doth *Galen* place, beside that in the heart, another hearth as it were of the inbred heate, and these are the houshould Goddes which doe blesse and warme the whole bodye" (241). Finally, "in excellency the Testicles are like vnto the heart; for that Cordial *Epithymations* [small plasters] applyed to the Testicles in great languishments of the spirits doe little lesse auail, then if they were applied to the heart itself" (207). Crooke of course is talking about the male testicles: "The Testicles in men are larger and of a hotter nature then in women; not so much by reason of their scituation, as because of the temperament of the whole body, which in women is colder, in men hotter" (204).

"Harvey"'s final metaphor for the heart, echoing at once the older language of Crooke and the Anglican marriage service, is at once divine and domestic: "this familiar house-hold god doth his duty to the whole body, by nourishing, cherishing, and vegetating, being the foundation of life, and author of all" (59–60).[40] Galen's sensuous image of the invisible "kissing" of the blood vessels gives way to "Harvey"'s implied allegory of an erotic and divine harmony between the husband heart and the bodily wife, an internalized version of the bridegroom's vow in earlier versions of the marriage service, "with my body I thee worship." The circuit of the blood on these terms is a perpetual intercourse between the heart and its parts via the precious lifestream of the blood, an internal mirror of the ongoing human cycle between life and death illustrated most memorably in Harvey's writings in Exercise 28 of *De generatione* (1653 trans.):

the same *Species* may be prolonged, though by the ruine and obsequies of the Authors . . . the *Males* when they arm themselves, and are in all respects well appointed for Loves encounter, how strangly [*sic*] doth the potent *Cupid* heighten their enflamed spirits, how spruce are they, how do they pride it; how vigorous, how testy are they, and prone to conflicts! But when this office and performance ceaseth: oh! how soon doth their force abate, and their late fury coole! how doe they hale in all their swelling sails, and check their darings? Nay even while this jocund *Sacrifice* to *Venus* is in season, no sooner is the act performed, but they grow tame and pusillanimous: as if it were then deep printed in their thoughts, that while they impart a life to others, they are in full career to their own urnes.[41]

The householder heart, like a husband, does his duty to the body, recalling the *debitum conjugale* of 1 Cor. 7.3, but he is also a powerful god impelling his "spirit" forces in the blood to replenish and recreate the body, then return home to the household or "mansion" of the heart (61). There is an implicit allusion to the Pauline Christ and his relation to the spiritual body of his church, and the heart and the blood in this narrative seem to be analogous to the Father and Son/Holy Spirit in the Christian drama of the ever-active Trinity. The heart is like the Father whose house has many mansions. The blood with its "vital spirit" cherishing the body is like the Son who through the Holy Spirit ministers to the body of his church. The blood in this allegory undergoes a continuous process of death and resurrection in the body, with the Father-heart as source and resurrector. Near the end the narrator also describes how "the principality" of the heart, "the first subsistent" or prime mover of life in its embryonic form, is "a sort of internal *animal*" ("the original and foundation" of all animal—i.e., spiritual—power), which makes, nourishes, preserves, and perfects "the whole animal" who comes after it, a power again analogous to the creator Christ who makes the world. At the conclusion of the treatise, we learn that "the body of the *heart* is made with severall draughts of *fibers* streight, thwart, and crooked" (114), a textus reminiscent of the warp and woof of a loom. The heart is finally a kind of internal loom of human fate.

The narrator assigns the word "author" both to the heart (59) and to himself. As we look back over the text of *The Motion of the Heart*, certain correspondences come to life. We may now see (to use "Harvey"'s favorite verb of sensation) in the paradigm of the explorer-narrator going deeply into the dark labyrinth of the body and returning with his discovery an analogue to that discovery itself: the cycle of the blood venturing to the outermost parts of the body and returning to the heart. We may now also see what the narrator-anatomist does in his experiments with the heart—a process of alternately observing the action of the heart and then manipulating it—is analogous to what the heart does to and with the blood—alternately receiving and then dispensing it. Both of these authors, the anatomist and his subject, coexist in a dynamic textual interplay, mutually creating each other. Finally, "Harvey" (combining the implicit roles of professor, philosopher, physician, anatomist, fate, priest, wizard, author), allied with "divine Nature," and the author-heart, whom he has personified as a "Prince," may be seen in the English version of *De motu cordis* as a united heroic pair who have replaced the divine Charles as the champions of a newly "invented" or discovered heart.

Harvey and the Novel

It has often been noted that what sets Harvey apart from earlier anatomists is his emphasis on physiological process instead of morphological definition. It is precisely this emphasis and quality of mind that help ally him with subsequent artists of narrative fictions. Harvey is interested in describing the constitution of the heart only insofar as that description will explain its "motion," "use," and "function." It might be said that the heart and the blood together—a figurative child, virtually a new being, which "Harvey" names "Circulation of the Blood" (145)—were for Harvey what Robinson Crusoe was to be for Defoe and what Clarissa was to be for Richardson.

Harvey has long been called a "vitalist." In all his writings, he is preoccupied with movement, growth, development, transition, process—life processes. In this he anticipates that tenacity for exploring quotidian, transient, intermittent reality evident in certain eighteenth-century novelists, particularly Defoe, with his untiring and inventive accounts of how Robinson Crusoe and Moll Flanders perform activities that promote their survival as extraordinary individuals, Richardson with his minute recording of his characters' evolving and intermeshing moment-to-moment experience in life's "womb of fate," Sterne with his fragmentary and indelible evocation of gesture and bodily transition.

Recent discussions of the origins of the English novel have begun to pay more attention to the possible influence of "scientific"/medical narrative on the development of novelistic themes and discourse in the fiction of such writers as Behn, Defoe, Richardson, Fielding, Sterne, and Smollett.[42] Mikhail Bakhtin, in his continually suggestive *Dialogic Imagination*, notes that in the Socratic dialogues "we possess a remarkable document that reflects the simultaneous birth of scientific thinking and of a new artistic-prose model for the novel." Although Bakhtin is more concerned with the emergence of the novel in the second half of the eighteenth century than in the first half, a similar observation might be made for the rise of the English novel occurring not long after the scientific revolution in empirical method that Harvey did so much to bring about in experimental practice and—what has not been sufficiently discussed—in *fash-*

ioning a language to describe his practice. The most important aspect of Bakhtin's new genre of "becoming," the modern novel, is "an indeterminacy, a certain semantic openendedness, a living contact with unfinished, still-evolving contemporary reality," words that might also describe the experimental method of Harvey and modern science. Bakhtin concludes, "when the novel becomes the dominant genre, epistemology becomes the dominant discipline."[43] I contend that the English expository narratives of Harvey's work on the heart and on sexual generation have suggestive points of contact with Defoe, Richardson, and Sterne in particular and, in combination with the writings of those seventeenth-century physiologists influenced by Harvey, have exerted indirect cultural if not direct textual influence on the early development of the English novel.

The essence of narrative, it might be said, is the discourse of motion—motion from one place to another, from one moment to another. As I have already indicated, readers of Harvey's two major works, *The Motion of the Heart* and *De generatione*, are struck by his preoccupation with describing the function of the life-originating and life-maintaining parts of the animal body. In *The Motion of the Heart*, it is not the constitution of the heart and blood he is interested in so much as the question, what is their activity and function in the human body? He was always aware that "the blood must be continuously moving somewhere,"[44] and this phrase is also an apt description of his own narrative style as it translates into English. The overriding question for Harvey, in all of his works was, how does one thing get to another thing in the body? In *The Motion of the Heart*, how does the blood get around in the body, and finally, in *De generatione*, how does the semen get into the womb? The question has to do with the nature of the motion of key elements in the body, and that motion, like the motion of life itself, is always in one direction. Harvey's work is a "history" of such motion—the record of moving, living bodies and their interaction—and thus a paradigmatic, or primordial, novelistic narrative, for the novel records the passage of the protagonist *from one condition to another*, and each of the most memorable narrative authorial styles in the early modern period has its own unique kind and pace of movement.

Aphra Behn's eager, fast-paced style in her culminating novel, *Oroonoko* (the "Transactions" of whose hero she purports to describe in the opening paragraphs), partakes of the diction and the circumstantiality of detail to be found in the early volumes of the *Philosophical Transactions* of the Royal Society. Defoe shares with Harvey a particularly precise and animated quality of describing how complicated things work, how the human subject under consideration (e.g., Crusoe or Moll Flanders or Roxana) begins, develops, changes, and of delineating the nature of the critical moments in its passage. Richardson refines this narrative mode as the master of momentary narrative, of "writing to the moment," which culminates in the minute rendering of a dramatic series of critical moments in the lives of his protagonists, and Sterne develops a highly suggestive and complex representation of arrested moments of comic futility in his elaboration of the thesis that "attitudes are nothing, madam . . . 'tis the transition from one attitude to another . . . which is all in all."[45]

Closely allied with Harvey's narrative of motion and function is the eroticizing of the action of the heart and blood in *The Motion of the Heart*, what might be called the "sexuality" of the inner body in the interplay of heart, blood, and body parts, and his lifelong preoccupation with and quest for the secret of life's origin in male and female generation, expressed most fully in *De generatione*. As we have seen, *The Motion of the Heart* records a kind of dialogue between the masculinized heart/blood and the feminized outer body. The discourse of seventeenth-century science arises in part from the *discourse of gender conflict* in the encounter between the masculine natural philosopher and a feminized "Nature." One of the essential features of the early novel is its vivid and varied representation of new forms of courtship and marital dialogue between men and women extending in prose a rich and constant motif evolving from Chaucerian verse-narrative into Spenser's, and thence into the drama of the Renaissance and the Restoration.

Moreover, *The Motion of the Heart* conveys an ever-probing, dynamic representation of life and death processes—a uniquely Harveian kind of "vitalism." I have shown in *Mother Midnight* how a great deal of eighteenth-century fiction, influenced in part by popular "scientific" ideas of generation and by the pervasive rhetoric of human creation and generation in the Authorized Version of the Old Testament, gives a powerful and compelling depiction of human fate in relation to birth and sexuality, as well as death and closure. "William Harvey," the autobiographical "I"-witness of the English versions of his two major works, a kind of male fate figure sewing, tying, reconstituting, and rewriting the human body, shares the first-person mode of narration with the invented protagonists in the major fiction of Behn, Defoe, Richardson, and Sterne.[46] He presents himself with his own fears and anxieties, as do these protagonists, and he describes his own experience in terms of empirical self-experiments.[47] He and they are intimately concerned with describing life-and-death encounters in their narratives. Each develops a unique style of narrative "vitalism."

Perhaps the most intriguing feature *The Motion of the Heart* shares with major narratives of important early modern writers of fiction is the motif of heroic quest, encounter, and homecoming I have described here with respect to the motion of the heart and blood. The blood must come full circle back to its home and origin in the heart, hence the blood is a self-contained entity or "character," having a stable identity, and is not just a nourishing soup that is continually reconcocted, as in the Galenic model. In Harvey's narrative, the blood is always being renewed, not remade. In themselves, the complex interrelations of blood, heart, and body constitute a group of continuously interacting figures in a narrative within the "theater of the body," and the circulation of the blood mirrors the perpetual cycle of quest and homecoming as well as the ongoing cycle of life and death.

Of course, the homecoming motif in narrative is as old as the *Odyssey*, but Harvey's narrative—positioned between *Don Quixote* and the first English novels—gives new impetus to the motif. The life-plot of nearly all the major protagonists in English fiction from 1688 through 1750 repeats in its own way this basic "homecoming" paradigm, first seen in the two parts of *Don Quixote*. To give just a few examples: Aphra Behn's Oroonoko, at the end of his narrative, goes completely back to the primeval world of his origins when he renounces the slave name "Caesar" and reclaims his original African-American self epitomized in the name "Oroonoko." Defoe's Moll Flanders achieves a new self, a regenerated version of the innocent child (linked with the "grand Secret" of preserving her "True Name") after her experience in Newgate prison and her return to her mother's home in the new world of Virginia. Richardson's Pamela finally comes "home" to her parents when she can incorporate them into her new aristocratic world, but at enormous cost to her own autonomy as a free, self-directed person. After her prolonged and anguished spiritual quest, Clarissa comes back triumphantly to her "father's house" in her own hieroglyphic coffin-house. In the comic narrative tradition, Fielding's Abraham Adams returns home in a different kind of triumph of integrity, and Tom Jones's erratic everyman journey between country and town ends with his return to the Allworthy estate in which and from which he issued as the bastard and rejected son. *Tristram Shandy*'s conclusion, the story of the affair of Uncle Toby and the Widow Wadman, is a return to a subject the entire narrative keeps promising and enacting, the tragicomic incompatibility of the sexes in the Shandy world. Frances Burney's Evelina comes "home" to her real father, Sir John Belmont, when he recognizes her as his true heir. Variegated rhetorics, rooted in moment-to-moment experience, of the "life blood," "animal spirits," the complex figurative workings of the "heart," play prominently in all of these narratives. They each demonstrate a new and rich anatomy and language of the heart first explored in English, and literally described, in Harvey's little book.

3

The Heart of Eve
Satan and Eve in *Paradise Lost*

> That was not first which is spiritual, but that which is
> natural; and afterward that which is spiritual.
> —1 COR. 15.46

> Then cometh the devil, and taketh away the word out of
> their hearts.
> —LUKE 8.12

> He was a murderer from the beginning.
> —JOHN 8.44

> My heart a thousand ways he strove to win,
> Before it let the Charming Conqueror in.
> —APHRA BEHN, "Selinda and Cloris"

MY PURPOSE IN this chapter is to describe—in terms of the narrative and rhetoric of the heart—one of the chief actions in Milton's *Paradise Lost*: Satan's assault upon Eve.[1] The temptation or seduction of Eve (both terms are equally relevant) is not confined to the famous scene by the Tree of the Knowledge of Good and Evil in book 9 but takes place in a series of stages, beginning with Satan's intent visual apprehension of Eve's physical person, and his intent aural apprehension of Adam and Eve's first conversation. The whole process of Satan's relationship with Eve might be seen as an "anatomy," a dissection, a protracted rape, moving from the assault of his gaze to the violation, successively, of her "head" (in the dream he fashions for her [4.826]), of her "hand" (i.e., her handiwork or artistry after stalking her to her "Nursery" [8.46]), and finally of her "heart" (9.550, 733–34). Thus she is attacked three times by Satan in the poem, whereas Adam never even sees his opponent. She is the one exposed; Satan acts upon *her* body. She is the person most *acted upon* (or sinned against) in the poem, the figure most representative of the seventeenth-century sense of vulnerability to the external forces of life depicted in the Introduction. Milton's radical reimagining of the Fall underscores Satan's sin against Eve—not Eve's sin—as the primal crime. I am assuming in this discussion that Milton, though not a practitioner, was familiar with the new science of anatomy; he would have studied Galen at Cambridge, and probably such English anatomists as Crooke then or later; it is more likely that the anatomical knowledge he had was gained from books, but it is also just possible that he witnessed human anatomical dissection in Italy (during his Italian journey of 1638–39) or in England, and in that medical setting saw the inner constitution of a body literally tied and manacled together joint, limb, and ligament.[2]

As a corollary to my chief concern with the narrative of the heart in *Paradise Lost*, I hope to show that several key passages in Satan's assault upon Eden and upon Eve take on new meaning when examined in the context of early modern anatomical discourse. The anatomist invades the body, penetrates it, opens it, lays it bare, divides it up, inserts things into it, ties up vessels, inflates vessels and organs, performs experiments, draws pictures of the parts of the body, labels these parts in writing, and gives lectures to others about his work. By performing a kind of anatomical, oratorical, and inscriptive experiment on Eve—on her head, on her handiwork, on her heart—Satan functions as a perverse, demonic seventeenth-century anatomist. Though prevented from performing physical violence upon Eve, he invades her body and manipulates her mind and fancy in hopes of making her do what he wishes her to do.

Milton's God (like the Lord God of the Old Testament) also performs an anatomical experiment on Adam by surgically opening his chest, removing a rib, and fashioning it into the woman, Eve. Hence Eve is the product of an anatomical procedure, and she in turn is operated upon by Satan, the organic, instrumental adversary and unwitting accomplice of God the Father. In talking about Milton's "God" in this chapter, I assume a fundamentally dramatic nature of the interaction of the Father and the Son in the poem, with the role of the Spirit as a powerful personified presence not directly involved in the conversations of the Father and the Son, and I attempt to distinguish among the acting persons of this gendered Godhead in the commentary as the masculine Father and Son, and the androgynous Spirit.

It has not been customary to speak of Lucretius and Milton—much less Milton and Behn!—in the same breath, or even in the same context, but it seems to me high time we did so. Milton and Behn are both Restoration poets, and Behn, as well as Dryden, must have read Milton with great interest—there are echoes of "Lycidas" all through her poetry, for one thing—and more attention needs to be paid to the influence of Milton on Behn. But first, what of Lucretius's influence on Milton? Milton not only read Lucretius, he *taught* that "egregious" poet in the rigorous educational program Edward Phillips, his nephew, outlines in his famous early biography of Milton, and Milton himself mentions Lucretius as "one of those poets which are now counted most hard" who will become pleasant when read in the context of natural philosophy in his tract "Of Education."[3] Milton echoes Lucretius several times in *Paradise Lost* when accounting for the natural evolution of life and civilization.[4] As for Behn, we know that her reading of Lucretius in the translation of Thomas Creech in 1682 affected her strongly because she wrote a poem to Creech about the experience of reading his translation and she became well acquainted with Creech himself, who was a kind of mentor to her and wrote a commendatory poem to her, which we shall look at in the next chapter.

As I noted in the Introduction, book 4 of *De rerum natura* is especially relevant to seventeenth-century poetics because of its account of how we perceive the external world. Recent studies of *Paradise Lost* have encouraged us to read Milton more intensively as a Restoration poet and Milton's Satan more in the context of libertinism and phallic invasive power, but before exploring this theme further, we begin, as in the case of Harvey, with movement. Everything in Milton's Eden is in motion, and everything is *being seen*. Vision and perception as vital activities in the poem (and in life) are always in creative motion, but in *Paradise Lost*, as we shall see, there is a strongly Lucretian sense of individual persons and objects, such as Adam and Eve and their paradisal world itself, radiating powerful images perceived by various subjects within the poem and outside it. The viewers or gazers are first the fallen reader (Milton's idea of that reader and any mortal reader), then the narrator, then the Father, then Satan, the primary gazer in terms of what happens to Eve and Adam, who are gazing at each other. Book 3 opens with the Father bending down "his eye" on his newly created world (3.58), viewing his own works and their own workings—a continuously creative activity. The focus of his attention is

> Our two first Parents . . .
> . . . in the happy Garden plac't,
> Reaping immortal fruits of joy and love,
> Uninterruped joy, unrivall'd love
> In blissful solitude.
> (3.65–69)

The Father's gaze first dwells on Adam and Eve in their continuously joyful lovemaking before his survey turns to Satan coasting just under the wall of heaven.

The narrator, who through his invocation to Light in book 3 has gained access to the realm and mind of God, thus prepares the reader's first sight of Adam and Eve as one of bliss, through the eyes of the Father. Adam's first words will be about the infinite goodness of God, and God's goodness, for Adam and for the narrator, is his free, liberal, potent, generous, ongoing creativity. Goodness is all of these things *in action*. Milton's God, like the Lord of the Old Testament, is essentially a god of activity and process, a generous creator of ongoing fruition, an author, but also a destroyer and a torturer of the disobedient. *Paradise Lost* is the most complex and problematic of all creation myths, and it is an epic of the creative process in all its forms in the divine and human spheres. It is important for us to note at the outset then, as a prelude to our examination of Satan's assault upon Eve's "heart," the narrator's fervent incantation of the Father's and the reader's creative gaze upon Adam and Eve in their innocent lovemaking.

In Lucretius and Milton, perhaps even more than in Harvey or Richardson, there is a profound connection among sexuality, perception, language, and the "heart." What do we know of sex in Milton's epic cosmos before we encounter Adam and Eve? What do we know of the sexual life of Milton's triune God? As in the Authorized Version of the Old Testament, there are a variety of indications of male and female gender in Milton's God and in his cosmos before the begetting of the Son, or the conception of the female Sin in Satan's mind, or the creation of Adam and Eve as male and female in the image of God. Milton's cosmos is gendered. Heaven is a feminized place, and so is Hell (until book 10). Before Heaven was created there was Chaos and "eternal Night," male and female as they are personified in book 2. There Chaos is pictured as an infirm old man who can only be communicated with in the most strained and elliptical syntax. His realm is a world of total disorder, of turbulence in a huge force field of conflicting elements. "The wide womb of uncreated Night" appears to be the true opposite of a patriarchal almighty God. God and Night appear to be co-eternal in Milton's highly idiosyncratic reimagining of the Judeo-Christian myth and of orthodox Protestant Christianity. Adam seems to know that God and Night are involved in an eternal antagonism when he tells Eve that the heavenly bodies shine so that total darkness shall not regain by Night "Her old possession, and extinguish life / In Nature and all things" (4.666–67).

Night, in book 2, does not speak. Night is the uncreated and the unspoken. She is an enormous dark space that awaits silently the warm impulse that will create something out of her cold void, order out of the disorder of Chaos. The sexual life of God is first indicated in the poem by the Spirit that sat "brooding on the vast abyss" of Night, Space, Chaos, and "mad'st it pregnant" (1.21–22). God the Father, through the masculine agency of the Spirit as breath, wind, voice, impregnates the vast abyss and something grows out of it. I take this act of impregnation to be the primal generative act in Milton's cosmos, paradigmatic of all of God's acts of creation, preceding even the Son and Spirit's joint creation of the world, and presumably of the Son's creation of the angels and Heaven itself. In the beginning was the sexual act of the Spirit with the womb of Night, and Milton recreates that act in the opening lines of the poem by wedding the masculine Spirit with the feminine Muse Urania and indirectly imploring that androgynous Spirit to impregnate him so that what is dark may be illumined and he may transmit his vision to humankind.

How does Milton "write" the heart? To begin literally and quantitatively, the word "heart" occurs sixty-two times in *Paradise Lost*. As with the Authorized Version of the Bible, "heart" occurs more often than "spirit" (forty-four occurrences). Of these sixty-two usages, six refer to the heart experience of Satan, seventeen to that of Adam alone, nine to that of Eve alone, eleven to that of both Adam and Eve, eight to that of humankind, and three to that of the Father and the Son (excluding references to "bosom" or "breast"), and one all important reference to that of the narrator in the opening. Most of the allusions to the heart (twenty-eight) appear in the last three books, after the Fall, and allude to the mutual spiritual regeneration of Adam and Eve.

To consider Milton's writing of the heart more figuratively, just as God's speaking and writing is central to the master narrative of the heart in the Bible, so it cannot be stressed enough that *Paradise Lost* is an *oral* epic. But like all oral epics that survive, it had to be written down, and the blind Milton was forced to write it at one remove: someone else—Jeremy Picard, a recalcitrant daughter, another amanuensis—had to record the words spoken by him and repeat them back to him. (The labor, frustration, confusion, and sheer exasperation of this process is beyond our powers of reconstruction.) The narrator of *Paradise Lost* is the opposite and adversary of the original adversary, Satan, and they are both oral artists. Satan too must do his work at one remove: since he cannot use physical violence upon Adam and Eve—cannot even touch them—he must employ an instrument—a predatory animal, a toad, finally a serpent. Milton the poet spent a large part of his creative effort on the poem re-creating and re-imagining the Eve of Genesis, composing her unfolding character, molding her identity as the companion fashioned from Adam's heart region and as the "Mother of Mankind" (1.36). The narrator has the assistance of the Spirit in this creative process, the Spirit who is superior to Scripture and who writes on the heart, like the apostle Paul's "Spirit of the living God" who writes "not in tables of stone, but in fleshy tables of the heart" (2 Cor. 3.3). Paul's thorn in the flesh may have been eye disease (as Milton may have discerned), and he too used an amanuensis; when he did write in his own hand, the letters came out large (Gal. 6.11). Paul told his followers that he did not need letters of commendation from them because *they* were the letters themselves, written in the apostles' hearts and visible for all to see. In a sense, all of Milton's characters in the *Paradise Lost* narrative—but especially Adam and Eve—are his letters written in his heart and manifested for the reader to discern and decipher. Adam and Eve are his "letters of commendation" for what humankind was and may be again. The blind narrator must see to it that his words are inscribed and recorded, that they last, and he can only verify this record by constant oral and memorial repetition. Satan, having gradually been weakened by sin when he finally encounters Eve, is wholly dependent on oral transmission of the venom that must pollute her, that will stain and "deface" her and be passed on to Adam and their posterity. This stain is Satan's inscription on humankind, his final "writing" on Eve's heart. He is an anatomist who cannot touch the body, perverting the physician/anatomist's healing purpose by invading the body to infect it and set it on fire.

In devising his oral epic, Milton deliberately attempts to create an original Edenic unfallen language for his poem, a language akin to the first three chapters of Genesis. This is the culminating epic of origins, and the poet conceives *Paradise Lost* as the original epic, prior to Homer or even the epic narratives of Abraham and David in the Old Testament. Milton sets out to create his version of a sacred language that will release the kind of energy Northrop Frye intuits in the language of ancient poetry:

> I think we can see in most Greek literature before Plato, more especially in Homer, in the pre-Biblical cultures of the Near East, and in much of the Old Testament itself, a conception of language that is poetic and "hieroglyphic," not in the sense of sign-writing, but in the sense of using words as particular kinds of signs. In this period there is relatively little emphasis on a clear separation of subject and object: the emphasis falls rather on the feeling that subject and object are linked by a common power or energy. . . . The articulating of words may bring this common power into being; hence a magic develops in which verbal elements, "spell," and "charm," and the like, play a central role. Words in such a context are words of power or dynamic forces.[5]

To illustrate how Milton creates his own unique magical language of power in *Paradise Lost* we must take a close look at the opening invocation. As the stricken heir of Orpheus (the son of the Muse of epic poetry), the poet entreats and virtually demands, albeit with reverence, the "Heavn'ly Muse" Urania to sing about mankind's first disobedience and the fruit and fatal consequences of the Fall until the actions of the greater man, Jesus Christ, can restore fallen humans to Paradise. The strangely and perhaps self-consciously "wizard-like" anatomist Harvey begins his narrative of the heart with an entry into the twin labyrinths of "Mistress Antiquity" and the human body, trusting and cooperating with a feminized Nature; Milton begins his narrative of the heart with an appeal to the feminine Muse of the Heavens. He first posits the Muse's habitation not in Greece but in the most powerful scriptural site of God's interaction with man, on the top of Mount Horeb *or* of Mount Sinai. He is conjuring the Muse as would an ancient spiritual medium or wizard or seer or sibyl or shaman, male or female or both, when that intermediary attempts to bring hidden divine powers into activity in the human world. The poet is *not* an Old Testament prophet. The divine power is *not* coming to him unannounced and unaided, as is the case in every instance of God's interaction with his prophets in Scripture. He first calls *them*, they do not call him.[6]

As we noted in the first chapter, Milton believed profoundly, with many of his radical religious brethren, that "the spirit which is given to us is a more certain guide than scripture,"[7] but first the Spirit must be invoked. This may be the most difficult undertaking for the poet in *Paradise Lost*: Milton must create a space for the Spirit to manifest itself in. Harvey must locate the spaces and direction of the circulation of the blood; Milton must create a space for the Muse and bring her into it. The Spirit may have chosen Milton, but he must invite the Muse into his and the reader's experience in a fitting manner. The boldness of the invocation, as Alastair Fowler notes, was condemned by some of Milton's contemporaries.[8] In the Bible, only Job (who is not a prophet) has the radical temerity to call upon God to show himself to him. So Milton first invokes the power that came to Moses and inspired him to be a great oral teacher *and then* a writer of God's law. Milton's narrator enunciates the epic equivalent of "before Moses or Abraham were, I am" (compare John 8.58).

Then the voice pauses, as if waiting for a reply. None is forthcoming, and he shifts the scene, moving downward to a less lofty eminence, to Sion hill, Mount Zion in Jerusalem, near Siloa's brook, a site more reminiscent of the paradigmatic Greek locale for poetic/religious inspiration. Rather than remain in the Wilderness with the extreme Otherness of the God of Moses, the poet shifts to the God of David and Solomon and the Temple, the God of the established nation of Israel and its city Jerusalem, the personified woman and mother, an urban scene, a more civilized and human setting. The poet offers the Spirit a choice. If this scene is more acceptable to you, I invoke your aid from that place for a poetic song that intends to soar above Helicon, the home of the nine Muses, a song that is above any poetic utterance of the classical world. Still there is no answer.

The poet then moves away from the city and focuses his attention on the inward Spirit given to all human beings, the Holy Spirit who prefers "th' upright heart and pure" (1.18) before all man-made expressions of worship or devotion. Milton weds the "perfect and upright" person of Job (1.1) with "Blessed are the pure in heart: for they shall see God" (Matt. 5.8) to enable his narrator's access to the divine world. Hence there is strong biblical authority for a direct link between the pure heart and a true imagining of the world of God. The three-part climactic movement to the human heart in the Invocation we have just reviewed precedes the Satanic movement toward Eve's heart in Paradise. The Spirit was present from the first and is thus identified also with the Sister of Wisdom or Sophia in Proverbs 8 (the "Sister" who is also invoked at *Paradise Lost* 7.10), the feminine spirit who played in the Almighty Father's presence and who knows everything, the mighty spirit who like a dove brooded over the vast abyss and made it pregnant in the first act of creating the world. The image of the dove, recalling the female dove that informed Noah of the new world and the one that announced the greater man who would save mankind, is Milton's magical symbol for an androgynous spirit whom he indirectly invites to come and impregnate him with the power to tell and spell his vision.[9] As in folktale, the third appeal is the effectual one. The poet asks this Spirit to name the cause that moved our great parents to transgress—"Who first seduc'd them to that foul revolt?" (1.33). Who first led them astray— "seduced," not "tempted"—into illicit sexual intercourse and knowledge? He knows the answer, but the Spirit itself must respond. The poet pauses again, and this time a new voice enters the poem, the voice of the androgynous Spirit. It is this voice, speaking through the poet as if through a medium or actor, that marks the narrative beginning of *Paradise Lost*. How to re-create this voice is a supreme challenge to the reader of the poem, but it must be spoken, it must be uttered, it must be performed, or the poem is not really being "read."

Milton in the opening of *Paradise Lost* reimagines the Spirit he refused to speculate about in detail in the *Christian Doctrine*, a Spirit who combines the feminine inspiring and nurturing characteristics of the Greek Muses and the sister of scriptural Wisdom with the masculine impregnating power of the Son/Logos/Word. Nearly every abstraction in ancient thought goes back eventually to the body, and the body of Milton's God has male and female elements, no matter how many permutations of gender, sexuality, and the varieties of eroticism it goes through in the poem.[10] The creative power of Milton's God thus grows directly out of Gen. 1.27 and the *imago dei*: "So God created man in his own image, in the image of God created he him; male and female created he them." This image of divine sexual union/generation in Genesis leads at once to the binary commandment, "be fruitful and multiply/have dominion over." Human beings replicate the Creator in their nature and function, as sexual and verbal creators and rulers. Hence the *imago dei* in Genesis and for Milton is generative, both sexually and linguistically, and seems to be inherent in Milton's notion of "right reason" as the divinely implanted ability to distinguish right from wrong, to guide and rule oneself, and to respond to God with loving obedience.

An even more difficult question associated with the nature of the sexual life of Milton's God is the meaning of God's "bosom," referred to four times in the poem. Most of the uses of bosom in the Bible evoke maternal and sexual intimacy, and in *Paradise Lost* there are allusions to the bosoms of the great feminine personifications, Night (2.1036) and the Earth (7.319). But the bosom of the Father is a *paternal* source of creation.

Exploring another version of the biblical link between the heart and the eye by building on John 1.18, "No man hath seen God at any time; the only begotten Son, which is in the bosom of the Father, he hath declared him," Milton reiterates that the Son's "blissful" home or dwelling place is in the Father's bosom. The bosom of the Father is thus a dwelling place of bliss and glory. For Milton as for the early seventeenth-century Anglican divine Lancelot Andrewes, the Father's bosom is the eternal heart source of the divine paternal begetting of the Son. Put more simply, the Father's heart is the genital organ of the Son. Andrewes makes the divine/human nature of the Son clear by stressing that Christ was "made" from the womb of his mortal mother in the world whereas he was begotten by the Father from eternity. To be "made" as a creature, a product, is inferior to being begotten. Man is a fiction, "*Factum ex muliere*": "He [Christ] passed not *through Her, as water through a Conduit Pipe*, (as fondly dreameth the Anabaptist).... She ministered the matter, *Flesh of her flesh.*" Andrewes invokes the Greek physiology of female and male seed generating offspring: Christ as man was formed of "*Semen mulieris,* The seed; and, *Semen intimum substantiae*, that is, the principall and very inward cheefe part of the *substance*. Made of that, made of her very *substance*." In contrast to the mortal "making" process, the Son was begotten "from the *bosome of His Father*, before all worlds."[11] Andrewes then goes on to make a textual/oral distinction in this creative process in an explicit allusion to the heart of God: the "generation eternall" of Christ as "*Verbum Dei* . . . is, as the enditing of the *Word*, within the *heart*. His generation in time (*Verbum Caro*) is as the *uttering* it forth with the *voice*."[12] The bosom or heart of God precedes and produces the voice of God that creates the world. Thus God's bosom, for Andrewes and for Milton, is a male/paternal creative power (sexual and verbal) analogous to the royal phallic heart cherishing the feminine body in Harvey's *The Motion of the Heart*. The bosom of the Father might be referred to as the heart of Heaven, inhabited only by the Son.

Beginning then with this bosom intimacy of the Son with the Father, we note that there is a special emphasis on the "heart" region in all the important persons and locales in the cosmos of *Paradise Lost*. At the center of the bottom of Hell are "four infernal Rivers that disgorge / Into the burning Lake their baleful streams" (2.575–76), each river associated with one of the dark passions, hate, sorrow, lamentation, and rage. As we saw in the Introduction, the heart was thought to have four major vessels attached to it and to be the seat of the passions. Beelzebub has an initial sense of miserable subjection when he wonders what business God the victor has in store for them, "Here in the heart of Hell to work in Fire, / Or do his Errands in the gloomy Deep" (1.151–52). Following Gen. 2.10–14, Milton records four corresponding rivers issuing from Paradise mountain, the heart of Eden (4.223–33).

Eve's fondest memory in her account of her first day of life is Adam calling her to return to him: "to give thee being I lent / Out of my side to thee, nearest my heart / Substantial Life, to have thee by my side" (4.483–85). One of Milton's great innovations in his representation of Eve is that until Adam's misogynistic outburst at her after the Fall, she is repeatedly linked with Adam's side and heart, not his crooked rib. They make love "side by side" (4.741), heart by heart. She sees herself as the heart person—the one formed from Adam's heart. Though now a separate being, her image resides still in his bosom. God's ultimate gift to Adam is not the "equal" Adam seems to ask for but, in God's words, "thy fit help, thy other self, / Thy wish, exactly to thy heart's desire" (8.450–51). We noted how the God of the Old Testament took special interest in the womb and heart experience of woman. Similarly in *Paradise Lost*, more attention is paid to Eve's heart than to Adam's before the Fall, and afterward Milton focuses attention on the painful process of contrition of heart in both of them leading to the history of Adam's grieved and then joyful responses to the drama of his posterity, a history recorded in terms of his heart responses. Although angels do not have particularized internal organs ("All Heart they live, all Head, all Eye, all Ear, / All Intellect, all Sense" [6.350–51]), Satan has a heart that, when he surveys the "horrid front" of his reassembled battalion, "Distends with pride, and hard'ning in his strength / Glories" (1.572–73). We noted in the previous chapter that Harvey, in his effort to describe the motion of the heartbeat, delineated a complicated and deceptive systole/diastole, contracting/dilating rhythm. Milton, in his effort to describe the motion of the heart in Satan and Eve delineates a dialectic of heart-hardening in Satan (based on the scriptural motif of the hardened heart in Exodus and elsewhere) and of heart-softening in Eve, a pattern we shall note as their relationship unfolds.[13]

The Heart of Hell

At the end of book 3, after outwitting Uriel, the greatest of all God's watchful angels and "the sharpest-sighted Spirit of all in Heav'n" (3.691),

Satan lands upon Mount Niphates. Satan's attempt to seduce mankind is presented as something rolling, boiling, coming to birth out of his "tumultuous breast," and is compared to a "devilish Engine" (4.16–17), which, as in the Hobbesian dynamic of force impinging on the heart to create a "counterpressure," recoils back on itself. Satan had already invented cannonry in the War in Heaven, and that invention here becomes internally transformed into the phallic engine of his "dire attempt" on God's favored "new Race called *Man*" (2.348), whom he wishes, in the words of Beelzebub, to "seduce" to the demonic party.

This image of the devilish engine recalls the discussion of the phallic heart and the heat of the testicles in the previous chapter, and has its counterpart in the only mechanical simile Harvey employs in *The Motion of the Heart*. Harvey compares the "continued motion" of the "ears" (auricles) and ventricles of the heart to the apparently instantaneous action of "Engines, one wheel moving another," or as "in the lock of a piece [firearm], by the drawing of the spring, the flint falls, strikes the steel, fires the powder, enters the touch-hole, discharges, the balls fly out, pierces the mark, and all these motions, by reason of the swiftness of them, appear in the twinkling of an eye."[14] It is at this point as well that the rhetoric of the hot heart in Greek physiology as discussed in the Introduction is most relevant to *Paradise Lost*. The anatomist Helkiah Crooke (following Galen) stresses that the heart must be an extremely strong organ to contain the extraordinary heat of the vital spirit, a heat which he depicts in language (again going back to Plato's *Timaeus*) usually reserved for descriptions of the unruly phallus: "The vitall part is very hot, impetuous, raging, and in continuall motion. . . . The animall faculty required another temper in her organ [i.e., the brain], otherwise the motions would have been furious, the senses giddy and rash; Reason would continually haue erred, because the property of heate, is to confound and make a medley of all things."[15] The property of male heat, when generated in excess—as in Satan's turbulent breast—is ultimately destructive. In Harvey's anatomical version of the circulation of the blood, the phallic heart, even though its action is likened to that of a firearm, cherishes the femininized body. But the hot phallic heart had a much more immediate vitality and presence for at least some of Milton's readers, the "sons of Belial" whose phallicism as well as skeptical libertinism Milton incorporates into his all-intrusive Satan. Only a few years after the appearance of the second edition of *Paradise Lost*, John Wilmot, the second earl of Rochester, addressed these words to his unperforming penis, again in the context of Lucretius's erotics of sexual injury:

> This *Dart* of love, whose piercing point oft try'd,
> With *Virgin blood*, *Ten thousand Maids* has dy'd;
> Which *Nature* still directed with such *Art*,
> That it through ev'ry *Cunt* reacht every *Heart*.
> Stiffly resolv'd, twou'd carelessly invade,
> *Woman* or *Man*, nor ought its fury staid,
> Where e're it pierc'd, a *Cunt* it found or made
> . . . .
> Like a Rude roaring *Hector*, in the *Streets*,
> That Scuffles, Cuffs, and Ruffles all he meets,
> But if his *King*, or *Country*, claim his Aid,
> The *Rakehell Villain*, shrinks, and hides his head[16]

Satan is a much grander conception of the rakehell than any Restoration dramatist or libertine poet could construct, but I suggest that Satan's relations with Hell, Sin, and Eve must be viewed in the context of Rochester's rampant libertine phallicism as well as in the traditional theological contexts.

Some readers of Milton may take too insubstantial a view of Satan's body. It is described as an ethereal body, but it is still a *body* of enormous physical power until he is gradually enfeebled by Sin and Hell (9.486–88). The phallic, hostile, violent force of Satan is stressed from the beginning, in intellect and in body: his "fixt mind / And high disdain" (1.97), his "heart" distending with pride as he glories in his strength (1.571–72), his "shape and gesture proudly eminent" over the rest, standing "like a Tow'r" (1.590–91), his joyful impregnation of Sin (2.765–66), his bold exploration of Chaos, his fierce penetration of the "world" when he threw "Down right into the World's first Region . . . His flight precipitant" (3.562–63) and "Down from th' Ecliptic, sped with hop'd success . . . his steep flight in many an Aery wheel" (3.740–41). The hard heart of domineering strength in warlike pride and glory, seen in Satan and in his human counterpart Nimrod (the one who rises up "Of proud ambitious heart" [12.25]), is also the phallic heart of the compulsive rapist, fixed in destructive rage, which culminates in the erectile posture of Satan as predatory serpent. As the programmatic climax to the War in Heaven,

Satan was thrust by the victorious Son into the burning maw of a feminized Hell:

> Hell heard th'unsufferable noise, Hell saw
> Heav'n ruining from Heav'n, and would have fled
> Affrighted; but strict Fate had cast too deep
> Her dark foundations, and too fast had bound.
> . . . .
> ... Hell at last
> Yawning receiv'd them whole, and on them clos'd,
> Hell thir fit habitation fraught with fire
> Unquenchable, the house of woe and pain.
> (6.867–77)

Drawing upon the conventional anatomical image of the Galenic fiery heart, shaped like a cone, Milton creates his version of the phallic Satanic heart and at the same time reinvents and transforms his portrait of Hell, first described as "A Universe of death, which God by curse / Created evil" [2.622–23]), into a fiery house of woe and pain. As we noted in the Introduction, the central function of the Galenic heart is powerful *attraction* or suction. If Crooke (as we just noted) can make the vital heat of the heart sound like the activity of a raging phallus, Milton can elaborate his Hell, a powerful feminine construct in itself, into a gigantic, distorted variant of the classical Greek heart, with the addition of another Galenic characteristic of the heart we have so far left unexplored: irascibility. Anger, along with affection, is a driving force in the autonomous motion of the Galenic heart. To feel something deeply in the heart could partake of the sincerity of rage as well as love. Thus the male Satan and the female Hell are indissolubly united under the aspect of the Galenic heart.[17] Hell first swallows him up in her ferocious attractive heat, and he eventually internalizes Hell in a mock wedding vow:

>   hail
> Infernal world, and thou profoundest Hell
> Receive thy new Possessor: One who brings
> A mind not to be chang'd by Place or Time
> (1.250–53)

Hell becomes a death force internalized in Satan as, "inflam'd with rage," he stands now in the midst of a tumult of doubt and horror while his thoughts "stir" from the bottom this burning "Hell within him," which has now indeed become his heart partner, the true mate for his "dire attempt" (4.9–20). Hidden in the word "attempt" is the stark sense (even in present-day usage) of an attack on a person's life. The interaction of the attempt and of Hell will from this point continue to generate his assault upon the human pair.

Paradise

We do not see everything in Eden through Satan's eyes—we see through the narrator's eyes after our initial sharing of the view of Adam and Eve from the Father's eye. But before we see Adam and Eve again, the narrator confidently establishes the geography of Eden for us, and Satan moves over this new land as its first male invader and explorer. As Satan slowly swoops over this beautiful landscape toward Paradise, he meets purer and purer air, and the language invites us to think both his "heart" and the human heart of the reader are inspired with "Vernal delight and joy, able to drive / All sadness but despair," not simply Satan's despair (4.155–56). The following nineteen lines are devoted to the odors of Eden, in stark contrast to the sulfurous smells associated with the fiend. Fowler rightly points out the obvious: "*Paradise* is the garden situated within the land of Eden" (4.132 n) and, as many other readers have noted (following C. S. Lewis in *A Preface to Paradise Lost*), there are allusions to the sexual body in this passage (e.g., the mountain suggests the mount of Venus). But what is less obvious is that Satan's exploratory gaze is an epic parallel of the anatomist's investigation of the female body by means of a moving metal probe.

To see how this works, we must first look more closely at the Garden. The land of Eden is Milton's representation of an unfallen, feminine, maternal Nature, a multisensual version of the scriptural land flowing with milk and honey. Paradise crowns the head of a steep mountain:

> So on he fares, and to the border comes
> Of *Eden*, where delicious Paradise,
> Now nearer, Crowns with her enclosure green,
> As with a rural mound the champaign head
> Of a steep wilderness, whose hairy sides
> With thicket overgrown, grotesque and wild,
> Access deni'd
> (4.131–37)

As Satan continues his exploration, he is likened to predators, "a prowling Wolf" (4.183) and "a Thief" (4.188). Once in the midst of the Garden, near its fountain created "through veins / Of porous Earth with kindly thirst up-drawn" (4.227–28), he surveys the scene from its highest vantage point, the "Tree of Life" (4.194), and sees

> Groves whose rich Trees wept odorous Gums and Balm,
> Others whose fruit burnisht with Golden Rind
> Hung amiable....
> . . . .
> Betwixt them Lawns, or level Downs, and Flocks
> Grazing the tender herb, were interpos'd,
> Or palmy hillock, or the flow'ry lap
> Of some irriguous Valley spread her store,
> Flow'rs of all hue, and without Thorn the Rose.
> (4.248–56)

In his description of the female genitals, the anatomist Crooke gives this description of the vulva: "the rugous or plighted chinke or rifte . . . is placed as it were in the trench of the great Cleft, and like a narrow valley leadeth the way by a round cauitie into the inward parts" (236). He goes on to note that Galen calls the "womb . . . *pudendum muliebre*, the womans modesty," by others called "*Vulua*, as it were *vallis* a valley, or *Valua* a Flood-gate . . . We will call it the lappe" (237). The vulva is represented by a figure with two heart-shaped openings opposed to each other at the top (220, fig. 4). There follows a description of the nymphae: "These *Nymphae*, beside the great pleasure women haue by them in coition . . . have their name of Nymphes, because they ioyne vnto the passage of the urine, and the necke of the wombe; out of which, as out of fountaines (and the *Nymphes* are said to bee presedents or dieties of the fountaines) water and humours doe issue: and beside, because in them are the veneriall delicacies, for the Poets say that the Nymphes lasciuiously seeke out the Satyres among the woods and forrests" (237–38). The word "nymph" is used four times in *Paradise Lost*, and always in reference to Eve at a critical moment in the unfolding depiction of her sexuality and independence: in the first reference to the bower where she and Adam retire to make love (4.707), when Eve ministers naked to Raphael and Adam (5.381), when Eve takes leave of Adam to test her virtue (9.386), and just before her beauty renders Satan "stupidly good" (9.452).

Crooke says, "the extuberations . . . are called hillocks or mountainets (*Vesalius* calleth these extuberations *alae* or wings, the other *labia* or lippes) and the mount of *Venus*: these in mature or ripe women are adorned with haire, the bush of which is called *pubes*. . . . These hayres are in women more curled then in Virgins, and do reach as a covering vnto the lippes; the lippes were made for the ornament and for defence that the womb might be kept from refrigeration" (239). The female genitals are described in considerable geographical and mythological detail in the anatomies, but most important with regard to Satan's exploratory overview of Paradise is the steady, unhurried progression of the male anatomist's metal "probe" as he opens the secrets of the female body. Crooke continues: "in the demonstration of the wombe we will begin at the externall parts, wee must proceede by the guide of a vterine probe, and then the parts will thus arise. First the region of the share-bones, then the bush, the hillocks whereon the hayre growes, the two lips, the great outward fissure betweene the lippes . . . the two smaller clefts or fissures between the Nymphes, the two Nymphes themselues . . . the *Tentigo* or head or nutte of the *Clitoris* couered by the Nymphes as by a foreskin . . . all these may be seene without incision, the rest must be found by incision. And thus much of the parts of generation belonging to women" (239). The Miltonic terms "fountain," "delicious," "rural mound," "head," "hairy," "thicket," "hillock," "valley," and "lap" all have their counterparts in Crooke's anatomical discourse. Even the word "irriguous" has a strange similarity to "rugous" (ridged), and the reference to the thornless rose recalls the rose as sexual metaphor, to be discussed more fully later. Milton's language for Paradise makes the astonishing juxtaposition of a world of perfect vitality, sensuousness, and creativity observed by a figure from the "Universe of death," perched in the form of a greedy cormorant upon the "Tree of Life," whose moving gaze is implicitly analogous to the anatomist's probing of a female corpse. One recalls the slightly vertiginous spectator at the top of the Paduan anatomical theater.[18]

But the image of Paradise, though predominantly feminine, is both male and female interconnected, a geographical version of the *imago dei*. We see a feminine enclosure on top of a mountain, or mesa, under which a river flows, part of which is diverted upward into the fountain that waters the whole garden, then unites and forms a waterfall meeting the river, which issues out of a cavern at the base of the mountain, then divides into the four main rivers of Eden. The pulsating human heart and its four vessels is the deep underlying image of Milton's Paradise. Paradise mountain is God's special creation for humankind, a place whose own contours prefigure and enclose the dynamic of sexual and creative "delightful use" that is unfallen Adam and Eve's chief reason for being. We recall Harvey's similarly complex interweaving of heart, blood, and the feminized outer parts of the body working together in loving domestic harmony. Paradise mountain is a figure of the male and female human body interfused, with head and hair (and their sexual implications), fountain (a metonymy of male orgasm and of the heart), rivers, rills, and veins (the blood flowing or perhaps even circulating).[19] Hence, in the exceedingly rich prelude to the introduction of Adam and Eve in person in book 4, Milton features the sexually creative nature of the Paradise garden/mountain cradled within the largely feminine and maternal context of the land of Eden, the living feminine land created by God before he created Adam and Eve. Eden was rendered in English "delight," one of Milton's favorite words for the goodness and joy of human life, and it is mutual male and female delight.

The long passage (4.235–88) leading up to the entrance of Adam and Eve becomes ever more replete with the presence of a feminine Nature, with images of pagan goddesses, with proleptic suggestions of the unfallen and fallen Eve. The garden Paradise is a complicated text or *textus* (fabric) where mythic figures are interwoven with plants and animals. Nature's fertility is linked with an innate self-mirroring artistry as both activities are foregrounded together. Nature's "flowery lap"—with the specifically sexual meaning of "lap"—is a sexually receptive place; she spreads her store; the vine lays forth her grape; the lake holds up to a green bank her crystal mirror, and thus holds the bank in it. Here Milton's Nature is an innocent version of Shakespeare's "great creating Nature"; she is generous, abundant, receiving, flourishing, self-generating, and self-reflective. She has her attendants, like God. The birds supply her angel choir. In this respect, Nature prefigures Eve in Adam's confession to Raphael in book 8, Adam's book: Eve will become for him a goddess, a rival to God with her own angelic guard, her own grace, in the heaven of her own beautiful presence and the work of her hands.

The language of the Fall in book 9 seems to be built into the language of the garden and prefigured here, resulting in an interplay, in the reader's mind, of unfallen and fallen language. Though Milton himself is deprived of the visual reading experience, he expects his fit reader to have read the poem many times, to make connections, to remember how one part relates to another, to take the poignance of this interchange to heart. The crisped (curly) brooks rolling on sands of gold presage in their "mazy error" Eve's golden tresses, and we think of Eve when in this passage we see words like wept, vine, mirror, nice art, wanton, and coy. There is a sense all through the garden world of male and female interplay and intertwining, a sense of sexual pantheism, of polymorphous eroticism. The narrator sees the universal Pan himself, the primal Greek god of forests (and wood nymphs), of the wild, of fertility, a god who loves lechery and music, "knit" in dance with the Hours, the Graces, one of whom was the Mirth of "L'Allegro." The sorrowing Ceres (Demeter) searches for her beautiful daughter Proserpina (the virgin Persephone), the fair flower gathered by gloomy Dis (Pluto), recalling Eve as the fair flower unpropped by Adam (9.433).[20] This complicated prelude emphasizes timeless parental and filial sorrow—unhappy mother, subjugated daughter, anxious father, cursed son—encompassed within an overarching sense of the upsurge of the bountiful Earth, Nature, and maternal goddesses. We recall that Eve's first response after eating the fruit in book 9 is a maternal, nurturing one.

At this moment Adam and Eve first walk into the gaze of the "Fiend" (meaning "the one hating"), who sums up the whole "seeing" motif to this point in the poem when "To all delight of human sense expos'd" (4.206), he sees "undelighted all delight" (4.286), he who embodies the absolute opposite of Eden. In the first description of Adam and Eve, both together are given eight lines, then Adam is given six, and Eve nine. Both reflect their maker's image, both radiate truth, wisdom, sanctitude, true freedom, true authority (all of which virtues I take to refer to both of them). In what follows, I shall be talking about Adam and Eve as characters in an unfolding drama. Milton originally conceived the literary project of "Adam unparadiz'd" as a drama, and a great part of the poem's enduring power is its dramatic, dialogic interaction between Adam and Eve, between Adam and Raphael, between Gabriel and Satan, between Satan and Eve, even between the more static Father and Son. The poem was meant to be read aloud, enacted with the voice, or a group of voices.

As well as presenting his uniquely imagined versions of Adam and Eve as dramatic, lifelike characters in the drama of the Fall, there is little doubt that Milton also was consciously re-creating the human pair as new epic models of the Galenic soul, with Adam embodying an ambivalent version of the rational soul, allied with the "animal spirits" of the brain and nerves, and Eve embodying a complex version of the "Corporeal" or "Sensitive

Soul," allied with the vital spirits formed in the heart. I say ambivalent and complex because Adam, as we shall see, occasionally has more "heat" in his rational faculty than was considered desirable, and Eve has more "cool" in her vital heart.[21]

One of the fullest and most interesting accounts of the rational and corporeal souls in humankind is found in the work of another of Milton's contemporaries, the physician and anatomist Thomas Willis (1621–75), whose work represents seventeenth-century medical epistemology in its purest form. Willis's description of the work of the intellect is a good introduction to the mind of unfallen Adam: "But indeed, the Intellect presiding o'er the Imagination, beholds all the Species deposited in it self . . . formes universal things from singulars . . . so it speculates or Considers both the nature of every substance, and abstracted from the Individuals of Accident, viz: Humanity, Ratiotinality, Temperance, Fortitude, Corporeity, Spirituallity, Whiteness, and the like; besides, being carried higher, it Contemplates God, Angels, it self, Infinity, Eternity, and many other notions, far remote from Sense and Imagination."[22] But it is Willis's account of the twofold nature of the feminized Corporeal Soul, particularly as it relates to the activity of the "Praecordia" (the parts around the heart that separate it from the other internal organs), that I find especially relevant to Milton's Eve. Eve as a character has a more varied emotional response to her experience than does Adam, before and after the Fall. Under the influence of Satan she undergoes a pattern of exaltation and depression, before the Fall in the dream he gives her, and after the Fall in her falsely heightened consciousness and her mortification and despair. Later, away from the influence of Satan, she undergoes humiliation and a kind of regeneration, presented in terms of her experience of the heart. Willis sees the Corporeal Soul existing in one of two states, "tranquillity," which would correspond to Eve's experience in Eden before Satan gives her the dream, and "disturbance," corresponding to her experience after the dream. The "disturbed state" (following Galenic theory regarding irregular palpitation of the heart) is analogous to the systolic/diastolic motion of the heart because, according to Willis, it consists of either a dilation or a contraction. His description of this rhythm is an apt introduction to the heart experience of Eve as it will unfold under Satan's influence:

First, Sometimes this Soul, as it were leaping forth, erects and stretches out it self beyond measure, and so dilating . . . desires to reach it self beyond the bound of the Body . . . and as [the animal spirits] so shake the *Praecordia*, by a more full inflowing, they Compel the Blood therefore to be snatched together, and to be poured forth more freely into all the Parts. Secondly, Sometimes on the contrary, this Soul being struck, is more narrowly Compressed within it self . . . the *Praecordia* also being destitute of their due influx of Spirits, almost sink down, and suffer the Blood to stay too long there, and to stagnate oftentimes . . . either she stretches forth her self into a greater Compass, by profuse Pleasure, as if it affected to be dilated beyond the bounds of the Body: or being overthrown by Sorrow or Grief, she is contracted more narrowly . . . from this twofold Affection of the Sensitive Soul, all the other Passions take their Origine.[23]

We shall see another version of Eve and her relation to the Corporeal Soul at the conclusion of this chapter.

Returning now to Satan's and the reader's first view of Adam and Eve, one notes that they are "godlike," lords, not children, but innocent, primal, pristine. Even from this first description, we can discern the lineaments of Eve's Christian heroism, a developing moral faculty that emerges after the Fall superior even to Adam's. She is formed for "softness" (that is, compassion, mildness, tenderness, nurture, and self-givingness), an important word in the poem and one often misconstrued, and "grace," her human equivalent of the primary attribute of divine mercy. The ambivalence of her fate is signaled in the words "wanton" and "vine," applied to her hair. Her fall will come about in part because she is "wanton," heedless, unrestrained, unseeing, the victim of a figurative blindness that contrasts with (and parallels) the narrator's blindness leading to insight. Her veil of hair curls like the "vine," implying "subjection," evoking associations with "the fruitful wife" of Psalm 128, the "degenerate" vine of the harlot Jerusalem of Jer. 2.21, and Christ ("I am the vine, ye are the branches" [John 15.5]) who, as the Suffering Servant washing his disciples' feet, conveys the central heroic image—celebrated again and again in early Christian art—of patient martyrdom that the poem glorifies in the union of Man and God, an ideal that emerges quietly and gradually in the last six books.

Milton himself seems to have embraced the Christian ethic of patient fortitude in a profoundly active and vital way after the sudden succession of personal calamities in 1652. He became totally blind in February, suffered the loss of his wife Mary, who on May 5 died giving birth to Deborah, then the death of his only son John on June 16, and in August the most vicious personal attack on him yet to appear, the publication of *Regii Sanguinis Clamor*. Milton was left a blind widower with three daughters under the age of six, rooted even more humiliatingly in the mundane actual by an ongoing lawsuit with his mother-in-law. It was about this time that he seems to have begun the active planning and writing of his epic poem.

Satan's Gaze

The first physical description of Eve in book 4 moves immediately from her subjection to Adam to "those mysterious parts" (4.312) of the body consecrated to the sacred *mysteron*, or rite, of sexual delight and generation. Milton modifies for his own purposes the conventional blazon, or external top to toe description of the heroine in romance. The sweet, reluctant, amorously delayed movement of the descriptive language depicts both Adam and Eve, from head to hair to shoulders to waist, from male to female (echoing the movement of creation in Genesis 2), culminating with the mysterious parts and with Satan and the reader's perception of "the loveliest pair / That ever since in love's embraces met" (4.321–22), Adam the goodliest of men and Eve the fairest of her daughters. Repeatedly, the text insists upon the movement to the sacred sexual act, most memorably in the fact that Adam and Eve move directly to sexual consummation in the Bower after their creation, an act quintessentially debased in their mutually exploitative sex after the Fall. Adam and Eve in book 4, which is the book of Eve and Nature, are in love, mutually filling and fulfilling the world of the other, as all of Eden is in love with its own productions. A beautiful erotic sheen of loving interplay emanates from everything in the garden. All is sensualized, all is "sense." The narrator, the reader, Satan, and God all see them making love. They are always in the gaze, visualized, in motion, "passing on," like Dürer's vibrant and youthful Adam and Eve, reflecting the image of God. After their enjoyable toil they sit down by a fountain side and fall to their "Nectarine Fruits which the compliant boughs / Yielded them" (4.332–33), as round about all the animals play in concord, as if entertaining them.

And there is Satan looking on. Again, in order to establish more fully the context for Satan's assault upon Eve, we must reflect for a moment on the sexual life of Satan and further on the nature of sex in *Paradise Lost*. We learn from the narrator at 1.423 that "Spirits," which I take to be both unfallen and fallen angels, make love, and they can assume either sex or both in their lovemaking:

> For Spirits when they please
> Can either Sex assume, or both; so soft
> And uncompounded is their Essence pure,
> Not ti'd or manacl'd with joint or limb,
> Nor founded on the brittle strength of bones,
> Like cumbrous flesh; but in what shape they choose
> Dilated or condens'd, bright or obscure,
> Can execute their aery purposes,
> And works of love or enmity fulfill.
> (1.423–31)

Milton, like his older contemporary Harvey, had a keen sense of human anatomy and the material frailty, clumsiness, and vulnerability of the body. He seems at the same time to have been particularly aware of the beauty and vulnerability of his own well-proportioned body, which he took good care of in a long life.[24] We need to remind ourselves not only of Milton's interest in the human body and human anatomy but also that ordinary life in the seventeenth century afforded many more glimpses of all manner of torn, mutilated, and diseased bodies. The amiable angel Raphael, in his explanation to Adam of lovemaking in Heaven, elaborates further on the freedom of angelic sexual union:

> Whatever pure thou in the body enjoy'st
> (And pure thou wert created) we enjoy
> In eminence, and obstacle find none
> Of membrane, joint, or limb, exclusive bars:
> Easier than Air with Air, if Spirits embrace,
> Total they mix, union of pure with pure
> Desiring; nor restrain'd conveyance need
> As Flesh to mix with Flesh, or Soul with Soul.
> (8.622–29)

The emphasis is on a kind of totally pure interpenetration, as if pure desire were uniting with pure desire in a continuous ethereal orgasm. One cannot help but be reminded of the furious, desperate attempt of Lucretius's all too human lovers to "force their way to t'other's heart" in Dryden's stunning translation of book 4 of *De rerum natura* (quoted in the Introduction), or the frenzied interlocking limbs of Giulio Romano's drawings of lovers.[25] Adam, in his petulant and misogynistic grief after the Fall, seems to think that all the angels in heaven are male when, echoing Aristotle's definition of woman as "a deformed man," he laments:

> O why did God,
> Creator wise, that peopl'd highest Heav'n
> With Spirits Masculine, create at last
> This novelty on Earth, this fair defect
> Of Nature, and not fill the World at once
> With Men as Angels without Feminine,
> Or find some other way to generate
> Mankind?
> (10.888–95)

The angels who appear and speak in *Paradise Lost* all seem to be masculine in appearance and voice, but we can infer from these passages that angels are able to choose their gender and the style of lovemaking they wish, though masculine interpenetration seems to be the prevailing mode.

When Satan invents sin or ego rebellion in Heaven he reinvents angelic sex. Sin, his daughter-and-lover turned monster, whom he meets at Hell's gates, reminds him of her origin. When Lucifer and his subordinate angels met in their Assembly in the north to form their bold conspiracy, pain suddenly seized him, flames shot out of his head, and Sin followed, springing out as a beautiful goddess, fully armed, reflecting Lucifer's own bright image but in female form. The angelic host recoiled at first in fear, but Sin, through the art of pleasing by sweet attraction, won over her chief opponent, Satan, and they had sexual relations in secret that resulted in the birth of Death, an offspring mortally hostile to his own mother. Death raped Sin and engendered the terrible hellhounds who, in Sin's words, are

> hourly conceived
> And hourly born, with sorrow infinite
> To me, for when they list, into the womb
> That bred them they return, and howl and gnaw
> My Bowels.
> (2.796–800)

If Satan does not invent heterosexual relations when he produces Sin out of his rebellious intellect, he invents Satanic sex as opposed to what I have just described as angelic sex.

We may well remember at this point, with C. S. Lewis, the Augustinian definition of evil that informs Milton's representation of sin as disobedience in *Paradise Lost*: "What we call bad things are good things perverted. This perversion arises when a conscious creature becomes more interested in itself than in God, and wishes to exist 'on its own.' This is the sin of Pride. The first creature who ever committed it was Satan, the proud angel who turned from God to himself, not wishing to be a subject, but to rejoice like a tyrant in having subjects of his own."[26] Sin is initially egoistic, narcissistic, and militantly aggressive. Sin is partially female, but she is male-generated. She owes something to potent seventeenth-century Anglo-Puritan antifeminist doctrines, but Milton's allegory is more an expression of the *power* of female and male generative sexuality gone wrong, a paradigmatic emblem of the horror of fallen generation, a prefiguration of all the unhappy families of man where husbands and wives, parents and children, become monsters to each other. Hence Milton's Sin as the Mother of Death is an emblem of the origin of mortality or finiteness first authored by Satan.[27] In this respect, Satan and Sin are the forerunners of fallen humankind. They go through the experience of the Fall first. Satanic sex—invasive, possessive, exploitative, manipulative, self-gratifying, secretive, destructive—has all the earmarks of ego domination, of lust in action, as in Shakespeare's sonnet 129, "perjured, murd'rous, bloody, full of blame, / Savage, extreme, rude, cruel, not to trust"—a heaven that leads men to hell, as Sin begins in Heaven, sojourns in Hell, and finally fuses with humankind in the Fall. Hence Satanic sex—opposed to angelic sex and unfallen human sex—is the legacy of fallen human generation and history.

We return to Satan now gazing at Adam and Eve in book 4, the first of the two such major gaze scenes in the poem. At what point Satan decides to focus the force of his assault upon Eve instead of Adam is not an easy question. After he first distinguishes the beautiful human beings from the other creatures in the garden he, like the narrator guiding the reader, seems to take a long, admiring survey of their appearance and he is standing "still in gaze, as first he stood," almost unable to recover his failed speech, when the first word he utters is "O Hell!" (4.356–58). Satan thinks first of Hell because Hell—as I have suggested—has now become his intimate companion, his other self, a fit Hell mate, a compact version of "the heart of Hell" (1.151) right there within his own breast. He is speaking to the hot Hell that burns continually inside him, the partner whom he has exchanged for the sexual pleasures of Heaven and then of Sin. Satan immediately thinks of the contrast between Heaven and Hell and the bliss he has lost: "O Hell! what do mine eyes with grief behold, / Into our room of bliss thus high advanc't / Creatures of other mould" (4.358–60). Working from this passage alone, it is not difficult to see that most of the forty uses of "bliss" in *Paradise Lost* have a sexual or erotic significance.

Hell is Satan's internal sexual partner in burning torment, the unquenchable and unsatisfied "fierce desire" that is the direct opposite of the "pure desire" of good angels making the "bliss" of total sexual interpenetrability in Heaven as described by the angel Raphael. The fallen angels, on the other hand, have given up the voluntary harmonious bliss of heavenly lovemaking for the compulsory and cataclysmic Petrarchan extremes of heat and cold in their new habitation, hauled back and forth by "harpy-footed Furies":

> the parching Air
> Burns frore, and cold performs th' effect of Fire.
> . . . .
> [the damned] feel by turns the bitter change
> Of fierce extremes, extremes by change more fierce,
> From Beds of raging Fire to starve in Ice
> Thir soft Ethereal warmth, and there to pine
> Immovable, infixt, and frozen round,
> Periods of time, thence hurried back to fire.
> (2.594–603)

Satan eventually came to embrace and internalize Hell as the successor to his first sexual partner, Sin. Between them, Satan and Hell generate the psychological motivation of Milton's version of the compulsive rapist murderer. When at the end of his address to the Sun Satan says "Evil be thou my Good" (4.110), he reaffirms his marriage vow, in a highly personal sense, to Hell as the personification of the "Universe of Death." Milton reserves this superbly concise reformulation of Satan's thoughts in book 1 about his relation to God, good, and evil for precisely this moment.

In looking at the beautiful pair, Satan is struck especially by the "grace / The hand that form'd them on thir shape hath pour'd" (4.364–65). We recall the "attractive graces" of Sin, and the "sweet attractive Grace" (4.298) that the narrator attributes to Eve. "Grace" in Satan's mouth has its own peculiar ring, but there is no denying the potential for "love" and the beauty of Satan's great tribute to God's artistry in his words here. In order "to view his prey" more closely, Satan takes the form of various animals, ending as a tiger "who chose his ground / Whence rushing he might surest seize them both" (4.406–7). He is a predator choosing his ground for the attack, and from the first his assault is combined with desire. Satan seems to feel a sexual attraction to Eve from his first prolonged view of the human pair, and it would seem that his gaze lingers heavily and particularly upon her.

The construction of *Paradise Lost* as "a series of dramas within an epic" (Merritt Hughes's useful phrase) forces the reader, as William Empson emphasized, to pay as close attention to what each character in the contextual drama is saying as Satan pays to his potential victims. He apprehends everything they say and do *together* from 4.411 to 4.504, and only in this passage. He knows, like the devil in Revelation, or the anatomist who must do his grisly work quickly before the body decays, or the executioner of royalty, that he has not got much time. He has the strong advantage over Eve of having heard her account of her first day but not Adam's account of his first day (in book 8). What is it that Satan (literally the Accuser or Prosecutor) learns here about the human pair that will be used against them? He might observe that Adam stresses his similarities with his "Sole partner" (4.411—his first words in the poem), Eve, their differences. Modern biblical scholars point out that the Hebrew, *ezer kenegdo*, for Eve, may best be translated as "partner," a power equal to. In the words of R. David Freedman, biblical "woman was not intended to be merely man's helper. She was to be instead his partner." *Ezer*, as Milton the Hebraic scholar may well have known, combines two roots, to rescue, or save, and to be strong. The noun *ezer* occurs twenty-one times in the Hebrew Bible. Eight times it means savior; the other times it means strength, with the suggestion also at times of majesty.[28] All of this is relevant to Milton's Eve. Despite Eve's clear subordination to Adam, the sense of a *power equal to* is preserved in Milton's evolving representation of Eve in relation to Adam. When Eve gives her autobiographical sketch of her first day she is already characterized as a reflective subject. She is giving Adam an account of what she *was*; she already has a history.

In pondering, perhaps at a later time, the long account Eve gives of her first day, Satan would fasten upon her sense of wonder at her new world and her existence ("I first awak't, and found myself repos'd / Under a shade on flow'rs, much wondering where / And what I was" [4.450–52]), sensing that Eve's notion of her own identity, at the very beginning, does not encompass the idea of "who" she is. This is the key notion upon which he will build his attempt, and the decision to begin the "seduction" with her is probably made after hearing this speech. She acknowledges the strong influence upon her of the male voice (of God, for example, at 8.485), gently commanding her actions ("there I had fixt / Mine eyes till now, and pin'd with vain desire, / Had not a voice thus warn'd me" [4.65–67], "what could I do, / But follow straight, invisibly thus led?" [4.475–76]). Perhaps the dominant sense Satan has of her is of a creature influenced by outside forces: authoritative voices, the godlike one and Adam's, whose words she repeats, and images like the one in the water. Eve here has her first experience of the Other, or the Double, not knowing that the image in the water is her own. She is the first human artist, able to make a beautiful image appear by choice. She reflects Nature holding up her bank in her crystal mirror. Satan the narcissist responds deeply to Eve's innocent narcissism as she describes that "winning soft . . . amiably mild . . . smooth, wat'ry image" (4.479–80), one which he will endeavor with all of his own skill as a maker of images to replicate in his culminating attempt upon her.

As the preface to her account of all she remembers of her first day of life, Eve pays Adam the overwhelming compliment of being her "head," her "guide." She says in effect, "I was formed for you; you cannot find a consort like yourself." Her language here is similar to Adam's when he speaks to God in book 8. She is almost saying that Adam is her God. There seems to be a kind of innocent pride in her expressive self-presentation to him at the very moment she is displaying extreme self-abnegation. She says, "I am showing you how much I have learned, how much I owe to you. I am nothing compared to you." She literally denies her selfhood. It is as if the body were acting out its role for the benefit of the head, asserting the subjection of the flesh.

This subjection is carried over in the image—conveyed now to Satan and to the complicit fallen reader with almost Lucretian intensity—of her sexual submissiveness to Adam. This is also Milton's most Spenserian moment of illicit sexual perception. Eve's beautiful golden tresses are her original *textus*, the golden veil under which her "swelling breast" meets Adam's, and under the covering of which their pleasure takes place. Her hair is Nature's original work of art in her, and Eve's aesthetic handiwork in the garden will be an extension of this text. Satan reads beneath the text and moans with frustrated desire, defining the imagined paradise of Adam and Eve's intertwined bodies as "the happier Eden" where they enjoy complete, recurring, blissful sexual union while he is "thrust" into the infernal torments of "unfulfilled" sexual desire. The scene of Adam and Eve's connubial joy incorporating Eve's "first day" speech is framed in the way scriptural scenes are often framed—to accentuate the significance of what happens around and within them—by Satan's visual perceptions corroded by fierce desire: "O Hell! what do mine eyes with grief behold" (4.358) and

> Sight hateful, sight tormenting! thus these two
> Imparadis'd in one another's arms
> The happier *Eden*, shall enjoy thir fill
> Of bliss on bliss, while I to Hell am thrust,
> Where neither joy nor love, but fierce desire,
> Among our other torments not the least,
> Still unfulfill'd with pain of longing pines.
> (4.505–11)

Then he pulls himself back from these thoughts to focus on his mission: he will communicate his own desire to them, "excite their minds with more desire to know," and in the case of Eve, to teach her who she really is. What Satan must do is replace Adam as the source of Eve's being and he will do this by coming to her through *her own* world, through her head and later through her handiwork, in order to conquer her mind and her heart.

The Bower: Eve's Ear

Satan makes three temptation/seduction speeches to Eve in the poem, impersonating first Adam, then an angel, then a speaking serpent. The first two speeches take place in the dream he fashions while manipulating the organs of her fancy when he approaches the sleeping Eve in the Bower in the form of a toad. The third speech of course takes place in the final temptation in book 9. As in *Clarissa*, a novel that owes much to *Paradise Lost*— and which helps us to read *Paradise Lost* better—the seduction process is prolonged and protracted.

The Bower highlights the paramount significance of *place* in the poem. This is Adam and Eve's most important space before the Fall, their home. The Bower, made entirely of vegetation and chosen and formed by the "sovran Planter" himself "when he fram'd / All things to man's delightful use" (4.691–92), is a "Silvan Lodge" (5.377), or hut with walls of bushes, and planted inside with flowers that reflect the male/female interlace of the garden—tall iris, rose, and jessamine "Rear'd high their flourisht heads," low violet, crocus, and hyacinth embroider the ground with their "rich inlay" (4.699–701). The flowers recall the ones in Heaven but here there is more variety and color (3.352). There is a kind of dining area in the lodge, to which the sociable angel Raphael will be invited to a fruitarian supper, with a large, square grassy table and mossy seats. Further inside is the "inmost bower" (4.738), Adam and Eve's bedroom, in whose "close recess" (4.708), a term often used for the innermost parts of the womb in the midwife books of the time,[29] "Espoused *Eve*" first decorated "her Nuptial Bed" with a variety of flowers, garlands, and sweet smelling herbs. Eve continues where God the planter left off.

God framed the Bower for them and Eve elaborates and extends the creation in her own way in the "inmost bower" with God's approval, reminiscent of the intimate biblical God-Woman paradigm discussed in the first chapter. Eve the artist of flowers and floral arrangement presides over the marriage bed—"*her* bed"—and over the most important rites that Adam and Eve perform. While they sleep, serenaded by nightingales and distant angelic choirs, soft showers of rose petals float down upon their naked limbs from the roof of the Bower, a roof thickly "inwoven" also with the flowers of poetic honor, laurel and myrtle, which are an implicit tribute to the aesthetic achievements of Adam and Eve in their constant hymns to God's creative goodness and concern for their welfare. What is stressed here in the inmost bower is the thickness of the foliage, the protectedness of the place, the layers of beautiful color, the richness of the finely textured flowery inlay, the luxuriance, the concentrated appeal to the senses, especially to touch and to smell, the "thick-wovenness" (a term applied later to Eve's artistry in her Nursery, 9.437) and intricate textuality of the scene, the superlativeness of it all. In some deep sense this is Eve's place, her creative matrix framed solely and purely for Adam and Eve's "delightful use," in all the creative dimensions of that phrase. No "beast, bird, insect, or worm" dare enter (4.704). The inmost bower is the "Holy of Holies" in Milton's temple to the sacredness of the sexual act,[30] the place where Adam and Eve are closest to each other in verbal and sexual intercourse, where they "cleave" together, where they engage in as complete and pure a communion as unfallen human beings can attain, and it is here that Satan first penetrates. He comes between them. He becomes Adam's rival for Eve's attention.

Satan's manipulation of Eve's fancy, or imagination, in the dream he gives her is presented, in part, as a debased sexual act. Helkiah Crooke, in the midst of a meditation on sexual pleasure and "nocturnal pollutions," points out that "the imagination in sleepe is stronger than when wee are awake" (288). Something ugly enters Eve's ear. The toad, the witch's familiar by which she gains access to the devil as we saw in the story about William Harvey, is an emblem for the phallus. There is no better verbal context for this transaction than Shakespeare. In his much changed imagination, polluted by the demonic Iago, Othello's "heart," the "fountain" of his life force, has become "a cistern for foul toads / To knot and gender in" (4.2.56–61).[31] Satan attempts a perverse invocation of Eve as his Muse. In jolting contrast to Milton's initial entreaty of the divine Spirit to impregnate his poetic mind, to raise and support what in him is low, Satan wishes to impregnate Eve by "inspiring venom" in her fancy by which he might "taint / Th' animal spirits that from pure blood arise" and ultimately raise discontented thoughts "Blown up with high conceits ingend'ring pride" (4.804–9). In the Galenic system, "animal spirits" (or psychic pneuma) were the highest order of "spirits" in the body, generated from the vital pneuma formed in the heart, rarefied via the *rete mirabile*, the "marvellous network" of vessels at the base of the brain, and distributed by the nerves to give sensation and motion to the parts of the body as well as providing imagination and thought. Unfallen Eve would have the purest of pure blood. Since God had said that violence could not be used against Adam and Eve in the temptation (5.242, unlike the case of Job), Satan cannot *touch* Eve physically and must have recourse to the most ingenious "spiritual" and psychological means at his disposal to affect her will. In this regard, Satan's attempt to "blow up" ideas in Eve's fancy recalls one of the most delicate operations of the early modern anatomist on the human body. Crooke records in his inventory of necessary anatomical instruments "Glass-trunkes or hollow Bugles to blowe vp the parts" (27). Whether or not Satan does succeed in tainting Eve, or engendering something evil in her mind *in this operation*—and the issue is not at all self-evident—"Pride" is ultimately the true offspring of Satan and Eve, Eve's first birth.

In the rosy morn, Adam wakes first and wonders that Eve is still sleeping. Her discomposed tresses and glowing cheek are the external signs of Satan's visit, the first communication of his fire. Adam looks down at her with "cordial Love" (5.12), love from the heart, and we think again of how Eve in recounting her first day had recited his own words back to him, presumably just as he had spoken them, "to give thee being I lent / Out of my side to thee, nearest my heart / Substantial life" (4.483–85). Her looking at him at first "with startl'd eye" (5.26) is the first indication of fear and distrust in their world, because she heard his voice in her dream. From here on Eve's fear will grow until her encounter with the forbidden tree.

Many readers have noted that Eve's predominating sense is hearing, but an equally strong case might be made for her intent visual powers. I shall consider her visual orientation later, but at this point, I suggest that she is especially attuned to the male voice guiding her from her first moments of consciousness. Adam's waking her is a repetition of his voice in her dream: "Why sleep'st thou, *Eve*? now is the pleasant time" (5.38). Though Satan did not hear her question to Adam about why the stars shine, he heard enough from them both to have Adam give Eve an image of herself as "Nature's desire." In the dream, modeled in part on the two dreams in the Song of Solomon, she goes out looking for one who is not there. Satan is the Archimago of the voice, the manipulator of wonderfully lifelike replicas fashioned solely by the actor's mimicking skill. And then comes the angel's voice. We learn—and it comes as a slight shock—that the human pair often see angels in Paradise who exist, as Adam told her, along with those millions of spiritual creatures whom they cannot see but whose strange, ethereal songs they can hear. The angel murmurs to the forbidden tree as if it were his lover: "Deigns none to ease thy load and taste thy sweet?" (5.59). Knowledge becomes the object of sexual desire ("Hence I will excite their minds / With more desire to know" [4.522–23]). He tastes the fruit, addresses it but really its effect on him, then turns to her, as one angel to another ("fair Angelic *Eve*"), and calls her a "goddess" (5.78), the first use of that term for her in the poem. Satan will be her goddess maker, as Lovelace makes Clarissa into a "goddess" in his erotic imagination.[32] Then the angel comes close to her and holds the fruit right up to her mouth. The smell is irresistible and she "cannot but taste." He takes her up to the clouds in a repetition of Satan's great wheeling flights and the earth is outstretched below them, immense. She is exalted in an almost ecstatic flight, and then for the first time experiences frustration—her "guide" leaves her hanging, falling, sinking back down to sleep.

The Nursery: Eve's Hand

In the opening of book 9, Satan returns to Paradise at "midnight" after having fled the garden "by night." During the space of seven "nights," driven by anguish, "he rode / With darkness," keeping just ahead of the sun at the equator, and crossing "the Car of Night" four times from one pole to the other (9.58–66). Satan's "anguish" (9.62) is another literal form of his constricting, hardening, propulsive yet focused destructive power. Satan communes, in his desperate meditation of "Man's destruction," with the Uncreated, eternal Night. His is a seven-night anticreation agony, with no period of rest. His temporal anguish contrasts with the suspended time—perpetual summer—of Adam and Eve in Paradise. As book 9 opens, the fallen reader is still falling, drawn downward to darkness, like Eve from her exaltation in the dream: "No more of talk where God or Angel Guest / With man" (9.1–2). "The Sun was sunk" (9.48), "and now from end to end / Night's Hemisphere had veil'd the Horizon round" (9.51–52), a mood recalling Macbeth's nocturnal meditation that fates him for a murder which is also a rape:

> Now o'er the one half world
> Nature seems dead, and wicked dreams abuse
> The curtain'd sleep; witchcraft celebrates
> Pale Hecate's offerings; and withered murder,
> Alarum'd by his sentinel, the wolf
> . . . with his stealthy pace,
> With Tarquin's ravishing strides, towards his design
> Moves like a ghost. Thou sure and firm-set earth,
> Hear not my steps.
> (*Macbeth* 2.1.49–57)

Whereas Satan first entered Paradise leaping the verdant wall and entering Eve at her head, we are now drawn down with Satan to the "foot of Paradise" as he makes his new entrance in the upthrust fountain by the Tree of Life, polluting first the very heart current of the garden. The movement in book 9 is down with the narrator, and then up from below with Satan's serpentine point of view. He is bursting with "inward grief" and "passion" (9.97–98) in his long hymn to Earth. He begins with the poem's richest and most deeply felt appreciation of the beauty of the created Earth—and of the creative process that improves with practice: "as built / With second thoughts, reforming what was old" (9.100–101)—and he ends speaking in the cold, neutral tones of the driven murderer (in our language, the compulsive psychopath), abstracted from his own evil, like Macbeth at the end, with a final hint of the Hobbesian cardiac recoil effect:

> Who aspires must down as low
> As high he soar'd . . .
> . . . Revenge, at first though sweet,
> Bitter ere long back on itself recoils; [pause]
> Let it; I reck not, so it light well aimed.
> (9.169–73)

In Adam and Eve's early morning dialogue, the most important domestic conversation in English literature before the emergence of the novel, there is a new sense of urgency in Eve's voice, a new sense of anxiety. This motif of feminine anxiety will be expanded and complicated in the early novel from Behn to Defoe to its most profound representation in Richardson's Pamela and Clarissa.[33] The fear first indicated in Eve's startled response to Adam upon waking from her dream has intensified into

> If this be our condition, thus to dwell
> In narrow circuit strait'n'd by a Foe,
> Subtle or violent, we not endu'd
> Single with like defense, wherever met,
> How are we happy, still in fear of harm?
> (9.322–26)

Where does Eve go when she leaves Adam? I believe she goes to the same place she went when she withdrew herself in "lowliness Majestic" from the discourse of Raphael and Adam in book 8—to the fruits and flowers of her Nursery ("They at her coming sprung / And toucht by her fair tendance gladlier grew" [8.46–47]). One marvels at all the allusions in the poem to her hands and their magical touch. In book 9 she is carrying her gardening tools; she is compared again, with a variety of suggestions of her soft touch, to the goddesses who care for living and growing things (Pales, Pomona, and "Ceres in her prime," before she gave birth to Proserpine).

And we next hear of "ambush hid among sweet Flow'rs and Shades" waiting "with hellish rancor" to intercept her (9.408–9). Satan has stalked her to her most private place, and he emerges amidst Eve's own handiwork. He is "subtle" (9.307, 9.324, 10.20), the adjective from Genesis, and a favorite word of the anatomists for describing all manner of "spirits"—from angelic to demonic to the three spirits of the human soul. Another connection between seventeenth-century natural history and Milton is provided by Walter Charleton when he describes the "corporeal soul" as "composed of particles extremely small, subtil, and active . . . like fire."[34] Nicholas Udall's Geminus, following Galen in speaking of the right ventricle, says, "in hym is brought a great porcion of ye thyckest bloude therewith to nouryshe the Heart, and the resydue yt is lefte of this is made *subtyl* and thynner through the vertue of the Heart."[35] But the anatomists are describing the formation of pure, life-giving vital spirit; Milton draws on this language to depict just the opposite, and he employs the word "subtle" with great resource and resonance in this special context. The Latin *subtilis*—smooth, finespun, silky, like the spider's web—originally meant "closely woven," literally, "under the web" (*sub-tela*, from *texere*, to weave). The demonic spirit Satan as serpent strolling, upright, *is* the subtext here, literally moving *under* the text of Eve's artistry. As Adam says, "subtle he needs must be, who could seduce / Angels" (9.307–8).

Eve is now the fully developed artist in her prime, an accomplished gardener intent on the work springing up under her life-informing hands. The intensity of her auditory experience is equaled here by the visual and tactile concentration she brings to her work with flowers. In her nursery, caring for the flower children that will precede her human offspring and provide an experimental field preparatory to her primary role as the "Mother of all living," she is the preeminent goddess who makes life and beauty. When the fallen pair are evicted from Paradise by the angel Michael, it is this Nursery that the grief-stricken Eve thinks of first, and then her Bower:

>   O flow'rs,
> That never will in other Climate grow,
> My early visitation, and my last
> At Ev'n, which I bred up with tender hand
> From the first op'ning bud, and gave ye Names,
> Who now shall rear ye to the Sun, or rank
> Your Tribes, and water from th' ambrosial Fount?
> Thee lastly nuptial Bower, by mee adorn'd
> With what to sight or smell was sweet; from thee
> How shall I part . . . ?
> (11.273–82)

This speech is fallen Eve's pastoral elegy for her unfallen children and her life work—the work of her hands—in Paradise. It is her "Lycidas." The flowers will die without her. We learn from these lines that Eve as gardener is a naturalist as well as an artist—a classifier, a primordial creator of scientific as well as aesthetic order. In her mind the Nursery is an extension of the Bower, but in the prelapsarian context of book 9 there is a hint that the Nursery is now almost more important to Eve than the Bower. By this point in the history of Eve and Adam, the Nursery has become more *her* place, her own private creative space as she moves more and more toward a separate and distinct human identity, different from Adam's.

In this critical moment of Satan's attempt we see Eve as a beautiful woman learning to be a mother to her children. The flowers, as we noted, are linked with Adam and Eve's lovemaking in the Bower. There tall irises, roses, and jessamines rise up to shield them. In the Nursery, Eve is seen supporting and stroking the heads of her flowers. The upright serpent, moving unsuspected and hardly even noticed under her fingers, is her friend, like all the other animals. He fits right in with the entire scene, as everything fits with everything else in the communal erotic sheen of love and polymorphous generative vitality in Eden. Visually, he blends in perfectly with the beauty-making power of Eve's "ruddy and gold" world of roses and vegetative colors. Eve's wariness has ceased in the total concentration she brings to the moment of her nurturing activities in her own place in the garden. This undeviating absorption in her task is her strength and her weakness. She has recently heard all about Satan's heroic exploits in the War in Heaven. Surely he would not be so unheroic as to attack the weaker of the two human beings, and she seems to have put the danger out of her mind. There was another moment of such concentrated apprehension in Eve's experience:

> As I bent down to look, just opposite,
> A Shape within the wat'ry gleam appear'd
> Bending to look on me, I started back,
> It started back, but pleas'd I soon return'd,
> Pleas'd it return'd as soon with answering looks
> Of sympathy and love. . . .
> . . . .
> Till I espied thee, fair indeed and tall,
> . . . yet methought less fair,
> Less winning soft, less amiably mild,
> Than that smooth wat'ry image.
> (4.460–80)

The present scene in book 9 recapitulates the one at the pool in book 4. Satan as the serpent is now the beautiful image "floating" softly on the fringe of Eve's fluid consciousness, "now hid, now seen" (9.436). He has come strolling into her beautiful, thickset garden of "Roses" (9.426), "voluble and bold" in his quest, ever nearer his goal in a saturnine Miltonic parody of the romance knight's movement ever inward to his longed for Rose. The rose was not only an emblem of the female genitalia and of female modesty (pudendum), but was at the same time the flower of Venus, a sign of the Virgin Mary, with the red rose symbolizing mature female sexuality, and a symbol of the heart. The language of the rose is found in the oldest anatomies and midwife manuals, descriptions Milton was undoubtedly aware of: "The Matrix or chambre in woman is an official member . . . whan a woman doeth sprede her thighes, it altereth the ayre that entreth into the Matrix to moderate and temper the heate there. . . . Ferdermore, the necke . . . hath in her concavitie manye involutions and plightes or foldinges, rolled and pleited together in maner of rose leaves . . . before they be rype or spredde abrode."[36] Satan comes out of the "walks" among the stately trees directly into Eve's presence within the dense, thick-woven tapestry of "arborets and flowers" she has created. The serpent has now entered her "hand"—her handiwork, her art, her world, and her blind consciousness. The virtue that makes Eve such an expert and creative gardener—her capacity for intense concentration—is the very thing that prevents her from perceiving her present vulnerability and danger. Satan has moved from manipulating her fancy in the dream to this bold entrance into the *product* of her fancy, the burgeoning rose garden world of her Nursery:

> Veil'd in a Cloud of Fragrance, where she stood
> Half spi'd, so thick the Roses bushing round
> About her glow'd, oft stooping to support
> Each Flow'r of slender stalk, whose head though gay
> Carnation, Purple, Azure, or speckt with Gold,
> Hung drooping unsustain'd, them she upstays
> Gently with Myrtle band, mindless the while,
> Herself, though fairest unsupported Flow'r,
> From her best prop so far, and storm so nigh.
> (9.425–33)

From the erected serpent's point of view, Eve stoops invitingly as she props up and invigorates, with all the intricate skill of the supreme female gardener, the "head" of each slender flower, which she gently ties with bands from another flower sacred to Venus, while her own sexual partner and spiritual guide, Adam, is voluntarily absent from the scene, weaving (ironically) a garland for her. (Adam will later chastise himself for exposing her to danger [10.957]; since he failed to persuade her with right reason to stay with him, he could presumably have at least followed her at a distance to aid her.) The roses bush protectively thick around her like a hedge that Satan must pierce. Satan thus continues his role as Adam's sexual rival in the contest of who shall possess and guide Eve's "heart," her essence and being. Adam had indicated candidly to Raphael, who by that point in their conversation had virtually become a kind of marriage counselor to Adam, that Eve's power over him was like that of a goddess, almost (though Adam does not say it) a rival to the divine power of the Father and the Son:

> when I approach
> Her loveliness, so absolute she seems
> And in herself complete, so well to know
> Her own, that what she wills to do or say,
> Seems wisest, virtuousest, discreetest, best;
> All higher knowledge in her presence falls
> Degraded, Wisdom in discourse with her
> Loses discount'nanced, and like folly shows;
> Authority and Reason on her wait,
> As one intended first, not after made
> Occasionally; and to consummate all,
> Greatness of mind and nobleness thir seat
> Build in her loveliest, and create an awe
> About her, as a guard Angelic plac't.
> (8.546–59)

Here (as in the final books) the language of the heart in *Paradise Lost* seems central, elaborating the rich biblical contexture of the land, woman, and the heart, which we examined in Chapter 1. The text seems to be saying what Milton the narrator cannot say: that Adam, because of his relation to Earth, to Nature, to Eve, and to his own language, could hardly have done anything else but choose to fall with her. We must go back to his own account of his first day of life in book 8. Adam begins in "softness," the poem's key word for feminine nurture, on a flowery bank ("As new wak't from soundest sleep / Soft on the flowery herb I found me laid" [8.253–54]). He comes to consciousness in the "balmy sweat" of one who has emerged as from the travail of the earth, or his own exertions, steaming with vapors—visible spirits—which the Sun soon dries. There is no hint in this narrative account of God's forming activity. (Raphael's account of Adam's making [7.524–28] is almost a literal transcript of Gen. 2.7 with no Miltonic elaboration.) From Adam's viewpoint at that moment, Earth bore him; he began life from the maternal softness of the womb of Earth, not from the hand of the Father. He springs "upright" on his feet, and we recall the Spirit's preference for "the upright heart and pure," the condition to which the narrator aspires for proper reception of the Spirit in order to see into the divine world. For Adam, the heart feelings are first: "all things smiled, / With fragrance and with joy my heart o'erflowed" (8.265–66). The primary image is the fountain, as in Plato's description of the heart, and the prevalent image of the heart from the ancient world to the early modern era. It is perhaps at this moment (though there are others in the poem) that we know the deepest and most resonant human image in *Paradise Lost* is the heart, unfallen and fallen, here stirred by the fragrance of the earth, overflowing with joy.

The sequence of events now for Adam, so different from Eve's first moments, is first the sensation of the joyful heart, then perusal and exercise of the body, then the conviction that he must have a personal identity—but not knowing "who" that particular identity may be in relation to his surroundings (8.270). He at once exercises the primal, divine power of *speech*; she does not. The tone of Adam's account of his first day is proud confidence; the tone of Eve's account is wondering perplexity. The question of who she is does not even arise for her at her beginning; Adam figures out who he is. And yet Adam virtually tells Raphael that Eve has become his goddess, one whom he adores because she seems so "absolute" and complete in herself. But what is it that is so *good* about Eve for Adam? Again the answer seems to lie in the context of Adam's heart feelings of his first day, a heart feminized, receptive, soft, overflowing, joyful. It is not the crookedness of the rib that is accentuated in Milton's vision of Eve's creation, but the "cordial spirits warm, / And life blood streaming fresh" (8.466–67) that become *her* cordial spirits and warm life blood. As in Leviticus 17, the blood is the life. "She who makes live" emerges from the primal creative warmth of the divine impulse as Adam, in the darkness of his trancelike sleep (8.478), witnesses her creation in his "fancy."

Despite his characterization of Old Night as feminine and cold, Milton, like his budding contemporary Aphra Behn, does not endorse the prevailing medical view of women's essential physiological coldness, a view we encountered first in the Introduction and again in Chapter 2. Because she makes life, Milton's Eve is as physically warm and vital as his Adam, or as the feminized Earth being born from "the Womb . . . of Waters," when "over all the face of Earth / Main Ocean flowed, not idle, but with warm / Prolific humour soft'ning all her Globe" (7.276–80). Eve's original transformative power is affirmed when Adam first sees her after her "forming":

a Creature . . .
. . . so lovely fair,
That what seem'd fair in all the World, seem'd now
Mean, or in her summ'd up, in her contain'd
And in her looks.
(8.470–74)

The primal power of Eve is that she infuses "sweetness" into Adam's "heart" and the "spirit of love and amorous delight" (9.475–77) into all things, and this power is also the source of her creative artistry.

For Adam, Eve continues where the earth left off; he is encompassed by the feminine Earth and Eve. Eve "daily" re-creates in him the primacy of pure feeling that he puts into words when he inferred that some great maker had given him the gift "that thus I move and live, / And feel that I am happier than I know" (8.281–82). If Adam has learned, in his conversation with Raphael, that the "prime Wisdom" is to know what lies before us in daily life (8.192–94), Eve is the mediator of that wisdom. Adam is impressed with "Her virtue and the conscience of her worth" (8.502), a sense of "self-esteem" (8.572), which the troubled Raphael gently suggests Adam himself needs more of. Adam gives the fullest and deepest expression of his sense of Eve's goodness (which includes submissiveness as well as mutual love) when "half abash't" he corrects Raphael's disparagement of human sexual intercourse by affirming its sanctity and then explaining that it is not sex with Eve that delights him so much

>   as those graceful acts,
> Those thousand decencies that daily flow
> From all her words and actions, mixt with Love
> And sweet compliance, which declare unfeign'd
> Union of mind, or in us both one Soul.
> (8.600–604)

If Eve's anxiety inaugurates a great theme in the birth of the novel, Adam's definition of the "prime wisdom" might also be taken as a declaration of the paradigmatic subject of the early novel—the daily interaction of men and women in the empirical world.

Eve's primal wisdom of the body in the experience of "delight," as Adam has just defined it in its larger context, makes higher wisdom seem like folly. She reverses the Pauline formula: not the wisdom of the world is foolishness with God, but the wisdom of God is foolishness with Eve when Adam is in her powerful presence. She here becomes the rival of God's feminine playfellow Wisdom and thus of the Muse Urania, the sister of Wisdom. Adam knows the doctrine about male and female inequality ("her th' inferior, in the mind / And inward Faculties, which most excel" [8.541–42]), but he does not *feel* it. His deepest sense of life comes from the primacy of the heart's feelings, and these feelings are imbued with the female creativity of the earth, nature, and Eve. In Eve, God the Father gave Adam his wish exactly to his "heart's desire" (8.451)—that desire was the crucial element.

Despite his "higher intellectual," Milton's Adam is the original man of feeling, and Eve, who was formed from his heart region, is the beautiful externalization of his own heart. But here the ambivalence of the heart again asserts itself. If the heart was thought to be the seat of the passions, it is not surprising that in Eve's presence Adam first feels "passion" (8.530), and the hint of "vehement desire" (8.526). Adam may have exercised the divine gift of speech on his first day while Eve on hers did not, and he may have a higher power of language and expressiveness than she, but he says too much. In particular, he has a profound problem with the word "but." If he had stopped exhorting Eve to stay with him when he told her to approve her constancy and obedience, she might have stayed. "But if thou think . . . ," he went on, and virtually challenged her to leave. Like the biblical Samson, Adam utters the fatal words that will entrap him. Perhaps these words contribute to his "fall." Earlier Adam had tripped over the fatal word as he tried to explain to Raphael his feelings when in Eve's sexual presence in contrast to the sensory delights of Nature (enumerated as the "delicacies" of "Taste, Sight, Smell, Herbs, Fruits, and Flow'rs, / Walks, and the melody of Birds"):

> but here [with Eve]
> Far otherwise, transported I behold,
> Transported touch; here passion first I felt,
> Commotion strange, in all enjoyments else
> Superior and unmov'd, here only weak
> Against the charm of Beauty's powerful glance.
> (8.526–33)

He goes on to complain that Nature may have taken too much out of his side. The anatomist Crooke (following Galen) tried to explain how Nature, wishing her work to be immortal,

> hath infused into [the instruments of conception] a strange and violent kinde of delight, that none of the *kindes* of the creatures should perish but remayne ever after a sort immortal. And truely it was very necessary that there should be a kinde of pleasant force or violence in the Nature of mankinde to transport him out of him-selfe; or beside himself as it were, in the act of generation; to which otherwise being maister of himselfe he would hardly haue been drawne; which extasie, (for it is called a little *Epilepsie* or falling sicknes) is caused by the touch of the seede vpon the neruous and quicke sensed parts as it passeth by them. (238)

Despite his loving tribute to Eve and her "thousand decencies," Adam's "transport" is a kind of "falling sicknes," and his putting it into words is the prelude to the Fall.[37]

The Tree: Eve's Heart

As we return to Satan gazing at the "person" of the oblivious Eve in her rose garden, now in her special "Place" (9.444), her shaded, inner, private "sweet recess" (9.456), he has already had intimate communion with her in the dream he gave her. Now she is awake but not fully conscious, involved in a kind of rapt daydream with her flower children. Why, at this point, does Milton conjure one of his earliest and most intensely personal evocations of Nature and the beauty of womankind, encoded in the private yet conventional male language of Latin elegy, and exemplified in a young blonde woman with the complexion of Eve amid her flowers? Milton seems to be going back to his own origins as a poet, reimagining his first, freshest, and perhaps most intense vision of female eroticism. The seventeen-year-old boy, in his first year at Cambridge, has been suspended ("rusticated") from his college and sent to the country, outlawed in a sense, the alien visitor to a world of richly textured natural beauty—like Satan:

> I also am a visitor in the grove where the elms stand close together and in the magnificent shade of a place just beyond the city's confines. Here, like stars that breathe out soft flames, you may see groups of maidens go dancing past. Ah, how many times have I been struck dumb by the miraculous grace of a form [stupui miracula formae] which might make decrepit Jove young again! Ah, how many times have I seen eyes which outshine jewels and all the stars that wheel about either pole, necks which excel the arms of Pelops . . . and a brow of surpassing loveliness, and waving tresses which were golden nets flung by Cupid, the deceiver! How often have I seen seductive cheeks beside which the purple of the hyacinth and even the blush of your flower, Adonis, turn pale.[38]

Satan now coming upon Eve is compared to one who, having been pent up for a long time in a large city and assaulted by the smells of sewers and of people crowded too closely together, walks out into the country on a summer morning, as if released from prison, and delights in every sight and sound, and the fresh smells of grain, new mown hay set out to dry, and cattle. As in Adam's description of all the "delicacies" of Nature in contrast to Eve (8.526–27), all of the senses come into play. The parallel with Adam's experience continues when Satan reiterates the transcendent moment of Adam's first seeing Eve: "If chance with Nymph-like step fair Virgin pass, / What pleasing seem'd, for her now pleases more, / She most, and in her look sums all Delight" (9.452–54). The power of unfallen Eve's goodness to infuse and inspire the spirit of love and delight—beyond the capacity of even the most powerful of the classical Muses—stuns Satan, rendering him for a time "Stupidly good" (9.465). Her "rapine sweet bereav'd" (9.461) him temporarily of his fierce intent. The word "bereave" has its original force of bearing something violently away. Hence she "rapes" him before he seduces her, briefly takes him out of himself, divorces him, momentarily, from his Hell mate. "But the hot Hell that always in him burns . . . soon ended his delight" (9.467–68), and Hell reasserts her torturing presence. Satan is forcibly reminded for the third and last time of "pleasure not for him ordain'd" (9.470). He communes with his thoughts (as Adam will speak to himself first after meeting the fallen Eve), but he is also communing with Hell when he chides himself for being so "transported" (Adam's word and Crooke's denoting sexual ecstasy) "to forget / What hither brought *us*, hate, not love, nor hope / Of Paradise for Hell" (9.474–76, my emphasis). His only pleasure now is in destruction. He gathers himself together in hate and moves on, enfeebled by pain and reduced from the grandiose immensity of that standing "Tow'r" of 1.591 to the still potent but now insidious "Circular base of rising folds, that tow'r'd / Fold above fold a surging Maze, his head / Crested aloft" and with carbuncle red eyes and neck of "verdant gold" (9.498–501), the carefully contrived coloring that will mirror the gold and pink coloring of Eve and of her flowers, as if Satan had heeded Lady Macbeth's advice to her mate, "Look like the innocent flower, But be the serpent under't" (1.5.65–66).[39]

Satan has already penetrated Eve's head and her "hand." He knows that she is profoundly influenced by beautiful images and by the male voice commanding her. As he prepares for his third and final seduction assault, one in which he will construct a new image of her and persuade her to accept it, we must attempt to delineate the nature of Eve's unfallen "heart" as it has so far been represented in the poem. Her heart is partner to Adam's heart. She is his heart mate, made from his side, and his fit help. As his "heart's desire" (8.451) she is created to respond intensely and creatively to his emotional life. Eve's "heart" would seem to be not only the center of her mind and emotions, but the evolving source of her own "conscience" of her "beauty" and her "worth." Her worth is a continuous power of creating love and beauty in her world, a world centered in Adam and the floral beauty of her Nursery and her Bower. If Eve is the external image of Adam's heart, her Bower and Nursery are progressive external exfolliations of her own heart. Satan initially appeals to her beauty, and his words make their way into her heart (9.550). At the same time, Milton draws on the ancient image of the heart as the earth to forward Satan's appeal to Eve's "culture of the heart" (to use a term from Mary Wollstonecraft)[40]— to her authority and influence in *her own world* of beauty, to her developing mastery of the cultivation of plants, fruits, and flowers, to her love for growing things and her gift for making them grow, including her love for her flower children, for Adam, and for her children yet to be born.

Satan, who has constructed himself as a beautiful serpent, now constructs himself as an orator (9.667–78). Milton distills everything he knows about classical oratory, about the *impassioned* classical oration, and the skills of the seventeenth-century political orator/actor, in a complex figure of surpassing *oral* power—the power emanating from the mouth and tongue. One thinks of all the brilliant (and not so brilliant) speakers he was required to listen to (if not observe) in public and private presentations when he served as Cromwell's Latin Secretary. Satan's three carefully sequenced seduction speeches—each one longer than the one before—are an exploitative and ingenious adaptation of the seven parts of the classical oration, exordium or proem, narration, definition, proposition, confirmation, refutation, and conclusion. The Consult in Hell was certainly modeled to some extent on these experiences, but so is Satan's performance. The language here makes a special appeal to Milton's educated male contemporary reader, perhaps in part because he is trying to teach that reader the lesson that it is evil to talk to women in this way.

That Milton sees the initial temptation of Eve as a sexual as well as oratorical seduction is signaled by the narrator's comparison of Satan as serpent to the snake that Jove employed to sire Alexander and Scipio (9.508–10). Then Satan's serpent tongue prepares the ground for the attack. The "proem" (9.549), or entrance, or exordium (from *ordiri*, to lay the warp, again recalling the subtextual metaphor of "subtle"), is designed to gain the attention of the audience and to lay the groundwork or establish the principles from which the oration would proceed.[41] We begin again with the gaze, as Satan the oratorical actor gains Eve's attention by playing in front of her, attempting to lure her eye with a hypnotic curling of "many a wanton wreath" (9.517) (replicating the wanton ringlets of her own hair as absent Adam is apprehensively weaving his own garland for Eve), openly gazing on her with a gentle, dumb expression as he repeatedly bows his crest, and then orally but nonverbally encompassing her space (now more "innocently" than when he came unnoticed as a tiger or lion stalking his prey) by literally licking the ground she walks on as he circles around her. Milton stresses the instrumental ("organic") nature of the proceedings: Satan begins his fraudulent temptation "with Serpent Tongue / Organic, or impulse of vocal Air" (9.529–30). The phallic tongue within the erect serpent makes impulses of vocal air, pneumatic thrusts into Eve's open heart: "Into the heart of *Eve* his words made way" (9.550). In this manner (and only in this manner is it possible for him), Satan finally achieves sexual connection with Eve.

The groundwork that Satan attempts to establish in the proem is the notion in Eve's mind that she is the "sovereign mistress" of Paradise, that she is the truest image of her Creator, and that she should be seen and adored "daily" (9.548) as a goddess among gods by numberless angels (not simply by one man). The proem thus incorporates another element of the oration, the "definition" of the subject as a goddess who is out of place in her perfect garden world. She does not belong there—she belongs in Heaven. As we have noted, Milton's paralleling of Satan with Adam as Adam's sexual rival works on several planes, but the main point of the contrast is that Adam gives the angel Raphael his version of what Eve means to him as Satan gives Eve, the angelic woman, his version of what she should mean to herself. In this complex process of reshaping the mature Eve's image of herself, Satan appeals to three major areas of her experience and expertise (always centered of course on her essential relationship with Adam): her knowledge of horticulture, her knowledge of fruit and the pleasures of taste, and her knowledge of the rites and pleasures of sex.

When the angel Raphael visited, Eve sweetly contradicted Adam's command to "bring forth and pour / Abundance" of fruits on the table in the Bower by asserting that "small store will serve" when there is so much of everything, and she showed her developing mastery of the care of fruits by implying that some fruits are more nutritious because of "frugal storing" and drying (5.314–25). Eve is a mistress of hospitality (one of her strong ties with the heroic women of the Old Testament) and an artist of tastes, knowing which fruits are most "delicate," how to avoid inelegant mixing of tastes, and how best to order the serving of the fruits so that gustatory delight—"Taste after taste" (like "bliss upon bliss")—will be "upheld" in the most pleasurable and continuous sequence (5.331–36). When she is first led by her Maker to Adam, we learn that Eve is not "uninformed / Of nuptial Sanctity and marriage Rites" (8.486–87); presumably she is as expert in the arts of lovemaking as in cultivating fruits and flowers, and arranging the most exquisite series of "tastes." All these areas of expertise come into focus in the "narration," that part of the oration during which the serpent brings her to the tree of interdicted knowledge and describes how he ate the fruit and what effect it had on him.

Satan knows that Eve lives and moves in a world of "wonders" from her first moment of consciousness, "much wond'ring where / And what I was, whence thither brought, and how" (4.451–52). Wondering is a kind of thinking, but she senses herself as passive, one who is brought, one who is acted upon and led. We have seen a number of subsequent passages in which Eve's sense of wonder is paramount. In this mind-set of wonderment and bewilderment and in such a world of wonders where millions of spiritual creatures walk the earth unseen, it is not so surprising that Satan should create for her, in the speaking serpent, the penultimate wonder, and then tell her, in the serpent's first words, to "Wonder not," since she is the "sole Wonder" of her world (9.532–33). Eve's response to his first speech is a further stage of wonder—amazement. She had always thought that human speech had been denied to animals, but she had suspected that they could express something like human "sense" in their looks and gestures. She is someone who thinks and wonders plausibly about the given premises and postulates of God's world, and she had already told Adam that their happy state, and Eden itself, must be imperfect—and a source of intense anxiety inhabited now by a "Foe, / Subtle or violent"—if it is not "secure" to single, as to combined, virtue (9.323–24). Satan senses her anxiety and will manipulate it in his conversation with her. She says now that she always knew the serpent was the subtlest beast and asks him to "Redouble then this miracle" (9.562), recalling the magical redoubling of the fair image in the lake: "Say, for such wonder claims attention due" (9.566).

The prince of darkness is a gentleman. The serpent—perfect servant of love, perfect courtier to his queen—says that it is easy and proper to obey the commands of his empress, and now Satan first names her, "resplendent *Eve*." He will go on to call her "universal Dame" (9.612) and "Queen of this Universe" (9.684), in a gradual verbal elevation of her royal image, as he elevated her person in the dream flight, then was forced to leave her hanging. Eve and Adam had taken great pleasure in describing their first days of life; the serpent now has his chance to describe his first day as a new being. His narration of how he discovered the wonderful tree briefly recapitulates the sequence of Eve's narration of how she walked over to the sound of waters, lay down prone on the green bank and, bending down, found the fair image in the pool. The serpent says his thoughts were low and abject, only concerned with food and sex (two of the major preoccupations in Eve's empirical world), when he encountered the goodly tree laden with fruit of fairest colors, "Ruddy and Gold" (9.578), Eve's coloring.

The orality of the serpent, which began with licking the ground Eve walked on, now takes the form of sucking the full teats of ewes or goats at evening. He proceeds to describe having olfactory, culinary, and sexual intercourse with the tree all at once. God had said not to eat from the tree, nor to *touch* it, as Eve herself will reiterate the language of Genesis, where it is Eve only who mentions the prohibition against touching the fruit (9.651, 9.663; Gen. 3.3). Satan appeals vividly to taste and particularly, like Lucretius, to touch. His narrative proceeds to depict how the serpent wound himself around the tree's "mossy" trunk. The feel of moss, one of nature's more tactile productions, was familiar every day to Eve and Adam because the table and chairs in the dining area of their Bower were "mossy" (5.392). Moss is frequently associated with the female genitals in early modern erotica,[42] and Aphra Behn's lovers often make love on mossy banks. The tree described here is an inviting, domestic sort of tree. The serpent, like the prowling wolf "amid the field secure" (4.186), "Amid the Tree now got, where plenty hung / Tempting so nigh" (9.594–95), firmly mounted and fully involved, sates himself. Satan makes the tree stand for and epitomize everything important in Eve's world, and of course the full effect of the serpent's eating the fruit is to lead him to gaze upon and worship Eve, the one who epitomizes and unites everything "fair and good" in her world. Eve does not lose her head as the recipient of all this; she responds by recognizing the serpent's overpraising not of her, but of the fruit's effects.

Satan's third and final seduction speech includes a version of the rest of the parts of the formal oration—proposition, confirmation, refutation, and conclusion. Just before this speech Milton offers a brilliant epic simile of the classical orator:

> As when of old some Orator renown'd
> In *Athens* or free *Rome*, where Eloquence
> Flourish'd, since mute, to some great cause addrest,
> Stood in himself collected, while each part,
> Motion, each act won audience ere the tongue,
> Sometimes in hight began, as no delay
> Of Preface brooking through his Zeal of Right.
> So standing, moving, or to hight upgrown
> The Tempter all impassion'd thus began.
> (9.670–78)

Again, the tongue is central, accentuated not by its activity but by all the action going on around it before it moves. The serpent now directly addresses the tree, as if it were a living woman, the "Mother of Science" (9.680). Satan's task is to transfer his complex, concretely spiritual image of the tree directly to Eve's mind and heart, to make her accept and approve it as her goddess in place of God.

> O Sacred, Wise, and wisdom-giving Plant,
> Mother of Science, now I feel thy Power
> Within me clear, not only to discern

> Things in their Causes, but to trace the ways
> Of highest Agents, deemed however wise.
> (9.679–83)

The serpent is so successful in this particular move that if one were to ask a reader (a student, for example) to identify this passage, the reader would probably give it to Eve. Her first speech to the tree after eating the fruit echoes Satan's address (9.795–802). Satan's "proposition," that which must be proved, is that by eating this fruit Eve will overcome death and gain new life, a striking demonic parallel to the Christian promise of redemption and eternal life. The new knowledge Eve will enjoy will make her equal to the gods, who are not to be trusted, and who want to keep Eve and Adam low and ignorant, their slaves.

It would appear that Satan's overall strategy is to reconstruct Eve as the goddess superior to the gods and then to destroy the bond between Adam and God and that between Adam and Eve. The closest thing to a psychological counselor in seventeenth-century England was a close friend, a priest, a cunning man, or a cunning woman. Milton draws upon aspects of all of these figures—and upon the traditional view of the devil as a subtle interpreter of the human psyche—by giving Satan the accents of the outraged confidant. Responding to Eve's tone when she recites her version of the divine interdiction, Satan proceeds (rather like a modern therapist who deals with one fear at a time) to assuage first her apparent fear of God, and then her anxiety about death.

Satan says in effect, Queen of the Universe, don't believe those rigid threats of death. How *can* you die? By the fruit? It gives you life enabling you to know. By the Threatener? Look at me, who have touched and tasted, yet still live, and have gained more perfect life than was meant for me because I dared to go beyond myself. Shall humans be closed off from something given to beasts? (How can you truly have dominance over them if they can attain what you cannot?) Will God really be angry at such a petty transgression and not praise instead your heroic virtue, risking the pain of death, to achieve what might lead to happier life, knowledge of good and evil? If this is really knowledge of "good," how can God be just in denying it to you? If it is knowledge of evil—and evil is really real—why *shouldn't* it be known, since then it would be avoided more easily? Therefore God cannot harm you and still be a just or fair God. If he is not just, he is not God and not to be feared or obeyed. Your very fear of death removes any fear you should have of God. Maybe you *will* die, but it will be a death to be wished, putting off your human nature to put on the nature of a god. So even if death is threatened, nothing worse than this can happen. And what are the gods anyway that man can't become like them, eating their food? (Cf. 9.685–717.)

Eve had said that God's command about the tree was the "Sole Daughter of his voice" (9.653). Satan masterfully deconstructs, in Eve's mind, the idea of God into the "gods." He convinces her of this proposition by getting her to accept as real the image of the tree as the true source of knowledge, and by persuading her that she is the only daughter of the true Mother of Science, the original of true divinity. Satan's argument invokes the ancient tradition that the Mother Earth goddess is prior and superior to the "gods" because she is visibly productive:

> The Gods are first, and that advantage use
> On our belief, that all from them proceeds;
> I question it, for this fair Earth I see,
> Warm'd by the Sun, producing every kind,
> Them nothing . . .[43]
> (9.718–22)

In this final intimate oration—combining just the right elements of respectful distance and concerned familiarity—Satan confirms and supports his proposition, refutes all of Eve's questions and her reassertion of the divine prohibition, and concludes by affirming not just her desire for the fruit but her *need* for it. "He ended, and his words replete with guile / Into her heart too easy entrance won" (9.733–34). The oration is plentifully supplied, stuffed with everything designed to "entrance" Eve's heart—too easy an entrancement.

For Eve, the fruit becomes a kind of therapeutic cure for all her wonder, bewilderment, and anxiety. She is ultimately defined by Satan as the "Goddess humane" (9.732), the goddess who cares more about the human and the natural than about the gods. It is important to note, however, that Satan only gains entrance to her heart—he does not finally possess it. She must complete the sin by abandoning "right Reason" and consciously choosing to disobey the injunction. Still innocent, she stands gazing on the fruit, entranced in the gaze Satan has verbally transferred from his love-smitten serpent to her, and compelled by the noontide claims of her unfallen but human body. Satan convinces her that her obedience has been misplaced. She owes more to the maternal tree than to the threatening, forbidding Father God. Satan replaces God in her mind with the tree, and the Mother Tree, representing now for Eve all the creative forces of bountiful Nature and beautiful Earth, becomes the mother that Eve never had. The tree, heavy with fruit for her to eat and drink, has a new kind of lifegiving power. As mistress, empress, universal dame, goddess humane, she is the only begotten daughter of the "Mother of Science," begotten by Satan upon Eve's first and fundamental notion of her identity given to her by the voice of God at her creation: "What thou seest, What there thou seest fair creature is thyself . . . Mother of human race" (4.467–75). Accepting and approving the notion that she is the true daughter of the Mother Tree is the final offspring of Satan's attempt to engender "pride" in the dream he gave her (4.809), and constitutes Eve's sin before she tastes the apple.

Endeavors of the Heart

The entire subsequent relationship between Adam and Eve is best traced in the poem in terms of their heart responses. Adam feels heart "tremors" after Eve's heart has been won. He feels the "falt'ring measure" (9.846), as if his heart has momentarily stopped; he has a mild heart failure, a premonition, a human reverberation of the massive lethargy or stroke that afflicted Satan in the excruciating intellectual birth of Sin. The music of the heart, the perfect harmony of music and poetry in unison between Adam and Eve, has ceased. Eve now appears to Adam in the persona of a newly fledged actress; as in Boehme's version of all this, the new knowledge that Eve has attained is acute *self*-consciousness.[44] Satan has not only convinced her that she is the sole daughter of the Tree of Knowledge, but he has made an actress of her, a curious paradigm of the project that the *soi-disant* diabolist John Wilmot was to carry out with Elizabeth Barry. Milton's Eve becomes an epic counterpart to the advent of women on the public stage, a model for the Restoration actress. Milton was well aware of women acting in the accustomed hyperbolic manner in the London theater of the 1660s:

> in her face excuse
> Came Prologue, and Apology to prompt,
> Which with bland words at will she thus addrest.
> Hast thou not wondered, *Adam*, at my stay?
> Thee I have misst, and thought it long, depriv'd

> Thy presence, agony of love till now
> Not felt.
> (9.853–59)

"Wonder" again, but now self-manipulated wonder. Adam knows at once that Eve has fallen—has suffered a rape or violation—and that Paradise is indeed "lost," as he communes with himself before speaking to her: "How art thou lost, how on a sudden lost, / Defac't, deflow'r'd, and now to Death devote?" (9.900–901). Satan has de-faced her, but she now has a new "face," the face of those who know how to make a face for any occasion. The words "face" and "surface" have of course the same root, a derivation exploited best perhaps in the comic drama of Jonson and Sheridan, and Eve the actress is now attempting desperately to carry off a lighthearted improvisation. She gushes about the divine effect of the tree to open eyes. The Mother of Science has opened her eyes, dilated her spirits, and amplified her "Heart" (9.876), recalling the Father's idea of Satan's exalted heart (7.150). Eve has grown up to godhead; she has reached her maturity as the daughter of "Science." The maternal tree has brought her to a new birth. Satan's final entrance and entrancement—with her own active participation—has encompassed her heart and dilated it with his own toxic blood spirits. Adam and Eve both become "intoxicated" (9.1008).

Adam knows he is ruined because his heart tells him so. He could afford another rib but not another heart: "loss of thee / would never from my heart" (9.912–13). It is intriguing to speculate about what Adam could or should have done (whether he might have taken it upon himself to die *for* Eve, not simply with her), and obviously the narrator disapproves of his decision, but the point seems to be that his heart has made his decision for him.[45] It seems now as if austere Adam has himself caught the contagion of fallen Eve's theatricality. Eve is his heartmate and his soulmate, as she reaffirms, histrionically:

> but short
> Of thy perfection, how shall I attain,
> *Adam*, from whose dear side I boast me sprung,
> And gladly of our Union hear thee speak,
> One Heart, one Soul in both.
> (9.963–67)

Adam says, "I feel / The Link of Nature draw me" (9.913–14)—Nature now as a vital chain of fate, a bond shared by fallen human and fallen angelic creatures. Even Satan and Sin have a deep heart sympathy and resonance (10.357–58). Adam's mental recitation of the "one flesh" formula seals his original marriage vow to Eve, in "bliss or woe" (9.916), and then he restates the vow aloud to her:

> So forcible within my heart I feel
> The Bond of Nature draw me to my own,
> My own in thee, for what thou art is mine;
> Our State cannot be sever'd, we are one,
> One Flesh; to lose thee were to lose myself
> (9.955–59)

As book 10 opens, we move from the fallible human heart to the "Heart / Omniscient" of God (10.6–7). It would seem that the "heart" is the chief thing Milton's God and his human creatures have in common, that the heart is the source of creativity and love and regret, the true *imago dei*. Of course in biblical terms, the corrupted heart of mankind is the source as well of all evil. The stress in *Paradise Lost* is on Satan's "heinous and despiteful act" (10.1), not man's, and the wisdom of God's all-knowing heart, not mind. This is one of only two specific allusions to the "heart" of the Father (as opposed to the "bosom") in the poem; the other is at 11.887 when God, in language that echoes Gen. 6.6, was "Griev'd at his heart" because of the violence and corruption of Adam's progeny. The heart of the Father has ambivalent emotions toward man. As God again gazes upon man from Heaven, now fallen man, Milton might more conventionally have referred to the omniscient *mind* of God, and to Satan's attempt upon the "heart" of man, but the passage affirms the primacy of the heart feelings of the Creator/Author—a heart that loves and *cannot* be deceived—and of his heart bond with his fallible human creatures.

Milton underscores the heart bond of creature to creature in the subsequent reconciliation of Adam and Eve. Eve sitting desolate in her own affliction nevertheless arises and gently approaches Adam, who, lying outstretched on the ground, has just delivered himself of the longest speech in the poem, a 125-line self-pitying lament for the human condition and his posterity, modeled on Job but without Job's furious sense of his own integrity. She brings "Soft words to his fierce passion" (10.865), and Adam, seeing not Eve but the serpent who caused their fall, reviles her in a tirade remarkable for its vehement distillation of a number of seventeenth-century antifeminist clichés, then turns away from her, the only time he does so in the poem:

> He added not, and from her turn'd, but Eve
> Not so repulst, with Tears that ceas'd not flowing,
> And tresses all disorder'd, at his feet
> Fell humble, and embracing them, besought
> His peace, and thus proceeded in her plaint.
> Forsake me not thus, *Adam*, witness Heav'n
> What love sincere, and reverence in my heart
> I bear thee, and unweeting have offended,
> Unhappily deceiv'd. . . .
> (10.909–17)

In John 13, at the moment the devil is represented as putting "into the heart" of Judas Iscariot the notion of betraying him, Jesus rises from his last supper and, taking off his clothes in a gesture that reveals his human vulnerability and mortal bond with his disciples, girds himself with a towel. With the towel he washes his disciples' feet from a basin of water. After doing this, he tells them that he has given them "an example, that ye should do as I have done to you" (13.15). One of the disciples, "leaning on Jesus' bosom" (13.23), asks him who it is who shall betray him and after the sop is given to Judas, "Satan entered into him" (13.27), and Judas goes out into the night. Jesus then gives his disciples "a new commandment," "that ye love one another; as I have loved you. . . . Let not your heart be troubled; ye believe in God, believe also in me. In my Father's house are many mansions . . . I go to prepare a place for you" (13.34–14.2). Here Jesus seems to associate the heart and true belief.

Book 10 of *Paradise Lost*, the book that recounts the regeneration of Adam and Eve and God's revenge upon Satan, is framed by the divine image of the washing and embracing of the feet. When the Son is sent to judge Adam and Eve after their transgression, "pitying how they stood / Before him naked to the air," he "disdain'd not to begin / Thenceforth the form of servant to assume, / As when he wash'd his servants' feet" (10.210–15). The Son, generated from his Father's "bosom," here becomes the father of the man; he takes upon himself the role of the father of the human family, a far different image of "the father" from that of Milton's Almighty, and clothes the outward and inward nakedness of "his Enemies . . . from his Father's sight" (10.219–23) against the coming cold and the eventual hostility that will result in his crucifixion and death. When Eve comes with soft words to Adam, we recall her original "softness" and "grace" and the resonance of meaning in "softness" as gentleness, compassion, tenderness, nurture, as well as the resonance of human and divine "grace." We also might recall the passage in the Gospels where Jesus visits the house of the Pharisee, Simon. A "woman in the city, which was a sinner," came and stood at his feet behind Jesus "weeping, and began to wash his feet with tears, and did wipe them with the hairs of her head, and kissed his feet" (Luke 7.37–38). Simon, a shrewd man, quietly watches all this thinking that if Jesus were really a prophet, he would know what kind of woman she is. Jesus takes Simon aside, tells him a short parable, then asks him if he "sees" this woman. Adam and Simon, in these passages, do not see the women before them, only the troubled screen of their own presuppositions. Jesus tells Simon that the woman's sins, "which are many, are forgiven; for she loved much" (7.47).

The narrator unobtrusively spells the heroic virtues of his new epic in the final appeal to his "celestial Patroness" in the opening of book 9, the book of the Fall. In the context of imploring a maternal Muse, a divine figure of feminine spiritual wisdom who without his bidding now comes back to him night after night to nourish, inspire, and dictate his verse, Milton implies that the transcendent human virtue is "the better fortitude / Of Patience and Heroic Martyrdom" (9.31–32). This passage sets the terms and the tone for the greatest exertion of heroism in the poem, Eve's undaunted and loving return to Adam after his rejection of her, and her expression of her willingness to die for him. This effort is all the more heroic in the light of the divine judgment, when the same Son who will wash the disciples' feet says to Adam, in Eve's presence,

> Was shee thy God, that her thou didst obey
> Before his voice, or was she made thy guide,
> Superior, or but equal, that to her
> Thou didst resign thy Manhood, and the Place
> Wherein God set thee above her made of thee,
> And for thee, whose perfection far excell'd
> Hers in all real dignity: Adorn'd
> She was indeed, and lovely to attract
> Thy Love, not thy Subjection, and her Gifts
> Were such as under Government well seem'd,
> Unseemly to bear rule, which was thy part
> And person, hadst thou known thyself aright.
> (10.145–56)

I take it (with Fowler) that the Son is thinking of Eve's external royal dignity and the power of her feminine presence when with Adam, but this is the most terrible indictment of Eve in the poem. It comes not simply from God but from the mediating Son (who here sounds like the Father), and she is standing in the presence of the Son and of Adam.[46] The Son here shames Adam's manhood—his male sexuality—in the same breath that he shames his self-knowledge, and Eve is redefined in Adam's shame. She here experiences what it is like to be physically present and yet almost refined out of existence by divine exclusion. But she holds fast. She exercises that *active* "patience"—an achieved, experiential virtue, not one that is simply given, like the "Truth, Wisdom, Sanctitude severe" (4.293) of unfallen Adam and Eve—which the later Milton found so important but difficult to enact in his own life.[47] Eve returns to Adam and helps him to conquer his fear and hatred, virtually building him back up. She is lowlier than Adam, and thus by the logic of Jesus and Paul—that the last shall be first and the humble exalted—she will be greater than Adam. The twin themes of reversal of status and reversal of values are arguably the strongest and most consistent in the entire New Testament. Eve may be inferior to Adam in mind and dignity, but she acts with superior Christian virtue, according to Milton's understanding of the New Testament message.[48] She is the stronger. She will be the Mother of humankind. In her return to the afflicted Adam, blind in his rage, Eve is linked analogically with the feminine Spirit/Muse who feeds and inspires the blind poet's song, and perhaps also with Milton's first wife, Mary Powell, who returned to him, and to his nurturing third wife, Katharine Woodcock. The Spirit is further linked with the "Prevenient grace" (11.3) which comes to Adam and Eve when, with "hearts contrite" and in the lowliest sorrow, humiliation, and repentance, they prostrate themselves in the place where they were judged.

Adam and Eve's mutual interplay of regeneration has its parallel in the physician-psychologist Thomas Willis's account of how the "sacred Affections" in repentant men and women, when

> delivered from the Rational Soul into the Sensitive, do first employ the Brain with the Phantasie, then being transmitted from the Brain into the Breast, there, for that they produce in the Heart and Blood variety of Motions, receive their Complement or Perfection: Wherefore, in the Worship of God, Piety and Devotion are attributed very much to the Heart: Hence Repentance, the Love of God, and Hate of Sin, Hope of Salvation, Fear of Divine Vengeance, and many other acts of Religion, are wont to be ascribed to the work and endeavour of the Heart. The reason of which seems to be, for as much as the whole Corporeal Soul is Commanded by the Ratio-

nal Power, that in Adoring God, she should very much bow her self before the Deity, and as it were lye prostrate on the Ground.[49]

The term "endeavour of the heart" was also used by Hobbes in describing the counterpressure of the heart "to deliver itself" in response to the pressure of external stimuli,[50] but Willis—along with Milton and Puritan writers in particular—sees this "work and endeavour" of the heart as central to human religious experience. Willis's personification of the "Corporeal Soul" as a woman lying prostrate on the ground again recalls Eve's—and Adam's—prostration before the Almighty and their regenerative prayer and worship. Willis goes on to give a remarkable account, echoing the biblical language that equated blood and life, of how the blood supply to the heart and its adjacent regions ("the *Praecordia*") is increased during strong religious emotion and held there in a kind of sustained tension ("a continual *Systole*") or "long immolation" before it is "inlarged."[51] This account is a finite physiological counterpart to two of Milton's most cherished beliefs: first, the doctrine of greater poetic strength through deprivation evinced in his early poetics of chastity leading to the poetics of blindness, and second, to the dynamic of trial by "long obedience" (7.159) leading to the ultimate incarnation of God in humankind when, through the crucial intervention of the Son, "God shall be all in all" (3.315, 341).

The spiritual power of grace had removed "the stony from their hearts, and made new flesh / Regenerate grow instead" (11.4–5). In another replication of the Muse inspiring Milton with the unpremeditated verse that will enable the new heroism of patient but active self-sacrifice, grace now inspires them to breathe forth sighs "unutterable" in a new "Spirit of prayer" that flies to Heaven more speedily than any "Oratory" (11.6–8). After Satan's oratorical triumph, Adam and Eve achieve a greater nonverbal oratorical victory, a kind of ineffable language of prayer originating in hearts newly generated by the writing power of the Spirit of God. In response to Adam's later question concerning what will happen to the faithful after Christ reascends, Michael articulates this view of the power of the Spirit, which also serves as a divine response to Eve's and Adam's increasing anxieties and terrors in Eden:

> from Heav'n
> Hee to his own a Comforter will send,
> The promise of the Father, who shall dwell
> His Spirit within them, and the Law of Faith

> Working through love, upon thir hearts shall write,
> To guide them in all truth, and also arm
> With spiritual Armor, able to resist
> *Satan's* assaults, and quench his fiery darts,
> What Man can do against them, not afraid,
> Though to the death, against such cruelties
> With inward consolations recompens't
> (12.485–95)

God had implanted grace and right reason in human hearts, and Adam and Eve's prayers are the first fruits. Eve was the chief provider of care to the flowers and fruits of the garden and the one who initiated the process of regeneration in her humble reconciliation with Adam. Paradoxically, in the light of his terrible words about Eve, the Son—who in terms of the logic and chronology of *Paradise Lost* has yet to be tested as a mortal man—will follow her example more closely than Adam's in his own pastoral role on earth and in his ultimate and unexampled self-abasement. Because "man" is unskillful about which words to pray with, the Son says to the Father,

> let mee
> Interpret for him, mee his Advocate
> And propitiation, all his works on mee
> Good or not good ingraft, my Merit those
> Shall perfet, and for these my Death shall pay.
> (11.32–36)

The Son thus becomes the proleptic model for the kind of poet Milton the fledgling political writer hoped someday to become, "an interpreter and relater of the best and sagest things among mine own citizens . . . in the mother dialect,"[52] the English language and the language of the maternal Muses—divine and human—the "celestial Patroness" and mortal Eve. The Son and the poet will follow the path and discourse of the Mother of Mankind.

4

The Generous Heart
Aphra Behn, *Oroonoko*, and the Woman Writer

> All I ask is the Privilege for my masculine Part the Poet in
> me . . . to tread in those successful Paths my Predecessors
> have so long thrived in . . .
> —APHRA BEHN, *The Lucky Chance*

BECAUSE APHRA BEHN'S READING of Lucretius was a momentous event in her development as a poet, we begin with Behn and Lucretius. In the eight years between the second edition of *Paradise Lost* and her first reading of Lucretius's *De rerum natura* in the translation of Thomas Creech in 1682, she had written about sixteen plays and a fair amount of fiction, but had published very little poetry. Creech's translation of Lucretius's long poem into polished yet complex heroic couplets was immediately recognized as a major poetic achievement. Behn acknowledges its importance for her "humbler Muse" and for women in her poem "To the Unknown Daphnis on His Excellent Translation of *Lucretius*": "Thou by this *Translation* dost advance / Our Knowledge from the State of Ignorance; / And Equallst Us to Man!" She characterizes Creech as a demigod, and ends the poem with a blessing on his repose, his muse, and his mistress. We first encountered Creech's translation in the Introduction, and Lucretius has been an important presence in our reading of Harvey and Milton. In imagining how Behn read Lucretius, the following passage, which presents a vivid theatrical example of how human beings perceive external images, might have made a particular impression on her as a privileged observer of the flow of images penetrating a theatrical audience:

> Thus when pale Curtains, or the deeper Red,
> O're all the spacious *Theater* are spread,
> Which mighty *Masts* and sturdy *Pillars* bear,
> And the loose Curtains *wanton* in the Air;
> Whole Streams of *Colours* from the top do flow,
> The Rays *divide* them in their passage thro,

> And stain the Scenes, and Men, and Gods below:
> The more these Curtains spread, the pleasing *Dye*
> Rides on the beams the more, and courts the Eye;
> The gawdy *Colour* spreads o're every thing,
> All gay appear, each *Man* a *Purple* King.[1]

The streams of color coming through the curtains have an almost physical transformative power to stain and spread over the entire scene and audience, making everyone for the moment a purple king, and recall the "Rosie" irradiation of Crooke's internal "theater of the body," described in the Introduction. The Lucretian paradox of fluidity within stability also becomes a paradoxical principle in Behn's aesthetics, which combine an amazing verbal and stylistic fluency with a set of stable, recurring figural types, such as the image of the "Golden Age," riverbanks where lovers lie, or the predominant image of the passive male in repose, from Mars at the breast of Venus to Oroonoko at the place of execution. A Lucretian reading of Behn must begin, I suggest, with close attention to motion, rapidity, pace, to the variation of color in the theatrical scene, to "nature," human nature, and the divine.

In her poetry, Behn often seems to be having a conversation with the "gods," and they seem always to be the gods of love. Lucretius opens his great antireligious poem paradoxically with an invocation of the nurturing goddess Venus as the primary power behind Natura, a female god propelling the creative energies of maternal Nature herself. This magnificent opening seems to have had a special fascination for seventeenth-century women readers and writers, now given a new feminine model for inspiration and their own poetic endeavors. Richard Kroll points out that Lucy Hutchinson, the wife of the regicide, almost certainly made the first English translation of all of Lucretius's poem, and Mary Evelyn, the wife of John Evelyn, contributed a complexly gendered frontispiece to the edition of his translation of the first book of *De rerum natura* in 1656.[2] Aphra Behn's profound engagement with Lucretius thus seems to be the climactic moment in a tradition of women artists reinterpreting Lucretius's poem.

In the opening of *De rerum natura* in Creech's translation, the warm south wind "fans the Amorous fire," and soft love infuses the breasts of all creatures causing them to beget. Venus alone governs Nature, and the poet philosopher craves her as his "patron" and partner in writing the verses that he will fashion into the story of the nature of things. (This opening was also one of Milton's models for the poet/Muse relationship.) In language that Behn will appropriate into her own distinctive erotic voice, Lucretius imagines Mars refreshing himself in the Paphian court,

> Where on [Venus's] Bosom he supinely lies,
> And greedily drinks Love at both his Eyes;
> Till quite o'recome he snatches an *eager* kiss,
> And hastily goes on to greater Bliss.

The Roman male poet desires the preeminent female god as his "*Muse*," implying an erotic interplay—on the model of Venus intertwined with Mars—or the infusion of her generative power into him, so that he may rewrite Nature. He asks that she make his "Lines" her "choice . . . and most deserving Favorite"—their mutual product, the poem, an object of love.[3] Venus first brought forth Nature and now with her help Lucretius will redefine Nature in poetic verse.

All of this stands behind Behn's quintessential Lucretian poem, "To Lysander at the Musick Meeting." Lysander is usually identified as John Hoyle, the bisexual libertine advocate of Lucretian naturalistic philosophy, but Lysander may also incorporate an homage to Thomas Creech, the translator who surpasses even his divine subject in divinity. Both Hoyle and Creech take their place in Behn's poetic affections as successors to the most famous rake and erotic poet of the Restoration, her friend John Wilmot, the second earl of Rochester, who had died two years earlier, as Behn puts it in her elegy to him: "Large was his Fame, but short his Glorious Race, / Like young *Lucretius* and dy'd apace" (162).[4] Rochester also translated the opening lines of *De rerum natura*, and there are several allusions to the poet in his poems.[5] For Behn, Rochester is the first great libertine embodiment of Lucretius in her life.

If Milton in *Paradise Lost* is concerned with representing the complex figurative rape of a passive Eve by an active Satan who is forbidden to touch her, Behn in her poem to Lysander reverses the dynamic with a passive male invading the heart of a female gazer without ever touching her. Behn plunges the reader into an immediate apprehension of her sensual experience of receptivity, and establishes from the start a note of excess in the two predominating senses, sight and hearing: "It was too much, ye Gods, to see and hear; / Receiving wounds both from the Eye and Ear" (94). In his discussion of how all the senses perceive external stimuli, Lucretius stresses the wounding material power of sound:

> we *Sounds*, and Voice, and Noises hear,
> When *seeds* of Sound come in, and *strike* the Ear.
> All *Sound* is *Body*, for with painful force
> It moves the Sense....
> 'Tis certain then that *Voice*, that thus can wound,
> Is all *material*; *Body* every *Sound*.[6]

The speaker in Behn's poem is describing an experience of sensual ravishment wherein the doubled intensity of the impact visited from the object upon the senses raises the pleasure to "Extasie": "So Ravisht Lovers in each others Armes, / Faint with excess of Joy, excess of Charmes" (94). The speaker goes on to confess—in lines that recall Lucretius's Mars on the breast of Venus—that "Had I but gaz'd and fed my greedy Eyes," perhaps the source of her pleasure had been less, but the addition of music completed the conquest: "You storm'd without, and Harmony within." It is only later, after having read through the poem, that one realizes that all this sensual commotion has been engendered by a beautiful young man reclining passively, probably not even looking at her, and listening to music. But for the female gazer, his "Body easey and all tempting lay, / Inspiring wishes which the Eyes betray, / In all that have the fate to glance that way." As often in Behn, there is a strong imaginative equation of love and fate, but she goes on to elevate the subject to the status of an angel "raptured" upon a cloud, radiating his power from the top down as in Lucretius's theatrical example of the flow of colors descending upon the spectators. We also see in this poem the recurring motif of an ever-varying linkage between the eye and the heart in Behn's language of love. Behn the poet and gazer concludes that

> When from so many ways Loves Arrows storm,
> Who can the heedless Heart defend from harm?
> Beauty and *Musick* must the Soul disarme;
> Since Harmony, like Fire to Wax, does fit
> The softned Heart Impressions to admit.
> (94)

As Eve's heart is finally penetrated and vanquished by the visual and aural assault of Satan, so is the heart of Behn's active female gazer vanquished by the passive power of her male subject. In this poem Behn gives the reader a miniature version of the "story" of the speaker's heart. The trope of the "story of my Heart," or the "history of my Heart" occurs in her long translated poem "A Voyage to the Isle of Love" (247, 305), and "the Hearts fond story" comes up again in another poem "To J. H." (202). In terms of narrative, *Oroonoko* is her most extended and complex elaboration of "the story of the Heart," a phrase we shall encounter again in Steele's *The Conscious Lovers* (1722) when we consider the action of *Clarissa* in Chapter 5.

The Transcendent Muse

In this chapter, I concentrate on the rhetoric of the heart in the last eleven years of Behn's writing life, and she was writing more prolifically and with more fervor and urgency as her end approached.[7] Behn has two public poetic personae—the one she constructs, and the one male writers constructed for her. I shall focus on Behn's poetic self-inscriptions later, but we shall look first at how some contemporary male poets described her. Much has been said in recent commentary about the corrupt female "poetess" male satirists like Robert Gould and Matthew Prior made of her;[8] not enough has been said about the more positive poetic persona created by less well known writers like John Cooper and Daniel Kendrick.

In moving from Milton to a consideration of Behn's poetry, we shall reflect first upon how nine male poets (the number seems consciously to evoke the Nine Muses), in their dedicatory verses to her *Poems on Several Occasions* (1684), represented her poetic powers in relation to the male heart. The first three of these poets acknowledge her envied power to subdue the male heart and pen, to strike "Poetick fire" in every breast, and to tame the savage heart to the sweet captivity of her verse.[9] They also represent her as a new phenomenon in English poetry, the perfect androgynous union of, on the one hand, female sweetness (119), softness (117), tenderness, beauty, prophetic power (120), the influence of the Graces, and on the other, male thought and vigor, and "manly Grace" and beauty (119). Charles Gildon, invoking the Galenic sexual model, remarked in a preface to a play of Behn's published after her death that "to draw Mrs. Behn to the life one must write like her, that is, with all the softness of her sex and all the fire of ours."[10] The male poets liken Behn's androgynous beauty to that of young "*David's* face" (119), recalling the master delineator of the biblical heart in the Psalms. But going far beyond customary hyperbole is the dedicatory poets' attribution to Behn not only of the Lucretian power of expressing the beauty of Venus and the power of Mars in sexual union but of embodying the divine androgynous power of the male/female *imago dei* found in the hermeticist tradition. Combining classical and biblical allusions, they virtually make her the new female god of creation, replacing the male Father God in the Garden of Eden as she surveys her good works:

> With all the *thought* and *vigour* of our Sex
> The moving *softness* of your own you mix.
> The *Queen* of Beauty and the *God* of Wars
> Imbracing lie in thy due temper'd Verse,
> *Venus* her sweetness and the force of *Mars*.
> Thus thy luxuriant Muse her pleasure takes,
> As *God* of old in *Eden*'s blissful walks;
> The Beauties of her new Creation view'd,
> Full of content She sees that it is *good*.[11]
> (117–18)

Daniel Kendrick, in his dedicatory poem to Behn's prose translation of the French love allegorist Paul Tallemant, "Lycidus: Or, the Lover in Fashion," celebrates in Behn "A Brain so Glorious, and a Face so fair," the refined union of a Venerean body and a Minervan mind (296). Her "manly numbers" flow soft as her lips and charming as her eye. But Kendrick transcends praising the androgynous Behn to call her "more than Woman! more than man," a godlike creature, the contemporary equivalent of the Roman goddess Astraea.[12] By this time Behn's famous nom de plume was well established, but Kendrick gives Astraea the added dimension of possessing a familiarity with the Nine Muses that is denied to male poets. Whereas Milton in the opening of *Paradise Lost* struggles, as we have seen, to conjure the heavenly Muse to come to him and reveal the inner workings of the divine world, Behn is represented by this male poet as beyond gender but enjoying a special open and unreserved access to the Muses: "Upon her Pen await those Learned Nine" (297). Kendrick also rehearses the by now familiar image of Behn as prophetess, "Beauteous Prophetess" in the opening line, and at the end the "Mighty Prophetess" who has the power, like Ezekiel, to wave the "Mystick wand" of her pen and raise the dead (296, 298). Similarly, in her poem to the failed playwright Edward Howard, Behn herself enlists the feminine powers of the Muse to recuperate the phallic pen of her disgraced friend.[13] And we recall that the word "tread," in the epigraph for this chapter, has a male sexual connotation. The theme of resurrection takes many forms in Behn's writing and culminates, as we shall see, in *Oroonoko*.

In the anonymous nine-stanza dedicatory poem to the 1684 edition of her poems, Behn is contrasted with "bold Magicians in Philosophy" (124) who vainly attempt to conjure the angels down from heaven with fantastic charms and magic circles (barbaric alchemical counterparts to the conjuring poet Milton), whereas Behn is the "great Prophetess" whose "tuneful breast" is the wondrous storehouse and source (in the heart) of her godlike power to ravish her hearers (125). The poet invokes Urania and several other Muses by name to laud Behn as the master-Muse or universal poet whose "large capacious Brain" contains the images of all things, an image of "What Divine Nature can in Woman doe" (124). While the dull male sex has trod in beaten paths, she uses all her wit and strength to move at a different pace (127) and becomes the learned "Chymist" who can protect against the power of death and "raise the buried Man" (128). Again we hear the accents of a quasi-medical discourse directed toward Behn as female prophet of male resurrection.

We turn finally to the most important of the nine dedicatory poems in this volume, the one by Thomas Creech. Nineteen years her junior, he had recently published his translation of Lucretius and is the one male contributor to the commendatory verses of her 1684 volume to praise Behn for a new kind of writing of the heart. In a perfect Lucretian metaphor for Behn's poetics, Creech says she incorporates in one "rich and flowing stream" all the wealth of the Nine Muses, leaving them dry (121). The image evokes the stream of invisible particles constantly flowing in the Lucretian universe, as well as the particular poetic stream welling up from the Hippocrene of the erotic heart. She in fact *is* the new Muse. (Here let us recall that Milton had redefined the Muse for himself and for contemporary poets as his own personal, nurturing feminine provider, the Sister of Wisdom, who eventually came to him unbidden.) Creech then, in what Maureen Duffy calls "a small erotic masterpiece," describes how Behn as the ultimate Muse undertakes a "new way of Love" through her pen.[14] She has given Cupid a new weapon far more powerful than all of his darts, a *feminine* pen that disarms men and "massacres more Hearts" than Cupid ever could. Hence Behn replaces not only the Nine Muses but Cupid himself. For Creech, the brilliant translator of Lucretius's omnipotent Venus, Behn becomes a new goddess of poetic power and love. The ancient image of a sword cutting the heart to pieces—the original biblical and epic anatomy of the heart in war—is now transformed in Behn into an "easie softness" that steals into men's eyes, comes upon them unawares, and destroys them as the exterminating angel slew the Assyrians in the "silent night." She has the divine power of life and death in her pen. Creech is at one with the male voice of the Song of Solomon who implores his beloved, "Set me as a seal upon thine heart," for he knows that "love is strong as death" (8.6).[15] Oroonoko, Behn's godlike warrior and lover, will later retreat to his military camp after making love to the beautiful Imoinda "with a Heart sad as Death, dying Eyes, and sighing Soul."[16]

Creech goes on to say that this female-authored erotic verse has the power to bind all its male hearers in "inchanting Groves," leading them to fantasize rapturous lovemaking with her heroine in "the very Bower of Bliss" (evoking the bowers of Spenser and Milton) where the male listener/reader lies now "in the same Trance" with Behn's young lovers, "And in their amorous Ecstasies we die." For Creech, Behn rewrites the "Raptures" (121) of the erotic heart, going beyond Carew's notorious "A Rapture" and recalling Milton's earlier narrator of the companion poems who climaxes "Il Penseroso" with "Dissolve me into ecstasies," a quasi-erotic and sensual poetic plea for divine vision. In contrast to this dissolution, the magic "Philter" (or drug) of Behn's verse "trickles to the Heart" (122), recalling Lucretius's famous image in book 4 of *De rerum natura*, and her written raptures are transfused like a benevolent infection throughout the erotic body: "You Nymphs, who deaf to Love's soft lays have been, / Reade here, and suck the sweet destruction in" (122). The absorptive, concoctive Galenic body is female as well as male, which Creech says "burns with a constant flame, / Like what you write, and always is the same" (122). Behn will use the same image for the usurper "desire" in her great poem "On Desire," to be discussed later. Behn's writings burns like love—*her* act of writing is the act of love consuming itself in the world of fallen Adam and Eve. As the transcendent Muse, she excels even Orpheus (for Milton the type of the male poet) because she not only inspires the stones but strikes living fire from them. Behn is "Loves great *Sultana*" (recalling the idiomatic term for a royal mistress or courtesan), who, echoing Milton's serpent, says to all lovers, male and female, "you shall not die," having "ravisht" them "out of breath." Her "elevated poetry" has such power, Creech says, that Behn can massacre her lovers' hearts yet still resurrect those lovers out of a state of "black Despair" into a new dimension of life and harmony, a new poetic afterlife.

Uneasy Rage

In tracing Behn's representation of the gendered heart in her own imaginative writing, we turn first to "The Golden Age," a paraphrase of a French original by Tallemant. The narrative voice of this poem, a tantalizing evocation of female accents (addressing "Honour" as the "base Debaucher of the generous heart, / That teaches all our Looks and Actions Art" [34]) and of a conventionally *carpe diem* male lover's plea at the end ("Then let us *Sylvia* yet be wise, / And the Gay hasty minutes prize" [35]), is a choice example of how Behn blends and hybridizes female and male elements in her poetry and other writing. The voice is further complicated in that it may be androgynous, like the voice of Milton's Spirit in book 1 of *Paradise Lost*, or the voice speaking at the end could be—instead of male—that of a wiser female narrator instructing a less experienced younger woman. In any event, the predominating voice is female—that of the "generous heart"—and creates the male elements in the poem. At the start of the poem, Behn depicts a "Virgin Earth" whose teeming womb contains "all Nature and all sexes," a multisexual or pansexual source of life and new creation. For Behn, as for Lucretius (whose Venus first brings forth Nature), a Venerean Great Mother is the source of life and love "without the Aids of men" (31). Creech saw Behn as a transcendent Muse with the power of life and death in her pen—woman as man's fate. In Behn's paradise there is no prevailing male principle of action or of heat, but both sexes share the "Effect of kindling Flame." Both sexes meet "uncontroul'd" and every vow is inviolably true. Here there are no rapacious interventions of the male-constructed "Plough" (31) or of fond religious causes, or fopperies of the gown or "Politick Curbs to keep man in," and above all there is no "Honour," the cruel law devised by men that first damned woman to the sin of shame, a niggard Miser—like all the grasping, hoarding, invasive, proprietary old (and some young) men in Behn's comedies—who debauches the "generous heart" (34) of female erotic love.

We turn now to the rhetoric of the gendered heart in Behn's comedies. Her best known play, *The Rover* (part 1), was written and produced just a year after the spectacular debuts of Wycherley's *The Country Wife* and Etherege's *The Man of Mode* in 1675 and 1676. With the latter's glamorous yet satiric portrayal of Rochester as Dorimant, Behn gives her own version of Wilmot as the Rover, Willmore, and more important, offers a fascinating contrast between two versions of the female heart, two poles of her rich imaginary of the female spectrum, in Hellena and Angellica

Bianca. In fact, there is more talk about the heart in Behn's two *Rover* comedies—and in more varied Galenic permutations—than in *The Country Wife*, *The Man of Mode*, and Congreve's *The Way of the World* combined. Restoration comedies usually begin with men speaking, and women get their chance to open a scene later, often in the second act. Behn's comedy begins with women speaking. Hellena's elder sister Florinda initiates the complex sexual rhetoric of the heart in this play by saying that something "about [her] heart" pleads "kindly" for her lover Belvile, and no one else can "enter" there. "Kind" is Behn's favorite term for female sexual readiness and compliance.[17] Florinda's heart speaks within her, having its own autonomous voice as a kind of gatekeeper to the house of her heart, but this structure is under almost constant threat throughout the play. Florinda is saved by Belvile from the "licensed lust" of common soldiers before the action of the play begins, then subject to rape by the Rover, then by Blunt and Frederick, then by the English gang, and finally even by her own unwitting brother, Pedro.

Hellena is more assertive and luckier than her sister. A virtuous yet mischievous Spanish girl trying to elude confinement in a nunnery, she initiates a female masquerade in search of a man of her own choosing during carnival. Her memorable call to her sister, "We'll outwit twenty brothers, if you'll be ruled by me . . . let's ramble" (164), is an almost innocent rejoinder to Rochester's flagrantly obscene "A Ramble in St. James's Park." Like the female speaker in "To Lysander at the Musick Meeting," she has a wishing heart. She tells Florinda, "but since you have set my heart a-wishing—I am resolved to know for what. . . . I don't intend every he that likes me shall have me, but he that I like. . . . I came thence not . . . to take an eternal farewell of the world, but to love, and to be beloved, and I will be beloved" (189). Hellena's heart talk is pragmatic, funny, and erotic, as when she asks Willmore to "swear to keep [his] heart, and not bestow it between this and that" (171). Hellena is the prime example in Behn's comedies of the heroine who chooses her lover without losing her heart, and her "wishing" heart speech has a poignant resonance with Behn's own words to Lycidas (John Hoyle) in *Love Letters to a Gentleman*: "Confess you are the teasingest creature in the world, rather than suffer me to think you neglect me . . . that have chosen you from all the whole creation, to give my entire esteem to."[18]

Hellena is virginal in body, but curious and sexually experienced, adventurous, and experimental in mind and imagination. Her "humour" is gay, sanguine, warm-blooded, open, anything but that of the conventional Galenic cold or unresponsive female, and the words "humour" and "heart" abound in her speech. Her name clearly recalls Helen of Troy (and the "hell" wrought by that Helen), making the Rover Willmore her Paris. Instead of employing the male playwrights' device of a Medley (as in *The Man of Mode*) or a Horner to portray female beauty, Behn gives Hellena the remarkable gift of standing back from her own body and describing it as a vibrant and vivacious anatomical model of feminine eroticism: "have I not a world of youth? a humour gay? a beauty passable? a vigour desirable? well shaped? clean limbed? sweet breathed?" (160). Angellica Bianca, on the other hand, a somewhat older and exceedingly illustrious Neapolitan courtesan, has a wide experience of physical intercourse with men but possesses a "virgin heart" (213), which feels love for the first time in the physical presence of Willmore. Hellena the "wildcat" is a virgin in body but not imagination; Angellica Bianca the courtesan is an undefiled virgin in imagination but not in body. Behn plays upon the physiological and mental aspects of the female heart. For Hellena, the wishing heart is the Lucretian driving source of her physical and emotional being. For Angellica, the Galenic virgin heart is a special untouched space in her inmost being that is reserved for true love when she finds it.

In further contrast to Hellena, Angellica Bianca gives her "virgin heart" to Willmore. In Behn, as in her master Shakespeare, the heart in love is subject to transfer, manipulation, doubling, and all kinds of "transports." The male heart penetrates the female heart, the female heart becomes imprisoned in the male heart, hearts intermingle, exchange places in a shifting calculus of power relations, or become lost. As with Hellena, Willmore has three major dialogues with Angellica. The first reflects Behn's skill in dramatizing her figurative version of Lucretian mutual interpenetration of hearts. After putting a small erotic picture of Angellica in his breast so that it can interact with his injured heart ("I saw your charming picture and was wounded; quite through my soul each pointed beauty ran" [182]), Willmore turns the full force of his masculine presence upon her ("I will gaze—to let you see my strength") and she responds in an aside, "His words go through me to the very soul" (185). She tells him in blank verse that he has "a charm / In every word that draws [her] heart away" (187), presumably her "virgin heart" and her true love. She is in the same position as Astraea in *Love Letters to a Gentleman*, and as the speaker of Behn's late philosophical poem "On Desire," when she describes "desire" as "a new found pain" that has gained dominion in a part of her "unheeded and unguarded, heart" (281). One is reminded of Behn's epistemological proposition to the reader in *The Fair Jilt*: "I'll prove to you the strong effects of love in some unguarded and ungoverned hearts; where it rages beyond the inspirations of a god all soft and gentle, and reigns more like a Fury from Hell."[19] The demonically possessed Miranda of this novella is close in spirit to the Miltonic paradigm of Satan possessed by the Galenic "heart of hell" we explored in the last chapter. Behn the Lucretian anatomist of the usurped heart elaborates: "But Love, who had hitherto but played with her heart, and given it naught but pleasing, wanton wounds . . . sent an arrow dipped in the most tormenting flames that rage in hearts most sensible! He struck it home and deep, with all the malice of an angry god."[20] Or, as Ned Blunt, speaking of the magnificent courtesan La Nuche, puts it more bluntly in *The Rover* (part 2): "Look how Willmore eyes her, the Rogue's smitten heart deep—Whores."[21]

"Desire" comes upon the speaker of Behn's poem "On Desire" as a "mischievous usurper," as an inopportune "uneasy rage" that subdues the "glories" she has so far achieved in life and "the nobler fate" she has reason to expect. She knows that the "desire" which courses through her bloodstream like an infection, causing her "pleasing pain," is not a present or a future good. When she has previously conjured desire to appear it eluded her; now it is destroying her. The speaker of the poem might as well be Angellica Bianca or Aphra Behn, facing their respective "dear shepherds":

> Tell me, thou nimble fire, that dost dilate
> Thy mighty force thro every part,
> What God, or Human power did thee create
> In my, till now, unfacil heart?
> . . . .
> 'Tis thou that tremblest in my heart
> When the dear Shepherd do's appear,
> I faint, I dye with pleasing pain,
> My words intruding sighing break
> When e're I touch the charming swain
> When e're I gaze, when e're I speak.
> ("On Desire," 282–83)

The female heart in Behn is represented as unguarded, ungoverned, unheeded, unfacile until awakened by "desire," curiosity, "wishing," or a combination of these. This heart can be the "destinie" of all male hearts or the invader of those hearts, like Clemena in "A Pastoral Pindarick . . . Between Damon and Aminta" (276), but the female heart is usually receptive, "attractive" in the Galenic sense, drawing male language into its interior, for good or ill to the heart's subject, as in the words of Behn's Oenone (in "Oenone to Paris"):

> Quick to my Heart the perjur'd Accents ran,
> Which I took in, believ'd, and was undone.
> Vows are Loves poyson'd Arrows, & the heart
> So wounded, rarely finds a Cure in Art.
> At least this heart which Fate has destin'd yours,
> This heart unpractic'd in Loves mystick pow'rs,
> For I am soft, and young as *April* Flowers.
> (13–14)

These examples of the usurped or invaded female heart, but especially the complex transactions of Angellica's heart in relation to Willmore, form a case study in Behn's delineation of female "desire," a remarkable anticipation of how John Locke would define "desire" in terms of "uneasiness" just a year later in *An Essay Concerning Human Understanding*. Locke's meditation on desire attempts to answer the question, why do we act as we do? What is the fundamental motive of human action and agency? He then locates the primary motive for change in the human situation in discontent, dis-ease, discomfort, pain—what he defines as "uneasiness," what Behn defines more vividly as "uneasy rage," the power of desire. For Locke, will and desire are not the same thing. Will or power of volition is conversant only about our individual actions, whereas desire is the very state of uneasiness itself. "All pain of the body, of what sort soever, and disquiet of mind, is uneasiness," and until some form of relief or "ease" is attained, we remain in a state of desire or anxiety. As an extreme example of this desire, Locke cites the piercing cry of the barren Rachel to Jacob, "Give me children or I die!" (Gen. 30.1).[22] Locke links the cry of a woman with the fundamental meaning of desire, and fastens on a key element of Restoration anxiety, from the prevailing undercurrent of "unease" articulated in the resurgence of dramatic comedy to the growing uneasiness of Milton's heroic pair in *Paradise Lost*. And Locke's discourse on desire, ultimately an assertion of the underlying irrational ground of human motivation as he understood it, has profound relevance to the emergence of the drama and fiction of Aphra Behn, especially the writing of *Oroonoko*.

In the *Essay*, Locke talks all around the subject of sexual desire, alluding to it in the Rachel passage, hinting at it in a Galenic formulation when he refers to "other natural desires" that determine people's wills "for the preservation of themselves, and the continuation of their species," finally letting St. Paul say it: "'It is better to marry than to burn' . . . where we may see what it is that chiefly drives men into the enjoyments of a conjugal life. A little burning felt pushes us more powerfully than greater pleasures in prospect draw or allure." He explicitly argues, as Behn does implicitly, that the pressure of "present uneasiness" determines our actions far more directly than the attractions of "the greater good." And he reinforces this idea by quoting the most influential Roman love poet for the Restoration: "Video meliora, proboque, deteriora sequor [I see the good, and approve it, but follow the bad]," a sentiment that coincides with St. Paul's even more culturally influential, "For the good that I would I do not: but the evil which I would not that I do" (Rom. 7.19).[23]

What Locke goes on to say about passion is an apt description of Angellica Bianca's behavior for the rest of the play (reading "woman" for "man"): "Thus any vehement pain of the body; the ungovernable passion of a man violently in love; or the impatient desire of revenge, keeps the will steady and intent."[24] Angellica says "I am all rage!" and goes on to tell Moretta, her bawd, that if she had given Willmore all her earnings, she would not have lost a sigh:

> But I have given him my eternal rest,
> My whole repose, my future joys, my heart!
> My virgin heart, Moretta! Oh 'tis gone!
> (213)

We learn that Angellica's virgin heart, a uniquely special place in her being, has close affinities with an innocent, paradisiacal future life. Unfortunately for her, however, after inviting him into her chamber for two hours of love she gives him five hundred crowns, literally making him a "prostitute" by enabling him, in Moretta's words, "to *set himself out* for other lovers" (213, my emphasis). "Set himself out" suggests the Latin derivation of "prostitute" from to "stand before" or "stand out" for sale. Even her paying him "a heart entire" was not enough to raise him up to her level and make him "all soul . . . all soft and constant," so she reverts to violence, and in the final act stalks him around the stage with a pistol pointed at his heart: "Does not thy guilty blood run shivering through thy veins?" He replies with perfect Galenic male aplomb: "Faith, no child, my blood keeps its old ebbs and flows still, and that usual heat too, that could oblige thee with a kindness, had I but opportunity" (235).

If the female heart in Behn is at once warm, "tender," and receptive, as well as wishing and projective, the male heart, especially in the plays, is virtually an internal metonym for the phallus—generally hot, aggressive, and almost always ready to bestow a "kindness." In her first dialogue with Willmore, Hellena guesses he must have "a foolish inconstant English heart," that is, one that cannot contain or hold love. Willmore makes this clear by saying he has a world of love (or lust) "in store," as if his love were a quantifiable commodity pent up inside that must be discharged, as in Lucretius's graphic ejaculatory rhetoric as rendered by Dryden. His language of love sounds rather like the natural philosopher talking about fluids under pressure in containers, or Harvey on the measurable quantity of blood in any given body. Later Willmore tells Hellena he has "a heart with a hole quite thro'it," one that will not hold her in it for long (194). For Behn, in opposition to Dryden's Lucretius, men are "the leaky kind."

As she knowingly drew near the end of her productive life as a literary artist, and just two years before the composition of *Oroonoko*, Aphra Behn created a metaphor of the woman writer in the world by making Lady Fulbank, the most important character in her late, dark comedy *The Lucky Chance* (1686), the woman writer-in-the-play. Lady Fulbank—the young wife of Sir Cautious Fulbank, a rich old city alderman—writes and produces her own version of a masque of Eros to test the constancy of her libertine lover, Gayman. We can glimpse the emergence, in the Restoration, of the woman writer as a literary construct by briefly noting the contrast between Lady Fulbank as a playwright and Wycherley's brilliant characterization of Margery Pinchwife, the "country wife," as a writer of love letters from the heart and incipient dramatic scenarios. Her brutal and foolish husband, like Sir Cautious, equates women and money throughout the play, and in an indelible formulation that applies as aptly to *The Lucky Chance* as to *The Country Wife*, sees them both as objects that must be controlled by men at all times: "Our sisters and daughters, like usurers' money, are safest when put out; but our wives, like their writings, are never safe but in our closets under lock and key."[25] Sisters and daughters are best "put out" on the marriage market. "Put out" (like "set out" in relation to Willmore above) suggests the literal meaning of "prostitute."[26] An old usurer like Sir Cautious Fulbank is not at all averse to arranging the marriage for sale of his foppish nephew Bearjest to the daughter of his fellow alderman, and Sir Cautious will eventually preside over the prostitution of his own wife to Gayman for one night. The "writings" Pinchwife refers to are the usurer's legal and monetary documents that are safest in the bank. These writings are equated with women. Marriage settlements and documents fixed women, as long as they were married, into the status of legal nonentities, legal ciphers. It is the status of being fixed and "written" that Margery breaks out of when she literally comes out of the "closet" after *writing* her own letter to Horner, and it was Aphra Behn (whose first name, according to Angeline Goreau, was derived from a third-century Christian martyr converted from sacred prostitution) who first broke that barrier by putting herself out as a "published" writer in 1670.[27]

As everyone now knows, when she chose to make her fortune in the world by taking up her female pen—by writing for money—Behn crossed the line from respectable seventeenth-century womanhood into a more dangerous and disreputable realm. The ideal woman in early modern England was a silent text—fixed, written, layered, "covered" or "protected" by her husband (the wife as *femme couverte*, in legal terminology), effaced, veiled, or ornamented—in the literal sense of *textus* as a "woven fabric," a web, a clothed figure pictured in Nathan Bailey's later definitive (for the early eighteenth century) derivation of "Woman" from the Welsh *wan*, a "*Web* and *Man*, q.d. a weaving person."[28] Woman is also "Womb-man," and the womb was often imaged as spinning or sewing the child into being. Bailey's stress on a "weaving" rather than a "woven" person suggests woman's active ability to weave herself, and Behn (a country woman herself from the county of Kent) made the momentous transition from the realm of woman defined as a silent text and weaver-of-texts to individual woman putting together and putting forward her own fictional texts.[29]

Mistress Behn and the Royal Pair

Behn's novella *Oroonoko*, published in the explosive political atmosphere of 1688 (and a year before her death) is an even more thickly woven and delicately allusive verbal artifact than *The Lucky Chance*. Criticism on *Oroonoko*, though often too preoccupied with disparaging Behn's truth claims at the expense of considering the work as a fiction, has grown rapidly in breadth and complexity, with especially useful commentary on the historicity and historical context of the work.³⁰ In what follows, I have paid particular attention to the narrator of *Oroonoko*, to the epistle dedicatory, and to Behn's poetic self-inscription as it relates to *Oroonoko*.

At the time of writing this narrative, Behn was forty-eight, poor, sick, suffering from a variety of diseases, and actively and intently rereading the Bible.³¹ She was exactly double the age of her free-spirited and socially privileged and powerful "Eye-witness," the younger self-as-character who participates in the crucial historical events of the narrative (1). In this she prefigures Defoe's invention of the retrospective Moll Flanders looking back over an active and unconventional life—and *Oroonoko* is a vital text in the multifaceted birth of the novel—but part of Behn's purpose is to inscribe the experience and significance of her "Royal Slave" within her own closing life's circle. By looking closely at how Behn represents herself as the narrator in *Oroonoko*, I wish to call attention to the elegiac power of a narrative redolent of paradisal and gospel overtones as well as echoes from Behn's later royalist verse, a narrative in which the author preserves for "posterity" her godlike heroic pair with the reputation of her pen.³² At the same time she may in part alleviate her own sense of guilt in their demise while providing a cautionary literary and political fable for her dedicatee, the young nobleman Richard Maitland (nephew of the Lauderdale of Charles's Cabal) and his lady (another potentially important heroic pair), and for an England—and an English Catholic king—in crisis.

The title page of the first edition tells us that the author is "Mrs. A. Behn." Let us not take too modern an attitude to the prefix "Mrs.," or as it was pronounced in the seventeenth and early eighteenth centuries, Mistress. Although Aphra Behn almost always signs her name "A. Behn" in the epistles dedicatory to her works, the "Mrs." here, whether her own addition or most likely the bookseller's, conceals a wealth of meaning present to a late seventeenth-century audience.³³ "Mistress" was one of the few female words of power in this era, but of acutely ambivalent power. As the female equivalent of "master," "mistress" (according to the *OED*) meant the female head of a household or family ("mistress of the house"), the female governor of a state or territory, a goddess, a woman who has mastered an art or branch of study, a female teacher, an author or creator, a woman who has command over a man's heart and by extension, the more familiar sense of female paramour, as well as the conventional title of courtesy prefixed to the surname of a married or an unmarried woman in the seventeenth and eighteenth centuries. In 1688, Mistress Aphra Behn or her lively narrator can lay claim to nearly all these meanings. Mistress Behn has mastered the craft of playwriting as well as novel writing (as it was then understood), she was a well-known poet and an able translator, and insofar as we can determine from the evidence she was also, for a few months at least, a woman of considerable influence and authority in the British colony of Surinam, on the northern coast of South America, sometime around 1663. Her last great fictional character (and the only male protagonist in her novels), an idealized hero who shares in Mistress Behn's own physical demise, calls her "his *Great Mistress*" (46). Men give Aphra Behn the title of "Mistress" whether they be booksellers, husbands, fellow playwrights, or her own hero. She modestly does not claim the title for herself.

In the epistle dedicatory (printed only in the first edition of 1688) to Richard Maitland (1653–95), the former lord justice general of England in 1681 and the future fourth earl of Lauderdale, Mistress Behn gives an unusually sophisticated account of her development as a creative artist.[34] She compliments her noble dedicatee (and narratee) as a scholar well read in "innumerable volumes of Men and Books," and she appeals to his knowledge of the arts as a kind of ideal reader of the subsequent narrative. She likens her own inclusive creative method to that of a portrait painter who begins his creation by moving around and looking at the "face" of his subject from many angles to find the most agreeable aspect for depiction. The "face" and the "heart" will become the critical focal points in the relationship between Oroonoko and his true love, Imoinda, in the narrative proper. This narrative may be construed as the "story" of their hearts.

In the Restoration, of course, "poet" could still designate any writer of imaginative literature. "A Poet is a Painter" too, the dedicator goes on, but "we"—and now she equates herself with the verbal artist—draw to the life "in another kind; we draw the Nobler part, the Soul and Mind; the Pictures of the Pen shall out-last those of the Pencil, and even Worlds themselves." She begins with encompassing the outward image, and then goes deep inside. "Soul" and "mind" and "heart" are almost equivalent terms for Behn, as "mind" and "heart" are for Creech's Lucretius. In Aphra Behn's androgynously gendered presentation of her "self-as-writer," the poet—the "masculine Part" in her—can also be a "historian" of those lives of "Men of Eminent Parts," as exemplary as monarchs themselves, who might otherwise be forgotten.[35] Echoing the title page's "True History," she tells Maitland that "this is a true Story," one we know she told many times to her friends. Thomas Southerne in fact thought the oral version superior to the written one, and the narrative indeed shows signs of oral delivery, as in the occasionally confusing use of pronouns (1). She has told the story over and over; now she must preserve it in writing. The oral and the written telling are again aspects of her impulse toward inclusivity and preservation. She mixes the oral and written modes: "What I have *mentioned* I have taken care shou'd be Truth," though "I *writ* it in a few Hours," never resting her "Pen a Moment for Thought: Tis purely the Merit of my Slave that must render it worthy of the Honour it begs" (my emphasis).

She signs her name "A. Behn" and the next words of the narrative proper are, "I do not pretend." Despite this deceptively modest opening of her narrative, the author has moved now beyond the realm of the poet into the higher sphere of the pure "historian" by "relating the Truth" in such a way that the story "shall come simply into the World," like a natural birth, "recommended by its own proper Merits, and natural Intrigues." Like Truth, the proverbially elusive and beautiful woman who needs no adornment of any kind, the "history" of Oroonoko has its own merit and honor, as in Johnson's definition of "history": "a narration of events and facts delivered with dignity." The narrator subtly allies herself from the beginning with Nature, the preeminent and all-embracing feminine storyteller, and at the same time moves beyond history into myth. *Oroonoko* is a myth in the most basic sense of the term, *mythos* as word, and myth as the story of a god or godlike being. Mistress Behn in the epistle dedicatory and elsewhere stresses her identity as a teller and a writer, a verbal artist: when Oroonoko called her his "*Great Mistress,*" he also said her "Word would go a great way with him" (46). Behn's later writings show a consistent concern with her place in literary history, and she expects her "word" to take Oroonoko and Imoinda to literary immortality.

By claiming to be an "Eye-witness to a great part of what you will find here set down," and by claiming that what she did not see she "receiv'd from the Mouth" of the godlike hero himself (1), Mistress Behn implicitly invites comparison with New Testament authorities. Luke testifies to "those things which are most surely believed among us, Even as they delivered them unto us, which from the beginning were eyewitnesses, and ministers of the word" (1.1–2), and Peter disavows all artifice in his testimony: "For we have not followed cunningly devised fables, when we made known unto you the power and coming of our Lord Jesus Christ, but were eyewitnesses of his majesty" (2 Pet. 1.16). The narrator and a small group of her family and friends were the privileged few—distinguished from the "reader" unfamiliar with this strange new "other world"—"who were perfectly charm'd with the Character of this great Man, [and] were curious to gather every Circumstance of his Life" (1). The stress on "we" and "us" is also in the manner and tone of Gospel tidings.

The narrator thus represents her former self as an important and influential young Englishwoman who happened at that time to be living in the "best House" in the country, called "St. John's Hill." Besides Luke and Peter, her opening recalls the words of John 19.35: "And he that saw it bare record, and his record is true: and he knoweth that he saith true, that ye might believe." In terms that also recall Milton's description of Paradise, the house stood at the top of a huge rock of white marble, at the foot of which ran a river "a vast depth down" and the opposite bank was adorned with large quantities of different flowers eternally blowing (49).[36] Oroonoko is frequently linked with flowers, and the author gives her African hero the name of the great river of Caribbean South America, the one that Robinson Crusoe will eventually find himself in the mouth of. She will testify at length to Oroonoko's superhuman but also finite powers as a vulnerable hero of waters and the earth, Nature's own heroic god.

It is, then, in these contexts of social and mythic power that Mistress Behn presents her eyewitness account of the royal pair—the "Royal Slave" and his consort, Imoinda—a marvelously intricate, robust, and self-contained work of language and a creation story about a new black Adam and Eve as old as creation, written by a woman—male and female created she them ("Female to the noble Male" [9])—working in intimate touch with her own version of a multisexual Nature similar to that in "The Golden Age": virgin, predominantly female, fecund, all-inclusive, innocent—giving rise to "all sexes" and all forms of life. Nature is for Behn the original virtuous female libertine.

Like the island segment of *Robinson Crusoe, Oroonoko* is a peculiar kind of bipartite narrative, the second part (which recounts Oroonoko and Imoinda's career in South America, the American narrative) recapitulating the first (the African narrative of Oroonoko and Imoinda, ending with Oroonoko's arrival in Surinam near the midpoint of the narrative [37]). In both parts we have a luxuriant, highly visual and varicolored Lucretian evocation of the primeval world, the "New World" linked with "the Golden Age," set in South America. The voice and presence of the narrator is implicated in the re-creation of this other world, a scene of wonders, unheard of birds and animals, strange customs, miracle cures.

The opening description, after recounting the variety of Nature's productions in this new Eden, tells of the Indian aprons woven "very prettily in Flowers of several Colours" worn "as *Adam* and *Eve* did the Fig-leaves" (2). The Indians' faces are "painted in little Specks and Flowers here and there" (3). When the narrator meets Oroonoko and Imoinda in the second part, she records that Imoinda was "carved in fine Flowers and Birds all over her Body," and that Oroonoko was "carved with a little Flower, or Bird, at the sides of the Temples" (45). In a sensuous passage in the first description she prefigures the relationship between Oroonoko and Imoinda by noting how the Indians are so used to seeing each other naked, "so like our first Parents before the Fall, it seems as if they had no Wishes," and like Milton's prelapsarian Adam and Eve they have no bodily secrets, no lewdness or disguise, "but all you can see, you see at once, and every moment see" (3).[37] The Indians have no "desire" in the Lockean sense of "uneasiness" or in Behn's sense of the mischievous usurper of one's peace. The immediate, inclusive style of Edenic perception represented here (and contrasted with the painter's circumlinear sequence of viewpoints we noted in the epistle dedicatory) is re-echoed in the second part when Oroonoko recognizes Imoinda, who he thought was dead: "he soon saw *Imoinda* all over her; in a minute he saw her Face, her Shape, her Air, her Modesty" (43). Such is the unmediated vision of true love for Aphra Behn, one that incorporates innocence, wholeness, integrity. The face is mentioned first, but the face and the heart—the external image and internal architecture of memory and desire—are inextricably bound together.

The world of the Indians and the world of Coramantien (historically, Koromantine), Oroonoko and Imoinda's native country on the African Gold Coast, share certain values. Both are warrior cultures whose primary ethic of the inviolability of the spoken word (34) places the preservation of personal honor over life itself. (This theme will take on major significance in the two woman-centered novels of Richardson, *Pamela* and *Clarissa*.) Oroonoko's personal virtues are those of the traditional noble warrior, courage, honor, generosity, but he also demonstrates the feminine virtue of softness (the first attribute of Milton's Eve) making him "capable of the highest Passions of Love and Gallantry" (7). "Softness" for Milton (as we have seen in the case of Eve) and for Behn in the contexts we have noted signifies not weakness but mildness, tenderness, considerateness, compassion, "consciousness" in the emerging sense of shared perception of one another's feelings. Imoinda, in the mold of Lucretian female power, radiates beauty and softness, embodying "the silent language of newborn

Love," but she will also show herself a heroic warrior alongside Oroonoko in the slave revolt of the second part when she wounds the villainous deputy governor, Byam.

It is clear then that Oroonoko and Imoinda participate in the same primeval Edenic world of the Indians with its postlapsarian component of extreme violence. There is an essential continuity between the African and the American pagan worlds in *Oroonoko* set against the depiction of a European-Christian world that consistently distorts the principle of the inviolability of the spoken vow. The narrator goes so far, indeed, in the early description, as to declare that "these People represented to me an absolute *Idea* of the first State of Innocence, before *Man* knew how to sin: And 'tis most evident and plain, that simple Nature is the most harmless, inoffensive and vertuous Mistress. 'Tis she alone, if she were permitted, that better instructs the World, than all the Inventions of Man" (3). In her own way, the role of instructor is the one that Behn as Mistress Nature's handmaid aspires to; she is the author and narrator of a unique "novel," an implicit gospel of the religion of innocent Nature, with Oroonoko and Imoinda as her godlike heroes. But this role is fraught with tension and contradictions because, while allying herself with the primal creative power of a virtuous female Nature, Aphra Behn in *Oroonoko* also represents poignantly and acutely her subordinate status as a seventeenth-century woman, despite her "masculine Part" and her brief moment of power in the government of Surinam.[38]

When Oroonoko finds himself betrayed by the English captain and sold as a slave, his new owner, the plantation manager Trefry, gives him the slave name of "Caesar." As in Scripture, a new name means a new destiny. The masculine power structure gives him a new identity and fate in this dangerous and "obscure World" of Surinam where the Dutch will soon dispose of all the males who could have told his story (reminiscent of the biblical male annihilation motif of Exodus 1), and he is "afforded only a Female Pen to celebrate his Fame" (40), as if Aphra Behn—like the messenger in Job—were escaped alone to tell it. Oroonoko, Imoinda, and the narrator are all represented in the narrative as the last of their kind.

Behn's ambivalence about her role as a woman and a writer carries over to her account of her involvement in the critical period before Oroonoko masterminds the slave revolt that leads to his downfall. The narrator now enters the action of the narrative as a key character. I will call her Aphra to distinguish her from Mistress Behn, the narrator. The narrator describes how at the critical moment when Caesar is bargaining for his release, she herself is called in by the English powers-that-be to negotiate with him, as a kind of mediator, to buy time and prevent a mutiny. The author of *Oroonoko* devises a remarkable contrast between the twenty-four-year-old oral storyteller Aphra and the forty-eight-year-old Mistress Behn, the writer, as narrators. Aphra, working as an agent of the English colonialists, becomes the official entertainer of Oroonoko and Imoinda at her home and the three are together virtually every hour of the day (46). As the daughter of the "Lieutenant-General" who died at sea and as the chief resident of St. John's Hill, Aphra has easy access to the young lovers, Caesar and Clemene (Imoinda's slave name); she forms a friendship with Caesar and feels she has the authority to assure him of his liberty as soon as the absent "Lord Governour" will arrive. Aphra is characterized as a gifted teller of literary tales. She narrates the love stories of the "*Romans*," Romanizing (and romanticizing) the newly named Caesar even further, which "charmed him to my Company" (46). At the same time, she teaches Imoinda all the "pretty Works" of literature she is "Mistress" of, trying to Christianize her. Caesar balks at this (he has difficulty with the concept of the Trinity), but he acquiesces in this learning environment, preferring the company of women, presumably including Aphra's mother, sister, and female servant, above that of men. It is as if Aphra is trying to bring Oroonoko and Imoinda within the "compass" (48) of her feminine spellbinding powers, and thus further within the control of the English governors. At this point Oroonoko praises Aphra as his "*Great Mistress*," a kind of *magna mater*, protector, nourisher, instructor, and one who will (unknown to him) become—as the older narrator, Mistress Behn—his biographer and virtual apostle. Mistress Behn, now finally writing down the narrative she has told and retold to such universal admiration, conveys the sense that her relationship with these two beautiful creatures, each one inscribed on their bodies with indecipherable hieroglyphs of the natural world, was far more important than she recognized at the time. She is now, at the time of writing, in a position somewhat analogous to that of Onahal, the "decayed Beauty" who instructed the young concubines in the old king's "Otan" (seraglio) in "all those wanton Arts of Love" (18). Onahal, an early representative of the Mother Midnight figure (a kind of bawd, matchmaker, and agent of fate combined), played a crucial part in originally bringing the young lovers together. The decayed beauty Mistress Behn now writes the narrative of how as a younger woman she helped to determine the outcome of their lives. At this moment Aphra Behn as character and narrator incorporates many of the influential roles of "Mistress," and here as a character in her own fiction she becomes Oroonoko and Imoinda's living fate. At the same time she is, in her own view, only a woman, and Caesar and Clemene are only slaves. The three are bonded in subservient roles, and much of the enduring power of this text is its confederacy of the paradoxical pair—woman author and royal slave—attempting to overcome their bondage.

But Aphra, though in a position of apparent power, is further characterized by her narrator as a cautious and timorous woman: she does not trust Caesar. Before they part, she gets his promise to wait patiently a little longer for the arrival of the lord governor. Her next sentence, "After this, I neither thought it convenient to trust him much out of our view" (48), reinforces her caution, and later, when the news of his revolt is brought to her, "we [women] were possess'd with extreme Fear . . . that he would secure himself till night, and then, that he would come down and cut all our Throats" (68). Thus the narrator's anxieties about her female pen are augmented with visions of female terror. Whether Aphra's fears for the women are justified or not, there is no question that Oroonoko's deepening melancholy finds expression in a darker dimension of his own heart rhetoric and that of the narrator with regard to him. Whereas earlier there was an emphasis on his open, generous heart, there is now an obsession with revenge. Oroonoko now reflects the ambivalence of the biblical heart. He struggles between revenge and love for "the Victory of his Heart," repenting his softness for Imoinda. Imagining her being raped by "*every Brute*" in the colony before she is shamefully killed, "his great Heart could not endure that Thought. . . . These were . . . his silent Arguments with his Heart, as he told us afterwards . . . pleasing his great Heart with the fancy'd Slaughter he should make over the whole face of the Plantation" (71). He resolves to take Imoinda's life.

The sacrifice of Imoinda "to [his] Revenge" is one of the most remarkable episodes in the history of the royal slave. It is prefigured by Caesar's killing of the great she-tiger in the Indian rain forests. The narrator says, "when the Heart of this courageous Animal was taken out, there were seven Bullets of Lead in it, the Wound seam'd up with great Scars, and she liv'd with the Bullets a great while . . . This Heart the Conqueror brought up to us, and 'twas a very great Curiosity, which all the Country came to see" (52–53). Here a woman tells a new "truth" to men about the vital power at the heart of innocent female Nature. Nature's strengthening, invigorating support is crucial to Behn's depiction of creative organic life.

Nature is innocent teacher, nurturer, and supporting force behind all male and female desire figured in the generous heart of the great woman or the great man.[39] Caesar anatomizes the tiger and removes and displays her heart. By doing so he unwittingly reveals his own fate in the heart of an animal who exemplifies the superhuman life force in himself and his mate, but a force subject to his own will and the barbarous cruelty of others.

When Oroonoko married Imoinda in Coramantien he vowed, contrary to the practice of polygamy in his country, that "she shou'd be the only Woman he wou'd possess while he liv'd; that no Age or Wrinkles shou'd encline him to change; for her Soul wou'd be always fine, and always young; and he shou'd have an eternal *Idea* in his Mind of the Charms she now bore; and shou'd look into his Heart for that *Idea*, when he cou'd find it no longer in her Face" (11). The word "idea" here recalls the narrator's "*Idea* of the first State of Innocence" (3). We may presume that the idea of Imoinda's face resides in the heart of Caesar as she lays herself down before him "while he, with a hand resolved, and a heart-breaking within, gave the fatal Stroke, first cutting her Throat, and then severing her yet smiling Face from that delicate Body, pregnant as it was with the Fruits of tenderest Love" (72). As Caesar severs the "smiling Face" from the delicate body of Imoinda, he severs his own heart as well because her beautiful youthful image was preserved in his heart.[40] As before the old king of Coramantien had a "Bed of State made ready, with Sweets and Flowers" for his dalliance with the "trembling Victim," Imoinda (17), now Caesar lays the body of the "ador'd Victim . . . on Leaves and Flowers, of which he made a Bed, and conceal'd it under the same Cover-lid of Nature; only her Face he left yet bare to look on" (72). The fatal swiftness of the act recalls how "he ravish'd in a moment" her willing charms in his grandfather's otan (23). When he kills her, he kills his own strength. The older narrator's presence again hovers intimately, precariously, over this scene of tender carnage. We recall that it was Aphra herself who once feared that Oroonoko might cut all the women's throats (68).

A number of recent commentators on *Oroonoko* have offered ingenious political/allegorical readings of the protagonist, associating him with Stuart monarchs from Charles I to, in particular, James II. George Guffey, in "Aphra Behn's *Oroonoko*: Occasion and Accomplishment," a pioneering political interpretation of the work, notes that Behn refers to James as "Great Cesar" in her "Congratulatory Poem to Her Sacred Majesty Queen Mary, Upon Her Arrival in England" (1689), and that "Oroonoko, or Caesar, like Charles I . . . meets his executioner with grace and dignity. . . . Mrs. Behn, fearing that history might repeat itself in England, must have intended us to associate the unjust treatment of Caesar with the imperiled situation of James II during that summer of 1688." Maureen Duffy states unequivocally that "emotionally Orinooko, Imoinda and their unborn child are James, Mary [of Modena] and the unborn, while [Behn] was writing it, prince. Trefry, [Colonel George] Martin, and her family are the loyalists; Byam and Banister and their rabble are the opposition." Most recently, Laura Brown, analyzing the work in the context of early British imperialism, has reminded us that Behn's slave name for Oroonoko—Caesar—is the same she used for the Stuart monarchs Charles II and James II, and Brown makes an intriguing case for Oroonoko's heroism and tragic fate echoing that of Charles Stuart: "The sense of momentous loss that Behn's narrative generates on behalf of the 'royal slave' is the product of the hidden figuration in Oroonoko's death of the culminating moment of the English revolution."[41] I have no doubt that Oroonoko in some sense is designed to recall the virtues of the Stuart monarchs, as I attempt to illustrate further in the following pages, but though the foregoing conjectures are often informative, they are not particularly convincing in their specific details and at times ask for too narrow an "allegorical" construction.

The Excluded Prophet

In her later poetic celebration of the royal virtues of benevolent leadership, erotic creative force, compassion for one's subjects, protection, patience, suffering, humility, and divine power, Behn focuses on the two royal couples Charles II and his queen, Catherine (of Braganza), and James II and his queen, Mary (of Modena), but her fondness for noble pairings is evident also in her epistle dedicatory praising Lord and Lady Maitland in *Oroonoko* and achieves its most complex representation in the royal pair Oroonoko and Imoinda. I wish now to compare the rhetoric of the "royal" poems—largely the rhetoric of the heart—with that of *Oroonoko* in order to show more fully how the royal slave and his consort are deeply embedded in the verbal matrix of Behn's final, "royalist" poetic phase, celebrating at once the generous heart of royalty in the face of extreme adversity and the ambiguous role of the woman poet writing for immortality. Relevant passages from *Oroonoko* appear at appropriate junctures.

In 1685, Behn published "A Pindarick on the Death of Our Late Sovereign" and "A Poem Humbly Dedicated to . . . Catherine Queen Dowager," companion poems commemorating the death of Charles II and the queen's mourning for him. I do not suggest that Oroonoko and Imoinda are allegorical figures of Charles and Catherine, but it is worth noting that the royal slave and his consort belong in their own way to the "royal pindaric elegy" tradition crafted by Behn in her later poetry, and *Oroonoko* may plausibly be read as a prose "poem" within this tradition. The companion poems conventionally combine Christian and classical Greek elements. Behn explicitly compares the death of Charles to the death and resurrection of Christ, with Milton's "Lycidas" as the general model for this comparison. ("Lycidus" is one of Behn's favorite names for the ideal male lover in her poetry.)

The primary model in classical mythology for the controlling and shaping power of a woman over human life is the sewing (and later writing) Fate, as I have argued in *Mother Midnight*. There is a strong sense in this pindaric elegy of the sacred decrees of fate, and Behn, as a woman writer, subtly and indirectly assumes the role of a Fate, or secretary to the Fates. Charles in the poem is compared to Moses, and his brother James to Joshua, both laboring under the unalterable decrees of Fate. Behn is their sacred historian, recalling her adoption of the role of historian in the epistle dedicatory to *Oroonoko*. She now records how a combination of the powers of "Heaven and Nature" brought about the melancholy event of the king's death, and the poem ends with soft looks exchanged between Charles and James taking the place of the lamenting voice, and anguish the place of the heart, just before Charles dies. Again we see Behn's version of the link between heart and eye in the "anguish" of the heart and "languishment" of the eyes. Silence, death, and midnight hover around on every face as the poem extols the Miltonic epic virtues of patience, suffering, and humility.

The poem to the queen dowager moves from the pierced bleeding hearts of the mourners to the vast tide of woe that overflowed her "Royal *breaking Heart*," a far greater "Sacrifice" than that of the mourners. As in Psalm 51, "the sacrifices of God are a broken spirit, a broken and a contrite heart." The imperious force of the breaking heart almost overwhelms the "Banks of Life," and one recalls the compromised life force of a figure like Lady Fulbank. The image of a powerful flow of blood is reiterated when Catherine is compared to Christ. She has the patience of a suffering God. She disdains loud grief; her loss is "Fixt in the *heart*," with no outward sign remaining: "So the Blest Virgin at the worlds great loss, Came, and beheld, then *Fainted* at the *Cross*" (198). The comparison with Mary at the end of the Gospel of John is enhanced further by the picture of the Great Lord of Life laid upon her lap, "all wounded, Pale, and Dead." She is "transpierc'd" with anguish: "So His blest *Image* in Her Heart remain'd" (199).[42] The recurring image of the passive male love god in Behn's poetry enters a new religious register in this poem and in *Oroonoko*. As Imoinda's image remains in the breaking heart of Oroonoko, so Charles's image remains in the breaking heart of Catherine.

Heaven has blest you with a Lady [who] . . . as absolutely merits Respect from all the World as she does that Passion and Resignation she receives from your Lordship; and which is, on her part, with so much Tenderness return'd. . . . (Epistle dedicatory to *Oroonoko*)

The Prince softly waken'd *Imoinda* . . . I believe he omitted saying nothing to this young Maid, that might persuade her to suffer him to seize his own, and take the Rights of Love. And I believe she was not long resisting those Arms where she so long'd to be . . . he soon prevail'd, and ravished in a moment what his old Grandfather had been endeavouring for so many Months.
'Tis not to be imagined the Satisfaction of these two young Lovers. (23)

In the "Coronation" poem for James II, her most ambitious celebratory pindaric (in 785 lines), Behn represents herself as a female poet working in cooperation with a female Muse and with "soft Angels" (200) to evoke a biblical sense of creative sexual power worthy of her "Royal HERO" (James) and heroine, the "sacred LAURA" (Mary of Modena) (201). In stanza 5 the poet, joined with her Muse, issues a wake-up call to the royal pair to shake off their downy pleasure and rise from "the softest Charms of love. . . . From *joys* too fierce for *any* sense" but their own godlike and refined bodies (202). The poet, like the narrator of *Paradise Lost*, has the privileged position of witnessing this superhuman lovemaking, but in Behn's version the fair Laura embodies an erotic passion so intense and thunderous (like Jove with Semele, except that now a woman is Jovian), that only the king can sustain a force

> Fatal to *All* but Her Lov'd *Monarchs* heart,
> Who of the *same* Divine Materials wrought;
> Cou'd equally exchange the dart,
> Receive the wound with Life, with Life the wound impart;
> And mixt the Soul as gently as she thought:
> So the great *Thund'rer Semele* d'stroy'd,
> Whil'st only *Juno* cou'd embrace the *God*!
> (207)

These invincible royal hearts, exchanging wounds that impart life—a heart possessed equally by the female and male lovers—is one of Behn's most powerful expressions of fierce Lucretian eroticism attempting mutual interpenetration of the heart, and this passage is a capsule version of the prevailing theme in Behn's erotics of the woman *taming* and sublimating the violent Lucretian love play of mutual wounding into the softness of thought. The poet is blessed to be able to witness this power at a distance; as with the Israelites in the Wilderness, to approach too near "the sacred Mount was *Death*!" She finally counsels her impatient Muse to hold back, even though her eyes are loath to lose "the bliss," a synonym for orgasm in Behn's poetry even more explicitly insistent than in Milton's.[43] Then in her "own" voice, Behn utters, in a virtual hymn to the divine royal presence, one of her most moving self-inscriptions as a poet:

> I glide, and hover round the awful place,
>   Like Fantoms, where their hidden Treasure lies;
>   Or hoping Lovers who at distance gaze,
> And watch the tender Moments of their Mistress Eyes.
>   How e're I toil for Life all day,
>   With what e're cares my Soul's opprest,
>   'Tis in that Sun-shine still I play,
>   'Tis there my wearied Mind's at rest;
> But oh *Vicisitudes* of Night must come
> Between the rising Glories of the Sun!
> (212)

Behn evokes precisely this sense of her being a distant yet hovering, excluded yet intensely concerned prophetic witness to the royal action in her mature narrator's account of the lovemaking of Oroonoko and Imoinda, of the conception of their child, and of their individual deaths. There is a complex corresponding sequence to this account in the series of royal poems tracing the godlike lovemaking of James and Laura in the "Coronation" poem (1685), continuing with the conception and gestation of the "Royal Boy" in the "Congratulatory Poem to Her Most Sacred Majesty" (Mary of Modena) (a psalmic celebration, reminiscent of Psalm 139, of the work going on in the royal womb of her beautiful queen), and concluding with the "Congratulatory Poem . . . on the Happy Birth of the Prince of Wales" and the more somber "Congratulatory Poem to Her Sacred

Majesty Queen Mary" (Mary II) after the forced exile of James II in December of 1688.

> Methinks your tranquil Lives are an Image of the new Made and Beautiful Pair in Paradise . . . such humble Fruits as my Industry produces I lay at your Lordship's Feet. . . . The Royal Slave I had the Honour to know in my Travels to the other World; and though I had none above me in that Country yet I wanted power to preserve this Great Man. . . . 'Twill be no Commendation to the Book to assure your Lordship I writ it in a few Hours, though it may serve to Excuse some of its Faults of Connexion, for I never rested my Pen a Moment for Thought. (Epistle dedicatory to *Oroonoko*)

At the end of the royal "birth" poem, the speaker "lays [her] humble verses" at the feet of the queen and proclaims that they are

> Inspir'd by Nothing but *Prophetick Truth*,
> They Boast no other *Fire*, no other *Worth*.
> Full of the JOY, no LINES *Correct* can write,
> My *Pleasure*'s too Extream for *Thought* or Wit.
> (298)

In her welcoming poem to the *new* Queen Mary (Mary II, the Protestant daughter of James II), Behn's Muse, now retreated to the darkest covert of the wood, is sad, oppressed, and sighing with the heavy burden of "an Unhappy dearlov'd *Monarch*'s Fate" (304). She resolves to sing her fruitless songs on Britain's faithless shore no longer until suddenly she hears the "Sounds of Joy" accompanying the arrival of "Blest Maria." It is in this poem that Behn refers to her as "Great Cesar's Offspring" (307). In another idiosyncratic female/male role reversal, however, she restyles the queen as Moses descending from the Mountain of God with the power to reconcile the differing English multitudes. Finally, we should note that the succession of royal "Marys" seems to have stirred up in Behn images of the "Marys" in the Gospels, and of the "Stabat Mater," in these poems and in her meditation on the death of Oroonoko.

Gilbert Burnet, who became bishop of Salisbury in 1689 with the accession of William and Mary, appears to have asked Behn to write a poem commemorating the accession despite her well-known and ardent adherence to the Stuarts. In what might have been her last poem, "A Pindaric Poem to the Reverend Doctor Burnet on the Honour he did me of Enquiring after me and my Muse," Behn now compares *herself* (and not the queen) to Moses in this plaintive elegiac portrait:

> Thus while the Chosen Seed possess the Promis'd Land,
>   I like the Excluded Prophet stand,
>   The Fruitful Happy Soul can only see,
>   But am forbid by Fates Decree
> To share the triumph of the joyful Victory.
> (309)

Despite her frequent employment of "the topos of authorial modesty"[44] in her works (including this poem), it is remarkable that at the end of her life as a professional writer Behn should compare herself favorably (if ruefully) with the most important male depicted explicitly as a writer in the Old Testament, the author of the five books of Moses. Hence the account of Moses as a writer given in Chapter 1 comes back to qualify the emergence of the woman writer we have traced in this chapter.

Curiously enough, the poet Abraham Cowley (to whose heroic poems Behn pays compliment in the poem to Burnet) provides an intriguing link between William Harvey and Aphra Behn, and more significantly, a springboard for the further inscription of herself as a female poet who will endure. As we saw in the second chapter, Cowley's "Ode: *Upon* Dr. Harvey" represents the famous physician-anatomist in full pursuit of a mature virginal Nature who, "like Daphne," takes sanctuary in a tree. Harvey eventually surprises her hiding in the human heart and forces her to reveal all of her secrets. Sometime in the late 1680s (most likely), Behn translated *Sylva*, the sixth book of Cowley's *Plantarum* (Of plants), a royalist poem celebrating, in the words of Thomas Sprat, "the History of our late Troubles" and Charles II's "Affliction and Return."[45] This history is uttered by the goddess Dryas speaking the words of the ancient royal oak in which Charles as a young man took refuge during the Civil War. Again Cowley employs the metaphor of pursuing "hidden Nature" into a dark labyrinthine forest world, this time with his Muse as "Huntress": "Through all her Tracks let flying Truth be chas'd, / And seize her panting with her eager hast." As Janet Todd points out, "The oak had always been an emblem of strength and stability, and by the Restoration trees in general, and the oak in particular, had acquired extra political and ideological significance." John Evelyn dedicated his own *Sylva* to Charles II and believed the planting of forests by the king, in contrast to the destruction of forests by the late Parliamentarian "*Spoilers,*" provided a foundation for his power and the country's future wealth and safety: "The celebration of trees thus becomes an act of loyalty and a political statement."[46] Trees appear frequently in Behn's pastoral poetry, and the "Juniper Tree" in her poem of that title, a variant of the Tree of Life, functions as a masculinized protector and nurturer of the erotic love enacted under its canopy.

After cataloging a variety of tree goddesses in his *Sylva*, Cowley rehearses the story of Daphne, the beautiful nymph transformed into a laurel tree whose leaves become emblems of poetic inspiration and prophecy. Cowley's Phoebus adores her still, "and makes his Love his Prophetess" (line 566). The speaker of the poem addresses her as a "Princess," but if the goddess Dryas should not allow that title, surely she remains a "prophetess" from whose "triumphing Boughs . . . Poets claim a share." It is at this opportune moment in the context of poets and prophets that Behn "The translatress in her own Person speaks" (marginal note):

> Among that number, do not me disdain,
> Me, the most humble of that glorious Train.
> I by a double right thy Bounties claim,
> Both from my Sex, and in *Apollo*'s Name:
> Let me with *Sappho* and *Orinda* be
> Oh ever sacred Nymph, adorn'd by thee;
> And give my Verses Immortality.
> (335, lines 588–94)

Cowley was the masculinist-libertine poet par excellence (as *poet*), manipulating the paternal language of Latin (the linguistic vehicle reserved almost exclusively for male poets and scholars), with a skill rivaled only by the sixteenth-century George Buchanan, and by Milton, in the eyes of his contemporaries. Behn transcribes herself into this masculinized poetic context to assert her own identity as a female poet and prophet in a tradition linking the Greek Sappho to the seventeenth-century English poet Katherine Philips (Orinda). She asks Daphne to adorn her with laurels, the symbol of poetic immortality, and claims Daphne's poetic bounties by an androgynous "double right," by virtue of her being a woman at the end of a long line of female poets and in the name of masculine Apollo, the poetic and prophetic light bringer. By inserting her unique poetic identity into the poem at this point, she becomes the eloquent link between the sacred laurel tree (Daphne) and the sacred feminized oak tree, who through the voice of the prophetic Queen Dryas tells the story of the Civil War and the triumph of Charles II. Behn the poet thus inhabits the vital interior of the female royal oak and speaks Charles's fate who, as "a Captive-Slave exposed to Sale" (*Sylva*, 335, line 978), prefigures the royal slave Oroonoko.

They cut *Caesar* in Quarters, and sent them to several of the chief Plantations: One Quarter was sent to Colonel *Martin*; who refus'd it, and swore . . . that he could govern his *Negroes*, without terrifying and grieving them with frightful Spectacles of a mangled King.

    Thus died this great Man, worthy of a better Fate, and a more sublime Wit than mine to write his Praise: Yet, I hope, the Reputation of my pen is considerable enough to make his glorious Name to survive to all Ages, with that of the brave, the beautiful, and the constant *Imoinda*. (*Oroonoko*, 77–78)

The speaker of *Sylva*, who from the moment of the translatress's self-insertion now reflects her persona, wonders why s/he should reiterate the brave but futile deeds of illustrious men "Who did with thee [Charles II] deserve a kinder Fate," and then, in language that prefaces her/his account of the execution of Charles I, adumbrates Oroonoko's end as "a mangled King":

> Nor to your Griefs will this Addition bring,
> The sad Ideas of a Martyred King;
> A King who all the Wounds of Fortune bore,
> Nor will his mournful Funerals deplore;
> Lest that celestial Piety (of Fame
> O'er all the World) should my sad Accents blame
> (335–36)

In composing *Oroonoko*, Behn could leave the confines of the translatress's role and create her own royal myth of the generous and brave heart (male and female) ending in martyrdom, but even as translatress she seems to be trying to ward off blame for "sad accents" she would later characterize as the lesser work of "a female pen," and even implied blame for not saving Oroonoko from his butchers.

The Reputation of My Pen

In the sacrifice of Imoinda, Oroonoko preserves his native honor and that of his wife and unborn child, and reaffirms the vow he made after his first near-execution by the English: "Oroonoko *scorns to live with the Indignity that was put on* Caesar. All we could do, could get no more Words from him" (69). With this solemn pronouncement, he renounces the slave name and reclaims his original "African" and "American" self epitomized in the name given him by the narrator. Finally, as the narrator participated intimately in his original ravishing of Imoinda and his sacrifice of her, so she participates in the culmination of her heroes' descent into darkness, suggested in the literal blackness of "melancholy," a word that appears often in the final pages of the novel. After his second partial resurrection, she speaks with him like a parenthetical kindred ghost: "His Discourse was sad; and the earthy Smell about him so strong, that I was persuaded to leave the place for some time, (being myself but sickly, and very apt to fall into Fits of dangerous Illness upon any extraordinary Melancholy)" (76). The dying author (anticipated by her sickly narrator) and her slave go back to the earth together.[47]

At the end, Oroonoko, like the Indian warriors he esteemed who showed their royal courage by persevering in dismemberment contests, demonstrates a similar "passive Valour" (58). Behn's recurring image of the radiating power of the passive male lover, an image we have traced in her erotic poetry (especially "To Lysander at the Musick Meeting"), which appeared in a more elevated strain in her royal elegies (as, for example, in the depiction of Charles like Christ "all wounded, Pale, and Dead," laid upon the lap of his queen), culminates now in the quasi-biblical figure of Oroonoko, superhuman lover, sacrificial priest, executed criminal. Before the wild Irishman Banister (whose name recalls that of a famous sixteenth-century English anatomist) is allowed to exercise his "absolute Barbarity" in cutting off, in sequence, Oroonoko's genitals, ears, nose, and arms—as if chopping down a noble tree—the hero, smiling, blesses his executioners. The narrator remarks, "My Mother and Sister were by him all the while, but not suffer'd to save him" as "his Head sunk . . . and he gave up the Ghost, without a Groan" (77). The Gospel of Luke records Jesus' forgiveness of his executioners, and John testifies that "there stood by the cross of Jesus his mother, and his mother's sister . . . and Mary Magdalene" (19.25), who is an eyewitness to the post-Resurrection Jesus. Behn's hero and Jesus die within the grieving maternal presence of women. Jesus' last words in John are "It is finished: and he bowed his head, and gave up the ghost" (19.30).

Behn's non-Christian martyr smokes a pipe during the execution. His last heroic life act is more a symbol of pagan (or Lucretian) stoic resignation and possibly of friendship and peace than a sign of his Europeanization. But this is not the end. His body is divided into four "quarters," recalling the final stage in the prescribed narrative ritual of execution for high treason, and the parts are sent to the "chief Plantations," the centers of political power in the colony. This action is a deliberate allusion to one of the most appalling narratives in the Old Testament, the gang rape and murder of the Levite's concubine "from Bethlehem" in Judges 19, and the subsequent political statement of his dividing her body into twelve parts and sending them throughout Israel as a memorial of the crime and an incitement to revenge against the men of Benjamin. Behn's friend Colonel Martin says he would rather see the quarters of the colony's leaders on his plantation. I shall not speculate on the meaning of this final enigmatic allusion except to say that in the divided Oroonoko Behn seems to inscribe herself as his collaborative female victim. Oroonoko virtually comes back from death two times before his execution. Behn's preservation of him in her novella is his final resurrection.

We know that Aphra Behn wrote this narrative during a period of grave illness and anxiety and out of a compelling personal desire to make her hero and heroine live in a *written* narrative text that incorporates some of the dramatic fervor and idiom of her royal elegies and Pindarics, as well as that of Restoration tragedy. Created within a climactic cultural moment of great political uncertainty, the work itself conveys an indelible sense of anxiety in the fate of its heroes, both the explicit and the implicit ones. Out of her own philosophical articulation of "desire" as "uneasy rage," and from her precarious position as a woman who has gained some considerable "reputation" as well as notoriety for her pen, Mistress Behn can dedicate her novella about the Great Man Oroonoko to another Great Man, Richard Maitland. Theoretical concerns with epistolarity in fiction must also pay attention to epistles dedicatory. As we noted in connection with Harvey's dedicatory epistle to Charles I in *The Motion of the Heart*, a dedication (from *dedicare*) is originally a consecration, a setting apart for worship or devoting to a sacred purpose. For Mistress Behn at this point in her life an epistle dedicatory, particularly for *Oroonoko*, is a kind of last literary will and testament and an expiation. Maureen Duffy suggests the work "had been 'long expected.' . . . What other psychological impetus than the very deep one of solidifying her life for eternity in art could have prompted it?"[48]

In a last ambivalent gesture, Mistress Behn will put the story of the godlike Oroonoko and Imoinda into the protection of the one English aristocrat *and his lady* whom she most reveres and who, in the ever more threatening political atmosphere of 1688, must have seemed to Behn and to some of her readers the doomed European-Christian counterparts to her hero and heroine. Maitland, a Tory, a Roman Catholic, and a strong Jacobite, refused to accept the revolution settlement and became an exile with his king. His wife, Lady Agnes Campbell (1658–1734), was known for her Protestant sympathies. She was the second daughter of Archibald Campbell, ninth earl of Argyll (1629–85), who had been sentenced to death on a dubious charge of high treason in 1681. He escaped to Holland and joined Monmouth's conspiracy only to lead an abortive invasion of Scotland where he, following in the steps of his more famous father in 1661, was beheaded in Edinburgh. The doom of the Campbells was not for Aphra Behn (probably a Roman Catholic herself) a distant analogue to the apparent disaster overtaking the House of Stuart, and the violence of extraordinarily brutal execution was in the air she breathed from the judicial murder of at least thirty-five Roman Catholics in the Popish Plot of 1678 to the aftermath of the Rye House Plot and the reign of Judge Jeffreys in the "Bloody Assizes"—in which over one hundred persons were executed—after the defeat of Monmouth in 1685. Behn may well have been thinking too of James II and his queen with their unborn baby when she wrote of the fatal love between Oroonoko and the pregnant Imoinda, and she must have sensed (during the writing of *Oroonoko*) that her self-inscription as a royal prophetess was on the verge of bitter failure.

But her dedication of the work to Lord and Lady Maitland seems more literary and religious than political. She knows of Maitland's literary talents and aspirations—he was to become the translator, whom Dryden would commend, of another heroic work, Virgil's *Aeneid*. She praises him for youth, gaiety, wit, fine sense, morality, wisdom, generosity, and greatness of mind, all qualities exemplified in her hero. The metaphor of flowers is carried over from Oroonoko as Maitland is compared to the industrious bee returning from every flower with precious dew for the public good. The combination of his quality and the veneration paid to him by the people creates, like a primeval Oroonokan river, "flowing Plenty" in the barren soil of Scotland. Heaven has blessed him with a lady who is his feminine equal in youth, sweetness of nature, illustrious family, grace, beauty, virtue, and piety. Echoing the "tranquillity" of her idealized Indians in South America, Behn speculates that "your tranquil Lives are an Image of the new Made and Beautiful Pair in Paradise," recalling as well Oroonoko and Imoinda as the new black Adam and Eve.

The original Oroonoko was a man gallant enough to have merited

Maitland's protection, and if he had been so fortunate, he might not have made so inglorious an end. "Though I had none above me in that Country yet I wanted power to preserve this Great Man" (epistle dedicatory). Almost like an idealized literary executor, Maitland will protect the Oroonoko whom the young Aphra, working for her English masters, was not able to keep alive. There is a lingering sense of guilt adumbrated here and in the work itself for her role in Oroonoko's demise. In a sense, the whole narrative is an epistle dedicatory of Oroonoko to Lord Maitland and to posterity, the one way Mrs. Aphra Behn, the mistress and master of the art of dramatic narrative, has left to "preserve" both of these Great Men, and her own ambiguous sense of what is "great" about them.

Toward the end of her writing life—and for her the act of writing was living and dying—Aphra Behn inscribed herself into her work in a variety of ways: as the virtuous but duped Lady Fulbank, as the "Excluded Prophet" hovering over scenes of love, death, and political upheaval, as a female Moses, as the troubled, retrospective narrator of *Oroonoko*, as a female poet in an undying tradition that began with Sappho but was overshadowed by the masculine tradition. These self-inscriptions were all acts of writing that would preserve her as a character in her own imaginative work—the living body of her "poetry" in the largest sense of that term. She had been performing this act of self-transcription in all her work, most notably in her earlier dramatic phase as the character with her own initials and a gun (instead of a pen) pointed at the heart of her faithless male lover at the end of *The Rover*, but never so intently and so richly as in the final two years. All of these self-inscriptions are colored by ambivalence, failure, and defeat, except her assertion of poetic immortality. *Oroonoko* seems to embody all of Behn's anxieties about the Stuart kings, as well as those concerning her roles as female author, poet, prophet, and Fate. But the horrific death of Oroonoko is somehow counterbalanced by Behn's final representation of him within her affirmation of her ongoing poetic life.

As Oroonoko reclaimed his original name before his final ordeal, so Mistress Behn, now at the very end of her novella both confirming herself in her present role as author and complimenting the sagacity of her noble dedicatee (and her ideal reader), rises above ambivalence about her female pen by enclosing her "masculine Part" in a subliminal pun within her final feminine inscription to assert the hope that "the Reputation of my pen is considerable enough to make his glorious Name to survive to all Ages, with that of the brave, the beautiful, and the constant *Imoinda*" (78). For Behn at the end, the enigmatic biblical prophecy that "a woman shall compass a man" (Jer. 31.22) encloses "my pen is considerable." This claim for her reputation as a writer reverses her assertion in the epistle dedicatory that the merit of Oroonoko alone will render the narrative worthy of honor and stresses the equal claim to glory of the heroine. Oroonoko and Imoinda are united in the end, a heroic unit. The first and final words of the narrative refer to a woman as *Oroonoko* is enclosed in a feminine embrace, Nature's child laid to rest. One thinks of all the narratives in Western literature through the seventeenth century in which the woman martyr has suffered physical violation. Mistress Behn rewrites this tradition by making Oroonoko-Imoinda her creation, her black Adam and Eve, her king-queen, hero-heroine (yet slaves), and she tenderly but implacably—like an inscrutable Fate or that unheard of thing, a female anatomist—writes them to death, dismembers them with her "female pen," in order to affirm an alternate gospel of stoic martyrdom in the pancultural ("original," "innocent") heroic pair, the united male and female hero of "all Mankind."

We have traced Behn's depiction of the erotic and religious power of the passive male body and of the power of the female image, the "sign of Angellica," in a variety of figurative versions. We saw the power of the passive female body in the biblical stories of Sarah, Rebekah, Rachel, Hannah, Elisabeth and Mary, a power given new impetus from an entirely different source in Lucretius's representation of the force of a stream of minute material particles radiating from the beautiful female or male body. Milton incorporates the biblical and Lucretian dimensions of this motif in the spectacular image of Eve "ravishing" Satan, and now Richardson will take the image into a new and complex dimension in his interior portrait of Clarissa, a radiantly beautiful young woman who invests her entire being—her "heart"—in the medium of writing as act and artifact.

5

The Written Heart
Clarissa, Lovelace, and Scripture

> Theas rene sjel var i den bok. [Thea's pure soul was in that book.]
> —HENRIK IBSEN, *Hedda Gabler*

> Hearts are not had as a gift but hearts are earned.
> —WILLIAM BUTLER Yeats, "A Prayer for My Daughter"

THE LATE seventeenth-century English neo-Platonist John Norris, referred to by Clarissa's literary editor, John Belford, as "a poetical divine" and "an excellent Christian," was a writer much esteemed by Samuel Richardson in his own private meditations and alluded to in other significant ways in *Clarissa*. Norris makes a compelling transitional figure as we move from the language of the heart in Milton and Behn to the greatest work of narrative fiction in the eighteenth century, and the most complex imagining, by a male author, of the female act of writing in relation to the heart.[1] Norris, in *The Theory and Regulation of Love* (1688—the same year as the publication of *Oroonoko*), reworks the Augustinian (and Miltonic) notion of love as the motion of the soul toward good into the new "scientific" language (which we have traced from Hobbes to Willis, among others) of action upon the body and the body's reaction, making an analogy between the motion of physical gravity and the motion of the soul as he considers the similarity between the motion of love and the motion of the heart. I would like first to explore a few passages from this work that I think Richardson the reader would have found stimulating as he pondered the idea of "Clarissa" and ones that I find suggestive for a reading of the novel in the context of Lucretian materialism and the Hobbesian dialogue of force we noted in the Introduction and in certain of the narratives of the heart we have examined up to this point.

Milton's maternal Earth formed out of her own womb of waters becomes now for Norris the maternal emblem of Newtonian gravity, exerting an attractive force not unlike the terrific suction of the feminized Galenic Hell swallowing Satan and his fallen angels:

Having in the foregoing Section fix'd the general Idea of Love in the *Motion* of the Soul towards *good* . . . I thought it concern'd me to draw here a short Parallel between *Love* and *Physical Motion*. . . . Further therefore, as this Affection call'd *Gravity* in Bodys, is nothing else but that *first impression* or alteration made upon them by the various actings of those Effluviums or streams of Particles which issue out from the womb of the great Magnet, the *Earth* . . . so in the like manner this radical *Complacency* . . . of the Soul towards good (which I call her *Moral Gravity*) is nothing else but that first Alteration or Impression which is made upon her by the streaming influences of the Great and Supreme Magnet, *God*.[2]

Norris's discussion of the heart amalgamates the notion of the heart as a main component of the "Humane Machine" (which we have seen in writers as diverse as Crooke, Hobbes, and Charleton), with the traditional Platonic image of the heart as a natural fountain, the Aristotelian/Galenic stress on the heat of the heart, and the importance of the heart for Aristotle and Harvey as the first organ in the body to live and the last to die:

I have also another Parallel to make between Love and a *certain particular Motion*, namely that of the *Heart*. . . . First then we may Consider that the Heart is the great Wheel of the Humane Machine, the Spring of all Animal and vital Motion, and the Head-fountain of Life . . . and that its Motion is the First and Leading Motion of all, that it begins as soon as the Flame of Life is Kindled, and ends not till the *vital Congruity* be quite dissolv'd. (23)

He also gives a religious and ethical version of the significance of the double motion of the heart that we have considered throughout this study. I take "concupiscence" to mean erotic love and "benevolence" to mean charity:

And if we further Meditate upon the Motion of the Heart we shall find that it is not only an apt Embleme of *Love in General*, but that it also Mystically points out to us the *two great Species* of Love, *Concupiscence* and *Benevolence*. The Motion of the Heart we know is Double, *Dilatation* and *Contraction*. Dilatation whereby it receives blood into its Ventricles, and Contraction whereby it expels it out again. And is it not so also in this great Pulse of the Soul, *Love*? Is there not here also the like double Motion? For we *desire* good, which answers to the Dilatation and immission of the Blood, and we also *wish well to*, which answers to the Contraction and Emission of it. (29)

Norris goes on to say that as the arterial blood is transmitted to the brain by the pulse in order to generate "animal spirits" (the same animal spirits we examined in relation to Milton's Eve), which govern the action of the body (including the heart), so love, or the "moral gravity" of the soul, first moves the understanding that in turn moves the will, for the will and understanding move each other. This animal or spiritual circulation presides over the vital physical circulation, a discussion relevant to the moral psychology of *Clarissa*. He then gives the most explicit account I have found (by a writer who is not by profession a physician or "natural philosopher") of the circulation of the blood as it was understood and interpreted after Harvey and before Richardson:

Again as by the Continual Reciprocation of the *Pulse* there is caused a Circulation of the Blood, which is expell'd out of the Heart into the Arteries, out of these into the parts which are to be Nourish'd, from whence 'tis imbibed by the Capillary Veins, which lead it back to the Vena Cava and so into the Heart again; the same may in proportion be applied to Love. This is the *Great Pulse* of the *Body Politic*, as the other is of the *Body Natural*. 'Tis Love that begets and Keeps up the great Circulation and Mutual Dependence of Society, by this Men are inclined to maintain Mutual Commerce and intercourse with one another, and to distribute their Benefits and Kindnesses to all the parts of the Civil body, till at length they return again upon themselves in the *Circle* and *Reciprocation of Love*. (23–29)

One of the most difficult questions we face in attempting to delineate the "heart" of Clarissa is the nature and meaning of "love" in her experience, love as it is defined by Norris in its erotic and especially its "benevolent" and "emissive" spiritual senses.

Richardson as *Kardiognostes*

Discerning contemporaries well read in Richardson's fiction established what has come down to us as one of the most frequently invoked clichés of eighteenth-century literary history. In his novels, Richardson provided a masterly representation of human nature, and he was applauded particularly for his delineation of the human heart.[3] The association of the heart and the writing process was always a close one for Richardson. It begins with the heart as a storehouse of memory, an exceedingly sensitive instrument for receiving, recording, preserving, and expressing human experience. This image of the heart tends to stress the "feminine" component of the bisexual heart outlined in the Introduction, a highly refined version of the Galenic powers of attraction, reception, preservation, in a complex new public and textual or "print" dimension. In an analogy with the physiological operation of the circulatory system as it was understood after Harvey, in which the heart both receives and discharges the blood, the cultural ideal of the good woman or good man for Richardson and many of his contemporaries is represented by a friendly, undesigning, innocent, worthy, feeling heart (adjectives drawn from Richardson's correspondence), a heart capable of receiving the most refined impressions, but a heart that also hides nothing and that expresses itself with uncommon openness, spontaneity, and lucidity, whether speaking or writing—especially writing. The supreme goal for the Richardsonian correspondent was to transform human absence into presence by translating, faithfully, the life blood of intimate, natural, spoken conversation into written conversation. This pattern is a social repetition of the mutual movement from the spoken to the written/the written to the spoken, which we noted in Chapter 1. The intense epistolary correspondence Richardson describes is intimately connected with the receptive/expressive nature of the hearts of the writers and readers within his fictions and with the hearts of the outside readers of the fictions. Hence familiar letter writing is an ongoing expression of the heart of the writer and an impression on the heart of the reader, a circulatory system of receiving, expressing, and receiving again those impressions and ideas closest to the hearts of the individual correspondents.

Like Hobbes and Locke, but in a much more tangible personal sense, Richardson was acutely aware of *impressions*. For almost forty years he worked intimately with the process and business of printing and bookmaking—the messy literal business of print impression—before he wrote the first of his three novels. It is hard to imagine a more "bookish" writer than Richardson. He wrote books, he printed books, he collected books—he once even characterized himself as a book "taken up and laid down" by the ladies.[4] He was the only major English writer who made his living as a printer. Richardson's entire literary career might be seen as a recapitulation (and repetition) of the evolution from script to print. Printing, reading—and eventually writing—books was his life work, so it is not at all surprising that given his acute religious sensibility he should see his own life—and that of the fictional creation closest to his heart—under the aspect of God's "book of life," the register of those names enrolled for salvation at the last day, as discussed in the first chapter.[5]

Talking about the heart and nature was a way for Richardson and his contemporaries to express an awareness of his having provided in his fictions a new representation of inner experience, of the inner self, most notably the "passions," centering on that of love between men and women as expressed in his social world, but also considering love and friendship between women, and love and friendship between men.⁶ "All the letters are written," Richardson says in his preface, "while the hearts of the writers must be supposed to be wholly engaged in their subjects" so that the descriptions of "critical situations" as they arise are "brought home to the breast of the youthful reader" (1:xiv). It was customary in the eighteenth century to describe someone's being in love in terms of whether or not his or her heart was "engaged," and we still use the term "engaged" in a similar sense. But obviously the connection with love is not the only sense in which the heart can be "engaged," as we have seen in the previous chapters.

If ethical and religious experience is also taken to be, in the Protestant tradition especially, an expression of the inner life of humankind, Richardson's stress on inner experience is also a way of exploring certain religious states of mind and being. He first put this idea explicitly (and didactically) in the postscript to the first edition: the work "is designed to inculcate upon the human mind, under the guise of an amusement, the great lessons of Christianity."⁷ As he kept rereading and revising *Clarissa* through the first three editions (and all its "impressions"), the idea that the narrative had great religious import seems to have continued to work on him, but he came to express this idea more subtly. For example, in the preface to the third edition of *Clarissa* (1751), where after expressing his typical and no doubt deeply felt sense of the work's monitory function, he notes that "above all," he aimed in *Clarissa* "to investigate the highest and most important doctrines not only of morality, but of Christianity, by showing them thrown into action in the conduct of the worthy characters" and "the unworthy" (1:xv). This is Richardson's version of the emphasis on narrative *motion* we have been observing in the major texts treated in this study. Again, in the postscript to the third edition, in tones reminiscent of an Old Testament prophet, he amplifies in this age of "general depravity, when even the pulpit has lost great part of its weight," the "great end" he had in view in *Clarissa*. English "Puritan" and Anglican divines of the late seventeenth century—Thomas Watson, Stephen Charnock, John Norris, Robert South, John Tillotson, to name a few—seem closer to him in temperament than those of his own day, with a few exceptions, like his visionary friends Edward Young and William Law.⁸ "The author thought he should be able to answer it to his own heart [if] . . . he could steal in . . . and investigate the great doctrines of Christianity under the fashionable guise of an amusement" (4:553).⁹

The ambivalent word "investigate," which Richardson uses twice in describing his aim, does not occur in the preface or postscript to the first edition. For Samuel Johnson, to investigate means "to search out; to find out by rational disquisition"; investigation is "the act of the mind by which unknown truths are discovered" (*Dictionary*, 1755). The sense for both Richardson and Johnson seems to be in part an ongoing quasi-legal inquiry; it is a curiously "scientific" word for Richardson to use, and with it he can appeal to his more "philosophical" readers, even "deists." But the word also has the older etymological sense of "to trace or find out by steps, to search or inquire diligently," to trace (*vestigare*, track) something back to its source in order to achieve an original pristine meaning or state of being that has been lost or forgotten, as defined in Bailey's *Dictionnarium Britannicum* (1736). (This work was printed, in part, by Richardson.) One thinks of Aphra Behn's plaintive cry, "All I ask is the Privilege of my Masculine Part the Poet in me . . . to tread in those successful Paths my Predecessors have so long thrived in." If the act of writing is always an abbreviated form of treading, traveling, travailing, Aphra Behn's unconventional "female pen" broke ground not only for women writers, but for male-authored fictions about women writers in the early eighteenth century, especially those of Defoe and Richardson. In one sense, the history of Clarissa Harlowe is the tracing of her *vestigia*, of the tracks of her pen, translated into print, signifying the pure remembrances of trial and transcendence that her author (who chooses this way to walk in the ways of the Lord [Ps. 119.1–3]) wishes to impress upon his reader. Lovelace too, after the rape, meditates on Clarissa's "*vestigia*" (3:242) in relation to her broken heart.

Richardson may have been an orthodox, conservative Anglican with strong Puritan traits in the conduct of his day-to-day life, but his writing of *Clarissa* in the mid-1740s transformed his conventional religious ideology into a radical exploration and revision of the main doctrines of Protestant Christianity. On the vexed question of the meaning of the terms "Anglican" and "Puritan" as they relate in the ensuing commentary to English Protestant doctrine and practice, I am following, for the most part, the lead of Horton Davies who stresses the Puritans' preponderating concern with the individual's personal interpretation of the Holy Scripture and "interiority," with intense self-examination, with preaching, and with recording the intervention of divine grace in one's life, that is, with "witnessing," orally and in writing. The Puritan must have been one of the most discursive of all religious beings and Richardson is the end product of a long line of voluminous writers.[10] In his visionary, even apocalyptic, enterprise Richardson recalls Milton in *Paradise Lost*, and he has more in common—possibly via the influence of the ubiquitous William Law—with the author of "The Marriage of Heaven and Hell" (another self-educated English tradesman if only a part-time printer) than with his conventional Christian contemporaries. What were the doctrines Richardson wished to "investigate"? Whether he thought his program through in a systematic way or not (and Richardson the novelist is certainly not the religious ideologue Terry Eagleton makes him out to be), *Clarissa* was to emerge as the most profound and disturbing exploration in English fiction of the major religious issues in the Protestant tradition, primarily those of the meaning and nature of evil, the significance of the Fall, the conflict between the fallen world and the individual soul, the meaning of regeneration, the nature of Christian love and forgiveness, and the question of God's ultimate relationship to humankind.

It is not my purpose to explore these issues in detail. Rather, in this chapter, I shall focus particularly on Richardson's representation of the human heart as figured forth in Clarissa's experience—her "heart-workings," to borrow a term from the Puritan divines—in the context of representations of the heart in Scripture and devotional works as discussed in the Introduction and the first chapter that have the most bearing on his fiction. I want to suggest that the central dynamic of this enormously comprehensive novel is an extended parable of the trial and redemption of the heart. I suggested in Chapter 2 that trial is at the center of heroic narrative, secular and religious, in the dynamic of journey, quest, ordeal, travel and travail, new birth, self-overcoming, transcendence. We have seen unique versions of such trial and quest in narratives of the heart as diverse as *The Motion of the Heart, Paradise Lost*, and *Oroonoko*.[11] In *Clarissa*, Richardson imagines a new version of the traditional Christian account of how the Old Testament Law of the Father God gives way—in a regenerative process of unexampled trial and suffering for the new Christian hero, a woman and a writer—to a new covenant echoing the one first articulated, as we have seen, by Jeremiah in the apogee of Hebrew prophecy and reformulated by St. Paul in 2 Corinthians, a covenant written not in stone but in the tables of the heart—that is, in the book of the heart.[12]

The evidence for this discussion (in addition to the 1751 edition of *Clarissa*) will come from Richardson's own writing and reading, insofar as we know what he read, and from works that helped shape his Anglican/Puritan milieu and set of mind. In his correspondence, Richardson cultivated the pose of the nonreader, but we know that he read the Bible—frequently, carefully, devotedly—and in such a way as to make it a creative element of his fiction. His reading of the Bible was in some ways more characteristically Anglican than Puritan; Richardson should in this be counted with Harvey, and with Swift and Arbuthnot—the literary generation of Tory Anglicans in eclipse during the period of his full creative maturity. Richardson thought the Wisdom books of the Bible a "treasure of morality," notably Proverbs, and from the Apocrypha (still accepted as "inspired," especially for its moral instruction, by many eighteenth-century Christians), the Wisdom of Solomon and Ecclesiasticus. (The original 1611 edition of the Authorized Version contained the Apocrypha.) Lovelace has a great aversion to Proverbs because, when a boy, he never asked anything of his uncle, Lord M., "but out flew a *proverb*. . . . I made it a condition with my tutor, who was an honest parson, that I would not read my Bible at all, if he would not excuse me one of the wisest books in it. . . . And as for Solomon, he was then a hated character with me, not because of his polygamy, but because I had conceived him to be such another musty old fellow as my uncle" (2:329). Other books of the Bible most important to Richardson in the composition of *Clarissa* are Genesis, the Psalms, the Gospel narratives, the Pauline epistles (particularly 1 and 2 Corinthians), Revelation, and above all the Book of Job.

It is not too much to say that Richardson, in *Clarissa*, seems to be writing his own secular version of scripture. The "new" literary-historiographical approach to the Bible, exemplified in the work of Robert Alter and Meir Sternberg, has exciting possibilities in relation to a text like *Clarissa*. Starting with the similarity of sheer size (considering the King James Bible with the addition of the Apocrypha), the two works, *Clarissa* and the Bible, share certain features. For example, in each the narrative is a collection and series of smaller books (*ta biblia* / letters). Each work stresses narrative progression through dialogue and the development of unique kinds of "historicized prose fiction."[13] Each presents an extended and powerful early depiction of "family history" generating "family tragedy." Each poses a profound epistemological challenge to the reader. Making exceptions for Richardson's penchant for editorializing (especially in the later editions of the novel), I suggest that Sternberg could almost be talking about *Clarissa* when he says of the Bible,

the ubiquity of gaps about character and plot exposes to us our own ignorance: history unrolls as a continuum of discontinuities, a sequence of non sequiturs, which challenge us to repair the omissions by our native wit. Through a mimesis of real-life conditions of inference, we are surrounded by ambiguities, baffled and misled by appearances, reduced to piecing fragments together by trial and error, often left in the dark about essentials to the very end. Insofar as knowledge is true judgment, moreover, the scarcity of commentary forces us to evaluate the agent and action by appeal to norms that remain implicit, to clues that may have more than one face, to structures that turn on reconstruction, to voices partial in both senses. . . . With the narrative become an obstacle course, its reading turns into a drama of understanding—conflict between inferences, seesawing, reversal, discovery, and all. The only knowledge perfectly acquired is the knowledge of our limitations . . . to make sense of the discourse is to gain a sense of being human.[14]

There is no question that Richardson, despite his weak eyesight and modesty about his limited learning, was a diligent reader of the Bible and almost everything else. We know he read, in the line of duty, many of the works that were produced by his press, and as William Sale long ago showed us, "The clergy constituted the largest single group for which he printed."[15] And we know Richardson read himself. In the whole course of the tortuous evolution of *Clarissa*, he put himself through the same protracted physical writing and reading efforts he inflicted on his main characters—which included constant revising, transcribing for friends, re-transcribing, rereading both aloud and silently passages in the novel itself, and rereading his previous writing—and he did all this while attending to the business of his press, which was another way in which he read himself, or his own output.[16] Richardson loved to read his own writing but almost always, I think, with a view to revision, correction, and the additional sharpening of critical passages. It is hard to imagine Richardson reading anything without pen in hand, at his desk, "proofreading" in the literal sense of probing and testing for what he took to be the best representation of the "truth" about his characters in relation to themselves and to others.

I wish to suggest early in this chapter that Richardson continues the tradition of the narrative artist as "anatomist" or "*kardiognostes*" (to recall the Puritan Thomas Watson's terms), using the point of his pen as an anatomical instrument, not in the manner of Helkiah Crooke, nor in that of the inscrutable female Fate, Aphra Behn, who dismembers her male protagonist into a state of permanent remembrance, but delicately to sift, to probe, to "investigate," to "search" the hearts of his chief characters for the "truth" of their being. But he does this in a marvelously complex and indirect way, by casting his major, and some minor characters, in the role of anatomical "heart searchers" and "heart knowers." Anna Howe, for example, is represented by the literary critic Clarissa (in shivering accents of what I take to be erotic sublimation) as the best kind of satirist, one whose art is "founded in good nature, and directed by a right heart," who "makes one thankful for the wounds given by a true friend": "I am almost *afraid* to beg of you," writes Clarissa, "and yet I repeatedly *do*, to give way to that charming spirit whenever it rises to your pen, which smiles yet goes to the quick of one's fault. What patient shall be afraid of a probe in so delicate a hand." The final destination of this probe is of course the heart: "I may *feel* your edge, fine as it is; I may be pained . . . but after the first sensibility . . . I will love you the better, and my amended heart shall be all yours" (1:345). Within this playful use of the idiom of eighteenth-century surgical discourse and the conventional terms of heterosexual romance, Clarissa seems to be offering her heart to her lover.

If Anna the lover is Clarissa's best anatomist, Uncle Antony is her worst. After receiving Clarissa's desperate but ill-conceived letter denouncing her brother and Solmes, he assumes the role of the violently indignant Puritan preacher: "I will search your heart to the bottom; that is to say, if your letter be written from your heart. . . . So a noted whoremonger is to be chosen before a man who is a money-lover! . . . The devil's in your sex!" (1:160). As the relationship between Lovelace and Clarissa becomes more tortured after the departure from her father's house, Lovelace the tempter becomes the accuser, and in his great letter about testing Clarissa, he tries her heart by her own thoughts: "Well then, if love it be at bottom, is there not another fault lurking beneath the shadow of that love?—Has she not *affectation?*—or is it *pride of heart?* . . . is her virtue founded in *pride?*" (2:38). As we shall see, Clarissa becomes the courageous but ambiguous searcher of her own heart, and those of others, as she evolves into the quasi-divine female extension of her author.

If Richardson is "investigating" and rewriting Scripture for the edification of his own contemporaries, the trope of "searching the heart" may be the chief parallel between *Clarissa* and the Bible. Richardson, as modest as he appears to be, saw himself as part of a larger literary tradition (including Chaucer, Spenser, and Milton) in which the author or "maker" is at times an interpreter of God's word by means of his fictional creations. As such, he is a finite imitator of the Creator. Hence in Richardson's unique iteration of the divine creative process we examined in Psalm 139 (in the first chapter), his characters are first "written" in his manuscript and then "wrought" into books in the workshop of his printing press.

Richardson seems to have thought that his main contribution to the novel, his "new species of writing," was his representation of "writing to the moment," a talent for engaging his reader's heart by creating the illusion of the writing character's immediate and unfolding consciousness. In an age preoccupied with the artistic representation of "critical moments"—an attitude exemplified in the engravings of Hogarth—Richardson is the literary master of momentary narrative.[17] But all "moments" are by definition ephemeral. Richardson *did* finish the long labor of *Clarissa*, and with a finality many of his friends could hardly bear. For he did not lose sight of the final version of God's narrative for man in the Last Judgment and its bearing on his heroine's spiritual transformation.

Richardson's religious sensibility was especially attuned to the Puritan emphasis on the primacy of the Word of God in Scripture and the necessity for the Christian "professor" to read the Bible properly and to *write out* his or her relationship with God, whether by simply copying in a journal passages of Scripture particularly relevant to one's sense of one's own spiritual needs (or those of others) or by writing extensive "spiritual autobiographies," almost all of which could be described as conversion narratives.[18] The Puritan, more than any other Protestant believer, stood in a "writing" posture toward God and was supposed to be a living imitation of the Word made flesh, a living book of the Word, having transcribed him or herself into the proper relationship with God via Scripture. Now Richardson saw himself as a "common reader" of the Bible, not an expert in "opening" the text to elucidate doctrine. Because of his ill health and nervous disorders he was an infrequent churchgoer, but he read many sermons in the course of his professional career, and he was familiar with a wide range of Anglican and Puritan devotional literature.

A useful exposition of the idea of God as Author of humankind and the Puritan emphasis on the centrality of God's Word to all human existence, attitudes I believe Richardson shared, may be found in the nonconforming seventeenth-century divine Thomas Watson, whose discussion of God's "anatomy" of the heart we examined in the first chapter. Watson combines the trope of "writing in the heart" with epistolarity. For him, the Bible is a familiar letter, God's "golden epistle" sent expressly to mankind, and he gives explicit directions on how readers should "prepare [their] hearts" for receiving this "love-letter" from the Lord. "How doth one delight to read over his friend's letter! The word written is a divine treasury, or storehouse . . . to adorn 'the hidden man of the heart.'" One should labor to remember the Word, to get the Scriptures "by heart," to virtually *become* the Bible. The Roman lady Cecilia "made her breast *bibliothecam Christi*," the library of Christ, and all "Christians should be walking Bibles."[19] The great John Tillotson himself (whom Richardson quotes at the end of *Sir Charles Grandison*) had said that "No man can write after too perfect and good a copy," and the most perfect of all fair copies was thought to be Christ.[20] As Richard Steele (the divine) puts it in his sermon on the mutual duties of husband and wife, Christ " 'loved the church, and gave himself for it' . . . The husband must write after this copy. Not to love his wife in word and tongue only, but in deed and in truth; that if his heart were opened, her name might be found written there." We recall that the pagan Oroonoko said, "he shou'd have an eternal *Idea* in his Mind of the Charms [Imoinda] now bore; and shou'd look into his Heart for that *Idea*, when he cou'd find it no longer in her Face" (11). The true imitation of Christ is proper and virtuous "writing" after his example. "The purest love is written in prayer," and writing in the heart is the only sincere writing because it is the true union of word and deed—the writing of true virtue.[21]

Since the Bible is "the heart and soul of God" given to humankind, Watson implies that one should literally copy out the Word of God by hand, especially those parts that point directly to one's condition, putting a "special star" beside them, so that one can give the proper answer to these questions: "Are your hearts, as it were, a transcript and counterpane [a legal copy] of scripture? Is the word copied out into your hearts?" Watson's culminating exhortation, "Get the word transcribed into your hearts . . . Never leave till you are assimilated into the word," suggests that to the Puritan sensibility the best Christians are those who have best experienced the Word as readers, transcribers, and writers.[22]

Richardson read the Bible (in the Authorized Version) with the eyes of a master printer and with those of the female and male characters—all writers—he so brilliantly impersonated in his writing. In what follows (as in the first chapter), I ask the reader to help me "read" Richardson and Scripture with a similar act of empathetic impersonation. We shall turn first to the Old Testament. How would a Clarissa have read it? There is no more striking indication of Richardson's appeal to scriptural authority concerning a father's dealings with a daughter than Clarissa's invoking of Numbers 30 to rescind her promise to throw herself on the protection of Lovelace's family and meet him outside the garden door of "her father's house." Richardson the editor (in all the editions) appends a note that "the vows of a single woman, and of a wife, if the father of the one, or the husband of the other, disallow of them as soon as they know them, are to be of no force" (1:458).[23] This matter is so "highly necessary to be known by all young ladies especially" that the editor even quotes the four verses which particularly specify how the father's silence will affirm the vow by which the daughter "hath bound her soul," or how his breaking his peace will override and cancel her vow. Only the father's voice—speaking or even silent—is authentic. These verses may reinforce Clarissa's extraordinary deference to—and terror of—her father's voice.[24] Clarissa closes her "undigested self-reasonings" on her rash promise to Lovelace ("rather an *appointment* than a promise") and her strong bias against the odious Solmes by appealing to the authority of the heart: "the *heart* is, as I may say, *conscience*." She bases this appeal as well on scriptural authority, the "wise man" of Ecclesiasticus: "Let the counsel of thine own heart stand; for there is no man more faithful to thee, than it" (1:460, Ecclus. 37.13–14). Here then is a telling and poignant indication of Clarissa's early moral quandary. Asserting "the privilege of her sex" to change her mind, she can invoke, by way of Scripture, her father's authority to absolve her of a confirmed promise (1:443), while at the same time heroically defying his wishes for her marriage to Solmes, and then justify her action, again on scriptural authority, in the name of following the counsel of her own heart. If Clarissa can invoke a rather obscure passage from Numbers to support her position as a daughter making every dutiful obeisance to her parents short of self-sacrifice, we may accept that her reading of the rest of the Bible is at least attentive.

Inveterate Bible readers and letter writers and copiers like Aphra Behn (as we have seen) or Richardson (or Clarissa, or Anna Howe, or Pamela) would be unlikely to overlook the industrious scribal activities of a character like Moses in Exodus, and they would pay particular attention to the stories of women in the Bible and to references to the "book of life," as sketched in Chapter 1. The story of Hannah had particular interest for Richardson I believe partly because of his intense preoccupation with perpetuating his own given name. Six sons were born to the Richardsons (Richardson was married twice); all died in childbirth or early childhood, and *four* were named Samuel.[25] Richardson's own awareness, expressed with genuine modesty, of a talent for discerning the workings of the human heart, recalls Samuel as the agent for selecting "the Lord's anointed." Samuel learns to distrust appearances and follow God's direction to the inward truth, for "the Lord seeth not as man seeth; for man looketh on the outward appearance, but the Lord looketh on the heart" (1 Sam. 16.7). As I have shown in *Mother Midnight*, Richardson's more than ordinarily paternal interest in the experience of childbirth is evident all through his novels, but particularly in both parts of *Pamela* and in *Clarissa*, and he was no doubt aware that women's unique inwardness of experience is recognized repeatedly in Scripture, an experience related to their bearing of children.[26] As a close reader of the Bible, it is likely that he would have shared the sense, illustrated in Chapter 1, that woman's role as the preserver and nurturer of human seed relates to woman's experience of the heart.

In the late seventeenth and the first half of the eighteenth century—as is evident in the extracts quoted from Norris's *Theory and Regulation of Love*, to give just one example—the representation of the heart takes on new and more positive meaning as the source of circulatory power, vital equilibrium, and a variety of expressions of love. The heart, physiologically as well as in its contexts of mind, emotion, courage, integrity, inner religious conviction, and above all—by the mid-eighteenth century—sympathy, compassion, and "consciousness," comes to stand for the essential core of humanity. A memorable text depicting this transition in the early eighteenth century is Sir Richard Steele's *The Conscious Lovers*. Steele's young protagonist, Bevill Junior (secretly in love with Indiana), begins his day by putting on "an easy look with an aching heart," but prepares his spirit by reading Addison's *Spectator* 159, "The Vision of Mirzah," whose hero's heart, like an extension of Aphra Behn's Lycidus, melts away in secret raptures in the contemplation of Paradise. Bevill Junior tells the wise old servant Humphry "the story of [his] heart," which turns out to be a narrative of his beloved Indiana's tragic history. He is as "irrecoverably fixed upon this lady . . . '*as his vital life dwells in his heart*' "—that is, she is now *his* vital life, and they are "conscious" lovers because they have a preternatural awareness of each other's feelings.[27] They read each other's hearts. Bevill Junior does not have to wait to die for her face to be discovered in his heart; it is there every conscious moment of his existence. Steele's major concern in this play is to represent the mutuality of "conscious" love, of lovers constantly thinking about the beloved one's distress, internalizing it, making it one's own.

Such "consciousness" is a further extension of that limned by Congreve in the transitional "Restoration" comedy *The Way of the World*, in which his anatomistically inclined hero Mirabell "took [his mistress] to pieces; sifted her and separated her failings," and got them by rote till at length they were as familiar to him as his own frailties.[28] Indiana owes her life to young Bevill and must "suppress her heart . . . painfully divided between shame and love" out of her sex's natural decency and shame. She becomes an early eighteenth-century icon of the new passive woman whose sole purpose in life is "to please" her male savior, Bevill.²⁹ In Steele's melodramatic "bourgeois" comedy, the feeling heart becomes what it means to be human. When Clarissa says that Lovelace "wants a *heart*: and if he does, he wants everything" (1:202), she sums up in one simple phrase the richly evolving definition of the heart as an interlace of mutually shared associations against which her own heart experience must be measured.

Lovelace and the Male Heart

What does it mean that Lovelace wants a heart? What were the characteristics of the "good" masculine heart? Clarissa says early on that "whatever had been the *figure* of the man . . . the *heart* is what we women should judge by in the choice we make, as the best security for the party's good behaviour in every relation of life" (1:198). We can infer from a variety of contexts in the novel that the good masculine heart is kind, good-natured, generous, considerate, "conscious" in Steele's sense, and faithful. Anna Howe's Mr. Hickman has perhaps more of these traits (in varying degrees) than any of the other male characters in the novel. But it is Anna Howe and Clarissa who have the purest heart relationship as defined in terms of "consciousness," the capacity for mutually shared feeling, for entering deeply into the distresses of the other.

But if Lovelace "wants" the kind of heart that Clarissa and Anna Howe want to see in a man, he still (like Behn's Willmore) has a heart—a "bad heart," "a vile heart," a heart of "adamant," an "odious heart" (to rehearse some of the epithets for him used by women—and men—in the novel). There are almost as many allusions to Lovelace's heart as to Clarissa's, and Lovelace himself develops a rich imaginary and rhetoric for his own "masculine" heart. All through this study, beginning with Plato, we have seen examples of what might be called a "male heart function" in the discourse of the heart, and I would like here briefly to review our encounter with the multifaceted representation of the male heart. It is important to note that the same heart was thought to be operating in women and in men, but that the rhetoric of the heart often had a phallic bias. For Plato, the heart was a knot of veins producing a hot, racing fountain of blood, which guarded the power of feeling in the body against external dangers. The "Hippocratic" heart was a strong muscle with a large hot chamber housing the intelligent ruling principle of the soul, a view shared by Lucretius and the Stoics. In Aristotle's predominantly masculinist depiction of nature, the heart contains mental functions. It is the vehicle of the soul and thus the primary organ responsible for reproduction and movement.

Our survey of the biblical representation of the male heart focused on the "hardening of the heart" motif, especially God's hardening of Pharaoh's heart, on circumcision as a sign of God's power over the male source of generation, and on God's power over the "circumcision of the heart" in males and females. We noted how the boiling amorous heart of Lucretius's male lover causes him to roam restlessly "eager to inject" his seed into the "leaky kind," in Dryden's words. The earliest English anatomists saw the heart as virtually a genital organ, and Helkiah Crooke stressed the potentially destructive and unruly heat of the heart unless checked by reason. Crooke the traditional Galenic anatomist and Hobbes the new Lucretian-materialist philosopher of the body both characterized the heart as a strong engine or a mechanical spring, but it was William Harvey who was the first to *demonstrate* the tremendous systolic ejaculatory power of the human heart, especially the force of the left ventricle driving blood to the farthest reaches of what, in *The Motion of the Blood*, is a feminized body. Milton's Father God generates the Son from his eternally creative "bosom," and we saw how the "tumultuous breast" of Milton's Satan, like a "devilish engine" or cannon, recoils back on itself to produce his "dire attempt" against the human pair, exerting his full concentration on Eve, and culminating in the guileful oratory of an erect serpent whose words penetrate her entranced heart. In Behn's *The Rover*, Willmore's randomly aggressive male heart is subtly equated, in provocative dialogue with the wickedly virtuous Hellena, with the roving phallus. And Rochester, whom Behn honors as a "young Lucretius," conducts a graphic dialogue with his recalcitrant penis after it has failed to convey his "soul" up to the "heart" of his passionate mistress. This long and varied tradition of the rhetoric of the sexualized male heart reaches its eighteenth-century climax in Lovelace's dialogue with his own phallic heart in *Clarissa*.

Lovelace is introduced into the women's epistolary discourse as "a man of whose heart she could not be sure for one moment" by none other than Clarissa's envious sister (1:9). He is generally known as a man of "vivacity" and "courage," and Clarissa comments further on the "swift and surprising progress he made in all parts of literature" (1:14). Lovelace (like the young Cowley or his own namesake in the seventeenth century) is an aspiring *literatus*, a man of letters and a poet whose intellectual reputation, according to Clarissa's cousin, the worldly man of sense Colonel Morden, was tarnished in Florence and Rome by certain "liberties" he chose to indulge in. The conventional components of Restoration libertinism included an antirationalist skepticism, a revolt against conventional arranged marriage, the promotion of a varied and hedonistic sensualism, a predominant emphasis on Nature over Custom (as figured in "honor"), and on freedom of thought and expression, among other tenets.[30] This definition embraced a libertinism that included both Behn and Rochester as adherents. Colonel Morden provides the eloped Clarissa with his own idea of a "libertine," one which surpasses the Restoration model in the intensity of its mid-eighteenth-century "Richardsonian" cultural focus:

> A libertine, my dear cousin, a *plotting*, an *intriguing* libertine, must be generally *remorseless*. . . . The noble rule of doing to others what he would have done to himself is the first rule he breaks. . . . He has great contempt for your sex. . . . How will a young lady of your delicacy bear with so sensual a man? A man who makes a jest of his vows; and who perhaps will break your spirit by the most unmanly insults. To be a libertine . . . all compunction, all humanity, must be overcome. . . . I write what I know *has* been. (2:259–60)

Clarissa more than once expresses her apprehension of "these fierce, these masculine spirits" (1:22), which contend around her in Harlowe Place. Of these her brother is the most persevering and violent, he who "with such *masculine* passions, should endeavour to control and bear down an unhappy sister" (1:139). It is he whom the intrepid Lovelace wounds and disarms in a skirmish of swords. It hardly needs pointing out that the sword was an all too visible metaphor for the phallus in an age which might appropriately be named "The Reign of the Phallus" (to adapt Eva Keuls's title for her book on ancient Greek sexual culture)—beginning with the Restoration and continuing well into the eighteenth century—when gentlemen went armed in public, when duels were so frequent they provoked legislation against them, when male homosocial honor was upheld by the sword. Aphra Behn represents this cultural phenomenon with more psychological insight than most Restoration playwrights. Her male whore Gayman (in *The Lucky Chance*) is rendered momentarily impotent with shame in the presence of his monstrous landlady Gammer Grime when she says his "very Badge of Manhood's gone," meaning his "Silver Sword," pawned for an old-fashioned basket hilt.[31] Colley Cibber's Lord Foppington in *The Careless Husband* puts the case succinctly: "a man should no more give up his heart to a woman than his sword to a bully; they are both as insolent as the devil after it."[32] We should read Lovelace's talk about his heart in this verbal and cultural context of phallic violence, while at the same time recalling the idiom of Rochester's address to his "treacherous," "base," "recreant" penis, quoted and discussed in Chapter 3.

In his first letter to John Belford, his closest friend and a libertine, Lovelace quietly sets the tone: "Thou knowest my heart, if any living man does. As far as I know it myself, though knowest it. But 'tis a cursed deceiver; for it has many and many a time imposed upon its master—*master*, did I say? That am I not now; nor have I been from the moment I beheld this angel of a woman" (1:145). His heart not only deceives others, it has its own autonomy, and masters even its master. His heart, a self-fashioned construct that incorporates his fiery poetic imagination, has attached itself to Clarissa, whom Lovelace generally represents as "a charming frost piece," continuing the ancient Galenic stereotype of the cold, phlegmatic woman, and one who has an "inflexible heart," an "impenetrable heart" (1:148). Already his "heart rises at her preference" of her own family to him and "how much more will [his] heart rise with indignation against her" if she, "however persecuted," prefers the despised Solmes to himself (1:148). Such language sets the stage throughout the entire novel for Lovelace's dialogue with his heart, a dialogue central to his epistolary conversation with a fellow rake who both abhors what Lovelace is doing with Clarissa yet cannot wait to get the next installment—a remarkable surrogate reader for the reader.

After Lovelace has tricked and frightened Clarissa into leaving her father's house and has secured her in a London brothel, her "spotless heart"—combined with her youth, beauty, virtue, artless innocence—frequently overawes him in their verbal duels, occasionally surprising him into what he considers "a fit of unmanly weakness" (2:316). At least one model for such passages is Milton's unfallen Eve "ravishing" Satan momentarily of his fierce attempt, and Lovelace sees his own heart as satanic. At a later time he says "the devil indeed, as soon as my angel made her appearance, crept out of my heart; but he had left the door open and was no farther off than my elbow" (2:376). But her apparent "*indifference*" to him enrages him: "That she could resolve to sacrifice me to the malice of my enemies; and carry on the design in so clandestine a manner—yet love her, as I do, to frenzy! . . . These were the recollections with which I fortified my recreant heart against her" (2:316). "*Hard-heartedness*, as it is called, is an *essential* of the *libertine's character*" (2:315), and Clarissa will say only a few days later, to Anna, "I take Mr. Lovelace to be one of the most hard-hearted men in the world" (2:372). Here the hardening of the male heart, a theme so potent and manifold in the biblical rhetoric of the heart and in Milton's prose and in his final epic depiction of Satan's malice, takes a new turn. Lovelace must repeatedly "fortify" and "steel [his] own heart" (2:316) with increasing intensity as he moves toward the final rape of Clarissa. Before he can "steel" his phallus, he must "steel" his heart.

I would like to focus on one passage in particular to demonstrate how the phallus and the heart coincide at a climactic "satanic" moment in Lovelace's pursuit of Clarissa and in his personal rhetoric of the male heart, which are both really aspects of the same phenomenon. After Clarissa escapes from Mother Sinclair's brothel in Westminster, Lovelace laments, "What a void in my heart! what a chillness in my blood, as if its circulation were arrested!" (2:524). But with the help of his "villain," Will, he tracks Clarissa down to Goody Moore's rooming house in Hampstead and disguises himself as an old man in a greatcoat, which covers "even the pommel of his sword." He stoops himself in the shoulders and practices walking around in the shuffling gait of a gout-ridden man, mumbling half-intelligibly. The disguise amalgamates the image of Clarissa's gouty, tyrannical father with the "squatting," encroaching, semi-articulate image of her chief suitor, Solmes, the man her "heart . . . abhors" (1:67). Lovelace casts his account of how he discovers Clarissa as one act in a melodramatic bourgeois comedy within an overall narrative, packing this self-conscious literary exercise with all the resources at his command for Belford's edification and excitement. It is the "narrative of narratives," and incorporated in it is Lovelace's ongoing narrative representation of his heart, which includes his dialogue with his own heart in the theater of the male sexual body. He beholds a "piece" of Clarissa as he hobbles up the stairs to her room: "thou canst not imagine how my heart danced to my mouth at the very glimpse of her, so that I was afraid the thump, thump, thumping villain, which had so lately thumped as much to no purpose, would have choked me" (3:36). As he gets closer to her his heart again begins "to play its pug's tricks" (3:36). When he hears Clarissa speak, "Oh! how my heart bounded again! It even talked to me, in a manner; for I thought I *heard*, as well as *felt*, its unruly flutters; and every vein about me seemed a pulse" (3:40). When she actually appears he attempts to keep up his disguised voice but it slips and his rake's devilish heart seems to take over. He swears "like a puppy," Clarissa recognizes his voice, and she "starts" in terror. "I threw open my great-coat, and, like the devil in Milton [an odd comparison though!],

> I started up in my own form divine,
> Touched by the beam of her celestial eye,
> More potent than Ithuriel's spear!—" (3:41).

We recall that in *Paradise Lost* the two guardian angels found Satan "Squat like a toad" (4.800) at the ear of Eve trying to pollute the organs of her fancy, as discussed in Chapter 3:

> Him thus intent Ithuriel with his Spear
> Touch'd lightly, for no falsehood can endure
> Touch of Celestial temper. . . .
> . . . Up he starts
> Discover'd. . . .
> . . . .
> So started up in his own shape the Fiend
> (4.810–19)

We can see that Lovelace's adaptation of Milton is extremely free; the word "potent" is not used in the Miltonic passage, and Lovelace identifies himself with Satan, as he had earlier linked the devil with his heart (2:376). Lovelace's adaptation is unconsciously ambiguous, however, because it is not clear who is the more "potent," he or Clarissa. Lovelace is almost humbled by the Pauline paradox of Clarissa's strength in weakness: "Yet what a contradiction!—*Weakness of heart*, says she, with *such a strength of will!*— Oh Belford! she is a lion-hearted lady in every case where her honour, her punctilio rather, calls for spirit! (2:384).

We shall look further at the potency of Clarissa's heart later, but for now let us conclude with the trope of Lovelace's "villain" heart. He voices his desire that after the Hampstead episode he and Clarissa "shall be fast asleep in each other's arms in town—Lie still, villain, till the time comes. My heart, Jack; my heart! It is always thumping away on the remotest prospects of this nature" (3:172). This kind of talk has by now become a refrain for Lovelace in a variety of sexual contexts after Clarissa is in his power. Just after he gets her to London he asks, "What makes my heart beat so strong? Why rises it to my throat in such half-choking flutters? . . . I am hitherto resolved to be honest; and that increases my wonder at these involuntary commotions. 'Tis a plotting villain of heart. . . . Such a joy when any roguery is going forward!—I so little its master!—A head likewise so well turned to answer the triangular varlet's impulses." Then he directly addresses his heart: "No matter. I will have one struggle with thee, old friend; and if I cannot overcome thee now, I never will again attempt to conquer thee" (2:218). Most of Lovelace's allusions to his own heart characterize it as some sort of bounding, thumping "villain" who cannot be controlled, and who is at Lovelace's throat. Terry Castle, in her commentary on the tiny hands in the margin of Anna Howe's warning letter to Clarissa, notes that their "primary visual significance seems to be that they are suggestive, potential inserts in the *body* of the letter itself. They press in upon the text . . . [they are] an orthographic representation of the intruding phallus, according to the Freudian model of displacement upward."[33] She goes on to see this kind of intrusion operating in the rape of Clarissa: "simultaneously penetrated above and below, the heroine is robbed of utterance"; the rape is "a primal act of silencing."[34] We shall explore further the outcome of this act of silencing, but what is remarkable to me is that Lovelace's phallic heart all along seems to be trying to choke *him*, another kind of "displacement upward"; he seems to mimic the act of rape on himself. In some sense, when he rapes Clarissa, he also rapes himself with his own heart. The autonomous heart is always ambivalent, and some recess of Lovelace's "naked thinking heart" continually contemplates suicide. His death is in large part self-inflicted.

Clarissa and the Female Heart

Lovelace once says, speaking of a play, "does not the principal entertainment lie in the *first four acts*? Is not all in a manner over when you come to the *fifth*?" (2:274). The overall structure of *Clarissa* might be seen as a religious narrative drama moving in four stages through a series of English houses that gradually diminish in size but increase in symbolic power.[35] The first stage takes place almost entirely in Clarissa's father's house, an imposing and claustrophobic country mansion (to 1:471). The second stage (1:471–3:311) occurs largely in the elegant London townhouse of the demonic bawd Mother Sinclair. In the third stage (3:311–4:347), Clarissa, after sojourning in various London lodging houses, returns, in the fourth stage (her death at 4:347 to the end), to her father's house in her own "house," her carefully inscribed and embellished coffin. The fifth act is presumably Clarissa's assumption into her heavenly Father's house. Clarissa's progress is circular, and the Clarissa of the fourth stage, though dead in the eyes of the world that helped kill her, is a more powerful and influential character than she was while alive. Clarissa's circulation through these houses has a larger figurative and religious dimension. Within the overall movement of beginning and ending in her father's house (in the temporal and spiritual senses of the term), the heroine, after undergoing the loss of her chastity (her "honour") under the influence of a figurative second "mother" (the world as represented by the interlocking complex of London, Mother Sinclair, and her diabolic "son," Lovelace), and finally reclaiming her soul by achieving the religious single life she has wanted since the Solmes affair, is virtually defined in terms of the experiences of her heart.

In attempting at this point a brief historical summation of the "female heart function" as evidenced in this study (a more difficult task than that of recounting the male heart function in relation to Lovelace), let us again begin with the physiology of the Greeks and of Genesis, noting that in both a companionate counterpart to the "male" heart is stressed. In Plato, the cool lung supports and surrounds the hot heart; in "Hippocrates," a bladder of fluid cools the heart. In the Adam and Eve story, a rib protecting Adam's heart is fashioned into a woman helpmeet and, as Milton would emphasize, a heartmate. In these earliest narratives of the heart, the area *around* the "male" heart is associated with support and nurture. In Greek physiology, this area is linked to "female" coolness; in Hebrew physiology, with the "feminine" guardianship of the bones, as the Puritan Charnock noted. We saw that Galen continually characterized Nature as a purposive female agent, and his version of the action of the heart stressed powerful attraction of the blood in contrast to Harvey's emphasis on expulsion.

In Chapter 1, we focused on how the representation of the heart moves from Eve as the person formed from the rib to Eve as mother, and how the female heart and womb become the receptive and deeply internalized sacred space for God's creative communion with humankind and his ongoing generation of his people. Women like Samson's mother and Hannah know things in their heart about God that men are not given to know, or if men learn the secret—like Samson under the spell of another woman—they lose power. In the prophet Jeremiah's richly enigmatic phrase—my epigraph for the working of the female heart throughout this study—"the Lord hath created a new thing in the earth, A woman shall compass a man" (31.22). Following upon the motif in Genesis of the Lord's profound interaction within the heart and womb of selected strong women, Jeremiah uses this phrase to preface his version of God's "new covenant" with humankind in which he will put his law in their inward parts. Hence God's action of fruition and love within the feminine heart and womb in the Genesis narratives is the prototype of the creative reinscription of his law in the hearts of all humankind. In the transition from the "new covenant" to the "new testament," Elisabeth and Mary repeat the Genesis birth narratives in a new way, with Mary as the quiet, contemplative mother of a Savior who, like her, is "meek and lowly in heart" (Matt. 11.29). From womb travail to heart rejoicing to the sorrowful woman standing at the cross, Mary becomes for the Christian West the woman preserver of the living divine presence in the storehouse of her heart.

Recalling that for the anatomist Crooke the heart is the "*primum sensorium*," we noted Thomas Willis's account of the twofold nature of the feminized corporeal soul, especially the "Praecordia," the parts around the heart, and their relevance to the character and action of Milton's Eve. The "Praecordia" are comparable to the pericardium and "caul" of the heart in Bunyan's *Pilgrim's Progress*, the second part of which follows a woman's road to salvation. We noted further that the traditionally feminine biblical motifs of nurture, attraction, reception, inward communion, and meditation are carried over in a variety of ways into early modern Puritan versions of the action of the female heart, culminating in Milton's Eve, with the additional poetic elaboration of her heart—intimately tied to a luxuriant and abundant maternal earthly paradise—as the source of love, sweetness, softness, creativity, delight, and above all, spiritual regeneration after her symbolic rape by Satan, the quintessential figure of male hard-heartedness. Finally, before our encounter with the female heart in Steele and Richardson, we traced the "generous," capacious, radically unstable heart delineated in the works of Aphra Behn, a wishing heart in her pragmatic heroine Hellena, contrasted with the emblem of the heart as the source of "desire," or "uneasy rage," in Angellica Bianca. Angellica Bianca as a female victim of her own overwhelming desire and the predations of a phallic heart—one of Behn's most resonant self-inscriptions—makes a compelling transitional figure, along with Milton's Eve, to our final and most complex representative of the female heart.

The "history (or rather dramatic narrative) of Clarissa" (4:554)—to use Richardson's own description of the work—may be understood, in large part, as the story of assaults to her heart. In this respect, she is the novelistic successor to Milton's Eve. In the first part of the novel, the word "heart" is used most often in particularly emotional and crucial encounters between the heroine and her mother and father in neo-scriptural contexts of blessing and cursing. Her mother says, "I charge you . . . on my blessing, that you think of being Mrs. Solmes," the condition upon which the blessing will be given (the change from "Clarissa" to the hiss of "*Mrs. Solmes*" has the impact of a verbal blow, almost a curse: "what a denunciation was that!"), and Clarissa faints ("*There* went the dagger to my heart, and down I sunk" [1:71]). Her mother later says, "as you value your father's blessing and mine . . . resolve to comply" (1:74). Clarissa faints because, as a remarkably dutiful Christian daughter with a keen awareness of the Old Testament force of blessings—and withheld blessings—she places the highest value on her parents' combined verbal approval of her marriage, whenever it should come about. Her mother's revealing response to Clarissa's tears and anguish, "The heart, Clary, is what I want," tells us she craves (for a complex of reasons) Clarissa's complete submission, not her sincerity. Her words also convey again that profound equation in the English language between desire and nothingness in the word "want," an equation we have noted in Lovelace's "want" of a heart: Mrs. Harlowe unwittingly says she herself lacks a heart. We recall Locke's juxtaposing of "desire" and "uneasiness in the want of an absent good." In strict Puritan fashion, Clarissa examines herself: "is not vanity, or secret love of praise, a principal motive with me at bottom? Ought I not to suspect my own heart?" (1:92).

The conflict in the Harlowe family now has overtones of an ancient religious war. Uncle John Harlowe, speaking for the family, puts the situation squarely from the point of view of the three elderly Harlowe males and their sense of the binding force of the patriarchal word: "our promises and honour were engaged before we believed there could be so sturdy an opposition . . . we are an *embattled phalanx*" (1:154). Behind this mournful assertion lies the scriptural notion that once the paternal word has been formed and uttered, there can be no drawing back. After reminding her daughter that her refusal may shorten her father's already diseased life, Charlotte Harlowe asks her climactic question: "are you determined to brave your father's displeasure? . . . Do you choose to break with us all . . .?" And Clarissa phrases the central issue: "is not my sincerity, is not the integrity of my heart, concerned in my answer? May not my everlasting happiness be the sacrifice?" (1:103). Invoking the language of the Old Testament (the phrase "integrity of heart" is used in Genesis and 1 Kings in reference to royalty), she knows that marrying Solmes will violate her deepest sense of right and wrong and her self-respect; acceding to her parents' demands in this case is to commit a sin that may imperil her immortal soul. Hence

Clarissa, for the first time, links the integrity and purity of her heart with the preservation of her soul, her guiding religious principle to the end, however difficult it may be to follow. Clarissa's heart is a vehicle for her soul, a variation on the traditional Christian notion of the heart as the seat of the soul. Clarissa's heart is a vehicle in motion toward an unknown destiny.

Not long after her virtual abduction from her father's house, her spiteful sister Arabella sends a letter describing how her "father . . . on discovering your wicked . . . elopement, imprecated on his knees a fearful curse upon you . . . No less than 'that you may meet your punishment, both *here* and *hereafter*, by means of the very wretch in whom you have chosen to place your wicked confidence'" (2:170). After receiving this letter, Clarissa writes to Anna Howe: "O my best, my *only* friend! Now indeed is my heart broken! It has received a blow it never will recover" (2:169). She has heard about parental curses and she attributes great "weight" to them. The immensely wealthy house of Harlowe in Richardson's historicized version of the England of 1730 would seem to have its roots in Puritan culture, and the Harlowes are a picture of "the Puritan family" gone terribly wrong.[36]

What little we know about the background of James Harlowe Sr. and his two unmarried brothers suggests that the three sons had strongly biblical upbringings and there are indications that James, the *paterfamilias*, made much of the traditional paternal role of personally instructing his children in the moral lessons of the Bible, especially the Old Testament. Long after receiving her father's written curse (every syllable of which she carries with her like a weight on her heart), Clarissa, still suffering from the aftereffects of the violence done to her head and to her heart in the rape—a powerful reminder to us of Satan's practice with Eve in *Paradise Lost*—will recall the story of Rebekah's deception of Isaac and the father's misplaced blessing: "My father used, I remember, to enforce the doctrine deducible from it, on his children, by many arguments" (3:387). This doctrine would seem to be the irrevocable power of a father's blessing (or curse) and the rightness of God's will even in apparently unjust cases. In other words, James Harlowe Sr.—though exceedingly benevolent to his younger daughter until the Solmes affair—was one of those family tyrants who would resort to Scripture to uphold any of his actions. Clarissa's mother, bringing to mind the jealous God of the Old Testament, once reminds her daughter that she has "a jealous father, needlessly jealous . . . of the prerogatives of his sex . . . and still ten times more jealous of the authority of a father" (1:80). The old man is biblical to the last. His final message to Clarissa, not long before her death, is an extract from Ecclesiasticus (often regarded in the eighteenth century as the most virulently antifeminist book in the Bible) about a father's grief caused by a shameless daughter gotten with child in her father's house (chap. 42).[37] The passage has all the more impact on her since it was from the very book of Ecclesiasticus, as we have seen, that Clarissa justified opposing her father. This letter, like the curse, is also conveyed by another hand, here the officious Uncle Antony Harlowe, an old bachelor intimately conversant with the purple passages of Ecclesiasticus. He exhorts his niece "to lay it to heart," and provides a stinging commentary to each verse (4:105).

After learning from her Aunt Hervey that her father would have kneeled to her to oblige him on the Wednesday proposed for her marriage to Solmes, Clarissa responds, "I had deserved annihilation had I suffered my father to kneel in vain" (2:166). One recalls the verbal power of annihilation—both oral and written—in the Old Testament and how the force of this divine power, embodied in the father even when he is silent, permeates Clarissa's consciousness. Now from her sister she learns that he got down on his knees in the ritual posture of prayer to imprecate this horror on her head, and the worst of it is, "the curse extends to the life beyond this" (2:169). In the carefully circular balance of its parts, the curse seems to be formulaic, as if her father had learned it by heart from a book.

The mortal condition imposed by God on Eve in Gen. 3.16 was taken in the eighteenth century to be God's curse on woman, and like Clarissa's father's curse, it also has two parts. Any intelligent, marriageable young woman of Clarissa's time might be expected to have felt anxiety when reading the first part of this verse, and the ambiguity of "multiply thy sorrow and thy conception" seemed to imply repeated conceptions and repeated agony, as was indeed the case with nearly all fertile wives; as for the second part, she might well have been troubled about the idea of apparently inexorable "desire" for her husband-to-be, and the notion that he would "rule over" her seemed, as we saw in Chapter 1, to imply a master-servant relationship as well. Clarissa's cruel and self-righteous brother remarks on her "high notion of the matrimonial duty" (1:262), playing upon the proverbial sexual debt (the "due benevolence" passage in 1 Cor. 7.3) the husband owes the wife and the wife owes the husband—a debt usually construed as falling primarily upon the wife. Like the libertines he professes to despise, James has been nourished on Lucretian and other sexually explicit classical texts; he has already reminded his sister that she too is part of "the animal creation" (1:256), alluding to Dryden's translation of *Amor omnibus idem* in Virgil's third *Georgic* ("Thus every creature, and of every kind, /The secret joys of sweet coition find: / . . . For love is Lord of all, and is in all the same").[38]

Until her decline, Clarissa is represented in the novel as a nubile young woman of extraordinary vitality, beauty, and sexual allure whose presence exerts a profound physical attraction over Lovelace. To echo John Evelyn on his daughter Mary, "her extraordinary beauty was taken notice of." She makes clear her physical revulsion from Solmes, but in attempting to gauge her capacity for erotic love we can infer that she also seems to find Lovelace attractive physically and in other ways (though she often denies these effects on her) and she holds a traditional sense of a wife's subordination to her husband (1:101). But she holds an even stronger opinion of the efficacy of a curse. Nearly all the great curses by a father on a daughter in earlier English literature have sexual force or implication, and this effect, though muted, is not absent in Clarissa's father's curse. Besides Brabantio's curse on Desdemona and Lear's curse on Goneril, Richardson seems to have had in mind particularly Priuli's curse on his daughter Belvidera in Otway's *Venice Preserved* (1.1.50–58). Lovelace's vehement "*Oh, for a curse to kill with!*" when Clarissa makes her first escape from Mother Sinclair's (2:517) is a self-conscious echo of Jaffeir's curse on Priuli and the senators of Venice (2.2.57) in Otway's play. Lovelace will actually take Clarissa to a performance of this play in London, hoping that the woes of the heroine Belvidera will "unlock and open my charmer's heart. . . . The female heart (all gentleness and harmony by nature) expands, and forgets its forms, when its attention is carried out of itself at an agreeable or affecting entertainment" (2:342), and Clarissa describes herself as being "greatly moved" by the performance (2:372). Lovelace's description here of Clarissa's heart is one of the most explicit examples (in a literary context) of the female heart function recalling the essential action of the Galenic heart.

To someone so extraordinarily sensitive to the spoken and written word as Clarissa (almost superstitiously aware of the mysterious self-fulfilling power of language, especially of scriptural invocation), so highly verbal and articulate herself in all her dealings with others, so well instructed from an early age in the Bible and in the books of Anglican reflection by the ministers of religion with whom she corresponded (4:495) and by her nurse and spiritual mother Mrs. Norton (whose name recalls that of the religious writer John Norris, and who is herself the daughter of a divine

[4:66]), such a curse as this from her father, coming at a moment when Clarissa is attempting to collect all her fortitude and willpower to cope with her dangerous situation, has an actual physical impact on her. She is *"unhinged"* (2:176), and except for the ability to write, almost immobilized. Her response here prefigures her even more shattering collapse after the rape.

Behind Clarissa's simple "Now indeed is my heart broken" and the popular cliché—hackneyed even in the eighteenth century—of the heart broken for disappointed love, stands the far more vital and immediate religious significance of the image of the fleshy tables or tablets of the heart (2 Cor. 3.2–3), and within that image the breaking of the stone tables of the Law. This brilliant heroine is an exceptionally well read young woman with a profoundly sensitive religious sensibility. Because she is no ordinary "young lady" of privilege and wealth but "Clarissa," Richardson's female version of the learned and eminent "vir clarissimus"[39] (the courtesy title in use in the "republic of letters" during the early modern period), the entire network of associations we have traced in Chapter 1 pertaining to the breaking of the Mosaic tables qualifies her broken heart. We have noted Clarissa's ambivalent adherence to a father who, "according to the Old Law, [has] the *right* of *absolving* or *confirming* a child's promise" (1:458). Later, with Lovelace, she speculates "how shall I behave when got from him . . . if, like the Israelites of old, I shall be so meek as to wish to return to my Egyptian bondage?" (2:345). From the very first, it is her father, not Lovelace, who is Moses to Clarissa's Israel. Not Moses as the leader of the chosen people out of the Wilderness, but Moses conveying the anger of a superlatively jealous god. The tablets of her heart are now broken within her, as were the tables of the Law in Exodus, by the wrath of a father incensed at the disobedience of his children. "Don't let them break your heart," Anna Howe implores her friend (2:173). Clarissa's extraordinary book learning went into forming the book of her heart, and now her father's curse breaks that book. Anna comes to her friend's aid with consolatory advice and passages from the Gospels and Romans: "None but God can curse," "bless and curse not," "pray for them that persecute and curse us" (2:172); it is equally significant that at this point she also sends Clarissa, to assuage her grief, her personal copy of John Norris's *Miscellanies*, a popular book of meditations which was a cherished favorite of Richardson's. Clarissa returns the book. The damage has been done. From here to the end, the broken book of Clarissa's heart can be mended only through spiritual restoration.

The great gulf between Lovelace's heart and Clarissa's is apparent in their respective heart fortification exercises. In preparation for the ultimate assault upon her body, Lovelace (as we saw) "fortifies his recreant heart" (2:316) with repeated efforts to "steel" or harden it against the power of Clarissa's innocence and virtue. The representation of the process of Lovelace's heart-hardening seems to be a deliberate decision, on Richardson's part, to create a demonic parallel to the traditional Puritan "preparation of the heart" to receive God's grace. The rest of this chapter concentrates, in one way or another, on how Clarissa attempts to fortify the heart Lovelace and her family have broken.

A Right Heart

There is much cursing in Scripture, but no human father ever curses his daughter. If Miriam's father "had but spit in her face, should she not be ashamed seven days?" (Num. 12.14). The power of a father's curse in the biblical context would be almost unspeakable in its effect. Stoning would seem to have been a preferable alternative. A son or daughter who curses his parent is put to death (Lev. 20.9). "None but God can curse," and Clarissa's father is not God, but a father speaks with the sanction of the Lord, and even in the early eighteenth century, a father's word still had the reputed power of that sanction. It was a truism that, as the Puritan Richard Adams puts it, obedience "is the parents' due as in the place of God: they bear his image in their parental authority and relation."[40] Recalling the customary feminine gesture of holding a letter to the bosom, or inserting it into the bosom, Arabella says to her sister, "If all this is heavy, lay your hand to your heart and ask yourself why you have deserved it" (2:171). Bella tells Clarissa to take her crime and the words of this curse and press them down—seal them—into her heart, but there is little need to reinforce their impact with a physical gesture: "The contents of my sister's letter had pierced my heart" (2:181), and Clarissa falls gravely ill. Clarissa's father's curse shatters and pierces her heart in a combined evocation of the breaking of the Law and the Crucifixion. It is left for Lovelace to complete the breaking of her heart in her madness as a result of the rape.

In "the depth of vapourish despondency" after receiving her father's curse, Clarissa's relation to her broken heart becomes increasingly more complicated. Anna Howe is aware that all along in Clarissa's relationship with Lovelace, her friend has attempted to remain truthful to her, and to preserve the integrity of her heart: "I know the gentleness of your spirit; I know the laudable pride of your heart" (2:294). But Anna senses, though even she cannot say it outright, that she is not now simply trying to save her friend's peace of mind, or her reputation—she is trying to save Clarissa from destruction. Too much time has elapsed since she left her father's house. Clarissa must not stand on her delicacy and punctilio now, but "Give him the day" (2:295).

The advice of her friend prompts in Clarissa, despite her desponding spirits, a firm and clear reassertion of her sense of the integrity of her heart and the real meaning of her delicacy with regard to Lovelace. She will explain to her friend, once for all, that the motives for her behavior to Lovelace "arise principally from what offers to my own heart; respecting . . . its own *rectitude*, its own judgment of the *fit* and the *unfit*. . . . Principles that *are* in my mind; that I *found* there; implanted . . . by the first gracious Planter" (2:306). Clarissa here enunciates Richardson's version of "right reason"—another version of the *imago dei*—adapted from Milton. This version of right reason might also be compared with the revisionist version of Rochester in the *Satyr Against Mankind*, primarily an assertion of the true government of thought by action, of desire by will. Clarissa on the rectitude of her heart recalls her praise of Anna Howe's satirical powers stemming from "good nature . . . directed by a right heart" (1:345), and she makes a crucial connection here between reason and the heart, virtually centering, in biblical fashion, on the rational mind in the heart. Clarissa here articulates a traditional notion of conscience implanted in the heart, but her experience is moving her toward a more Lockean interpretation of conscience.

Locke, who generally avoids using "heart" language in his exposition of the understanding, asserts that there is no innate rule of virtue and that, not having conscience "written in their hearts, many men, by the same way that they come to the knowledge of other things, come to assent to several moral rules, and be convinced of their obligation. . . . conscience being nothing else but our own opinion or judgment of the moral rectitude or pravity of our own actions."[41] It is relevant to Richardson, the author as master printer, that all through the *Essay*, Locke uses the term "imprint," first to deny that innate ideas or principles are impressed by the "finger of God" into the mind or heart, then to indicate all the impressions made upon human sensation by the force of external objects. For Locke, "the person" is an accumulation of a multitude of imperfectly retained "imprints" from the external world and of ideas formed by internal reflection, analogous to a text (or "white paper") gradually accumulating more and more annotations.[42] Such a person is Clarissa, a developing and evolving moral agent suffering increasingly more violent "imprints" upon her body, heart, and mind. All this is another way of describing the process of the book of her heart being broken.

Despite Clarissa's affirmation of the "rectitude" of her heart, she is all too well aware, echoing Jeremiah and again invoking the image of Anna Howe's delicate "anatomical" probe, that "the heart is very deceitful: do you, my dear friend, lay mine open . . . and spare me not, if you think it culpable" (2:306). Clarissa is becoming more deeply aware of the ambivalence of her heart (and not just in love matters), an ambivalence rooted in the scriptural representation of the heart as discussed in the first chapter. The view that Clarissa believes in a transparent correlation between the "dictating heart" and language itself in her own discourse is an oversimplified interpretation of Clarissa's relation to her heart even in her more naive early phase in the novel. As she looks more deeply now within herself, Clarissa feels caught up in a virtual dilemma from which she can never fully escape as she attempts to reconcile the claims of a just and "laudable" pride of heart with a deceitful pride, the equally sincere emotions of loving and despising someone, strong prophetic "givings" (1:303) and misgivings about her fate, impulses of counsel and reproach, or forgiveness and self-justification.

On Sunday, July 23, the last day of her eighteenth year, Clarissa writes to Anna Howe the most important letter in the history of her heart suffering. Much earlier, she had identified herself with Israel in its wanderings (2:345). Now she identifies herself with David, the sweet singer of Israel, and Anna with Jonathan, as she reaffirms the sacred ties of pure friendship and explains to her friend for the last time why she cannot marry Lovelace. She will humbly attempt to imitate the "sublime Exemplar" in his resignation to the will of God, persuaded that she will not live much longer. The strong sense of her error, the loss of her reputation, the resentment of her family, and Lovelace's barbarous usage of her, culminating in her rape while drugged with laudanum, all "have seized upon [her] heart . . . before it was so well fortified by *religious considerations*," as she hopes it now is (3:522). In other words, before the rape her heart was not strong enough, in a religious sense, to enable her to survive the temptations and afflictions that were visited upon it. Here is a tacit admission that, as good a person as she knew herself to be, she was not good enough, in these terrible circumstances, to survive and live on her own high moral terms in the world in which she finds herself. That inability, and the related issue of Clarissa's capacity for "love" or charity, may constitute the real tragedy of Richardson's Clarissa.

Under these circumstances, how is Clarissa to be viewed as a moral exemplar to her sex? The novel is not telling young eighteenth-century women who have been wronged to curse men, forgive them, and die. In this sense Clarissa's death is no more an example to be followed than is Griselda's obedience to the Marquis Walter meant to be an example in Chaucer's "Clerk's Tale."[43] It is Clarissa as a warning and the Miltonic virtues of fortitude, piety, and heroic resignation with which Clarissa dies that are meant to be exemplary. For in this passage Clarissa also implies that between the rape and her writing of this letter, she has been able to "fortify" and restore her broken heart.

Even before she has fully regained her senses, Clarissa—unable to speak—engages successively in two separate and distinct acts of writing. This is where the biblical writing motif we have examined in the first chapter is most relevant to the action of the novel, and it is Clarissa's "critical moment." When she has lost almost everything—her honor, her speech, her senses—she still has the capacity to write, and even to love and to forgive, but in qualified ways. All along, we have been aware that Clarissa's primary life act is writing. For her, to live is to write.[44] From Genesis, she has learned that woman is created out of an act of mutilation, God's rebuilding or revising of Adam's rib into Eve. As we noted in the first chapter, God anatomizes Adam into Eve. From Psalm 139, she learned that humankind is written in God's book before being wrought in the womb. God writes humankind into being—writing precedes living. Clarissa may be considered a new model of Eve for eighteenth-century woman—not an Eve who bears sons but an Eve who writes—and a new Mary, not the one who bears the child redeemer but the woman writer who bears a new female version of the Word, a womanly hero of virtue and wisdom who combines in herself qualities of the two chief moral exemplars of Scripture, Job and Christ, with more of the former in her composition than the latter.

Partly as an act of revenge—on Clarissa, on her family, on womankind—Lovelace wounds her irreparably. It is the ultimate "wound" in the Lucretian love war. Clarissa is comatose for at least forty-eight hours after the rape, an act that Lovelace—the demonic anatomist in contrast to Anna Howe's benevolent one—justifies by a medical analogy as a kind of surgery necessary in "acute" cases, lamenting that "whatever the sex set their hearts upon, they make thorough work of it" (3:213–14). As she gradually attains intermittent consciousness, she attempts to write, but "what she writes she tears," throwing the fragments under the table, then trying to write again (3:204). These acts of writing are like the desperate survival gestures of a drowning person, the victim flailing about, attacking the destructive element. It is as if Clarissa and the Lovelace who has assaulted her in his sexual and literal inscription of her body go back to the origin of writing as considered in Chapter 1—writing as a hostile and divisive anatomy. But now it is herself she is marking, tearing, dissecting.

Clarissa begins her life after the rape by a kind of self-mutilation in her mad papers, torn fragments of her own written self. But shortly after the composition of the mad papers she begins a different kind of writing. This new writing is available to us both within and without the text of the novel in the book of Clarissa's *Meditations* Richardson had privately printed for friends. Clarissa seems to be tearing up the old raped self and beginning a new one *in writing*. The mad papers all refer to her own immediate experiences in relation to members of her family and to Lovelace and contain few biblical echoes. The new writing is an explicit transcription of Scripture. It is no longer writing as tearing but writing as ordering; one might call it Clarissa's new covenant or book of the heart written and remembered out of her own dismemberment and suffering. She does for herself what Aphra Behn represents herself as doing for Oroonoko.

Clarissa's little book of *Meditations* has a place of central importance in our experience of the novel. In adherence to good Puritan practice, Clarissa makes transcripts of those parts of the Bible she feels are especially relevant to her spiritual condition. But these are not simply copies—they are "collections," small anthologies, usually of half a page in length, of selected verses put into the writer's own order. Clarissa says, in her own preface to the collection, "*In some places I have taken the liberty of substituting the word* her *for* him, *and to make other such-like little changes of words.*"[45] These "little changes" are nothing less than a revision of patriarchal Scripture into her own person and gender, a move analogous to Aphra Behn's insertion of her poetic identity into Cowley's *Sylva*. According to the "Editor of the History of Clarissa," in his "Advertisement to the Reader" introducing the collection, thirty-six such "Meditations" were composed, four of which are inserted in the "history" (there are actually five). Richardson clearly implies in this "Advertisement" that he did not insert more of the meditations for fear of not engaging the attention of those readers (the light, the careless, and the gay) who stood most in need of instruction. Moreover, Richardson is remarkably sparing in scriptural allusions throughout *Clarissa*. He does not want the novel to sound like a tract, and his artistic restraint and skill in this respect are admirable. It is taken for granted that the heroine knows the Bible; it is her wide reading in literature and history that is stressed at various points in the novel (e.g., 4:504–5). The main thing is that after the rape, at the moment of deepest personal crisis, Clarissa really begins to read the Bible most deeply—to become truly "engaged" in it perhaps for the first time—as she transcribes and transforms it into her own spiritual autobiography, her own scripture, her new book of the heart.[46]

In the first three-quarters of the novel, Clarissa alludes to the Bible, directly or indirectly, only about fifteen times. Of these allusions, just four are to the New Testament, and one of these already shows Clarissa wittily adapting the Bible (here 1 Cor. 13.7) to her immediate needs. In her surprise meeting with Lovelace near the woodhouse, defending in great agitation her decision to remain in her father's house, she tells him "that it became me, ill as I was treated at present, to *hope* everything, to *bear* everything, and to *try* everything" (1:178). Of her remaining allusions, most are to the Old Testament, with Job predominating, and five are to Ecclesiasticus. Lovelace (who can almost always quote Scripture to his advantage) is not far behind Clarissa with about ten allusions. Again the Old Testament predominates, with his error in attributing "no wickedness is comparable to the wickedness of a woman" to either Socrates or Solomon caustically pointed out by the editor (2:56). In the last quarter of the novel, the balance of allusions naturally tips toward Clarissa largely because of her five meditations.

The first meditation (not in the text of the novel), dated "June 18," would have been written only five days after the rape and the self-mutilation of the mad papers when Clarissa, having been stopped by Mrs. Sinclair herself from escaping the house, retreats to her chamber (3:217: "Sunday Afternoon, 6 o'clock [June 18]"). Here, "in the anguish of her soul, she transcribes and adapts the curses of Job on his birth-day": "Let the day perish wherein I was born, and the night in which I was conceived." She substitutes a second "I" for "there was a man child" (Job 3.3).[47] She writes herself into the Book of Job and thereby into her own scripture, but by so doing she allows Scripture to influence her living experience in the most immediate form of writing to the moment. She must begin with a curse in which Job, innocent of intentional fault, brings down on himself what Clarissa's father has brought down on her. Everything in *Clarissa* comes back to that curse and its impact on her heart. As in the Bible and *Paradise*

Lost, the heart is central. The heroine unknowingly begins the restoration of her heart with a passage that in effect uncreates, undoes, the old Clarissa (a parallel to her self-mutilation in the mad papers) as she begins her new role—the one most compatible with her author's modest sense of his own talents as writer and printer—as copier, "collector," and composer of extracts, and "*when collected, the frequent recourse I had to them . . . gave me still greater comfort.*"[48] By collecting the biblical extracts, she re-"collects" herself—"writes" herself on paper and composes herself in person— so that she is supremely prepared for her head-to-head encounter with Lovelace and the women after the rape. Again, as in the Old Testament dynamic of the divine primacy of writing humanity into being, inscription precedes speech for Clarissa at the beginning of her restoration and her triumph.

Then follows her assessment of the hierarchy of evil authority poised against her. Her sacred "compact" is opposed to Lovelace's evil one: "Tell me . . . whether thou hast entered into a compact with the grand deceiver, in the person of his horrid agent in this house [i.e., Sinclair]; and if the ruin of my soul, that my father's curse may be fulfilled, is to complete the triumphs of so vile a confederacy?" (3:220). It is clear from this passage that Clarissa does not finally equate Lovelace with Satan, as others have argued. The rhetorical series of "whether . . . if . . . if" suggests that Clarissa already knows that the combined demonic power of "the grand deceiver" Satan acting through his agent Sinclair and their Faustian victim Lovelace cannot destroy her soul (the equivalent of the "second death" in Revelation, or being blotted out from the "book of life") so long as she chooses to accept God's forgiveness through grace. Clarissa in this great scene challenges Lovelace to speak and he is almost entirely incoherent (3:221). Her oral presence prevails over his, just as the "written mind" of her scriptural *Meditations* will prevail over his despairing correspondence.

The book of *Meditations* is especially important to an evaluation of the novel's religious meaning because, as Belford points out, Clarissa performed these exercises "to take off the edge of her repinings at hardships so disproportioned to her fault. . . . We may see by this the method she takes to fortify her mind" (4:96). This remark would seem to be Richardson's most pointed indication in the text of the significance of Clarissa's scriptural and scriptive activities in the heart-fortifying process. She eventually bequeaths the book of *Meditations* to her dear Mrs. Norton (4:423) and her mother finally wants to possess the book.

But the meditations are not meant finally for Clarissa's "friends"; they are written primarily for the God who alone can read the heart. Running throughout the meditations are several allusions to "the great day of account," and Clarissa clearly has the Day of Judgment—and her ultimate and final Reader—in mind as she reaps the comforts of transcribing the Wisdom books, concluding her book of *Meditations* with the Book of the Wisdom of Solomon, the fourth and fifth chapters. Her title, "*An Early Death not to be lamented*," alludes to Enoch (Gen. 5.24): "living among sinners, he was translated" (Wisd. 4.10; cf. Heb. 11.5). Her last transcribed words in the meditation are,

> And when they cast up accounts of their sins,
> They shall come with fear: and their own iniquities
> Shall convince them to their face.[49]

Thomas Watson points out in another representative Puritan sermon, "The Day of Judgment Asserted," two books will be opened at the trial of doom. The first is "*the book of God's omnisciency*" in which God has registered all of mankind's actions. This is God's "book of remembrance" (Mal. 3.16), the "book of life." The second book is the one each man and woman brings to be unclasped at the trial, one's "book of conscience" or one's writing in the heart, the trial testimony of word, thought, and deed. Watson puts his emphasis on the crimes that will be revealed: "The sins of men shall be written upon their foreheads with a pen of iron," but a divine like the Anglican Robert South notes that the book of life registers "all good and evil, whether done, spoken, consented to, or imagined" by humankind.[50]

In language that recalls the creation of woman out of the wound in Adam's breast, Watson—as we have seen in the first chapter—again represents Christ as "*kardiognostes*," "a Heart-Searcher" or "Heart-Knower," virtually a cardiac surgeon. He also represents the Holy Spirit writing "grace" in the heart, as in Milton's version of the divine writing in the heart: "Christ will at the day of judgment make a heart-anatomy; as a surgeon makes a dissection in the body, for it is not the most shining profession [which] Christ is taken with, unless he see the curious workmanship of grace in the heart, drawn by the pencil of the Holy Ghost . . . Nothing then will stand us in stead but sincerity," Clarissa's chief virtue and Lovelace's chief failing with respect to her.[51] Watson says "sincerity"; "charity" is the word one might have expected from a divine like Norris.

We might keep this passage in mind in assessing Clarissa's capacity for exercising the Christian virtues of charity and forgiveness. Whatever the nature of the new book of the heart being written in Clarissa, it does not seem to be the "generous heart" of charity, or of Milton's Eve.

Watson's emphasis on the divine "anatomy of the heart" is central to all representations of the heart in seventeenth- and eighteenth-century narrative. When one recalls that it was Christ who was imagined as the divine person actually creating woman in the original heart anatomy of Adam, womankind is seen to be a crucial element in the entire anatomizing process—one that involves creating, analyzing, "writing," judging—from the first day to the last. Although her heart is mortal, Clarissa's scriptural writings will, through the transformative power of divine grace, survive in the book of the heart—her "book of conscience," her "name"—which Christ will "open" and "confess" aloud at the last day when the elect are named (Rev. 20.12; 3.5). Adversity was Clarissa's "shining-time," but her radiant heroism was an expression in the visible world; all of her final scriptural activities are devoted to fortifying her heart, the inward realm and record of the spirit.

As Clarissa transcribes herself into Scripture, Scripture helps to guide her into the proper way to Christ. As she rewrites the Bible, it rewrites her. This ongoing process might best be described as one of mutual "translation," a more complicated version of what happens to Enoch. Clarissa is now attempting to do what her beloved Thomas à Kempis advises concerning spiritual consolation. Unfortunately, she was unable to heed this advice properly in order to save her life in the time of trial, but it is not now too late to save her soul. Thomas's Lord, represented as a "reader" of lessons, speaks to the faithful soul:

> Write then my Words in thy Heart; Grave them in deep and lasting Characters; Ponder them diligently, for thou shalt find them a seasonable Relief and necessary Support in the Day of Tryal and Adversity. What Reading only hath not taught thee, Affliction will interpret and make plain. For I do not always visit my Chosen alike. Sometimes the Comforts of my Grace are proper; at Others, the withdrawing those Comforts, and bringing their Patience and Constancy to the Touch, by Outward Calamities, and Inward Anguish of Spirit. Thus I daily train them up in Goodness, by chastising and making them hate their Sins, and cultivating and encouraging their Advancement in Virtue. The One Dispensation engages their Love of Me, the Other abates their Fondness for the World. But lost and wretched is that stupid Creature, upon whom these Methods make no Impression; for, *He that rejecteth Me, and receiveth not my Words, hath One that judgeth him in the last Day* [John 12.48].[52]

I submit that this passage may be considered a proof text for the action of *Clarissa* and one that completes, in a religious register, the dynamic interplay of inner and outer experience we have traced throughout this book. Richardson's heroine is a great reader of books, perhaps not so good a reader of persons, but according to Thomas she must learn to let her afflictions "read" her, "interpret and make plain" her path. One thing is clear. Clarissa warns Lovelace in her posthumous letter to him to take care lest he have "Not one good action in the hour of languishing to recollect, not one worthy intention to revolve, it will be all reproach and horror; and you will wish to have it in your power to compound for annihilation" (4:435–36). Again we return to the biblical theme of annihilation, of being written away or blotted out of the "book of life" with the stroke of a pen—"Write ye this man childless."

Clarissa's Compass

In the light of these passages concerning the "book of life" and the Last Judgment, we might say that Clarissa, like all humankind, is originally "written" by God in his book and "wrought" by God in the womb. As William B. Warner has said, "the Christian interpretive system gives Clarissa the idea of the self as a continuously unfolding history," or a book in the making.[53] Clarissa, fashioning the book of her works as the substance of her personal history, seeks to be recorded in God's book of life, and she uses the Bible to aid her in that endeavor. Within God's final application of the scriptural curse/blessing formula, Clarissa hopes ultimately to be one of those names called out by Christ in the absolution, as Robert South represents it, "Come, ye blessed of my Father," and not one of those in the denunciation, "Depart, ye cursed."[54] Clarissa's letters, brooding as they often are with a spirit of intense self-examination and the discovery of a "secret sin"—guilt-ridden and guilt-written—with an acute concern over the fallible body, with a sense of foreordained and individually signalized doom, are written almost daily, again like a Puritan diary or spiritual autobiography.[55] Moreover, Clarissa, like her author, is represented as constantly reading, rereading, and above all, transcribing copies of her own letters, and those of her correspondents. We think of the enormous expenditure of time involved, the *lived* time that goes into the first draft of a Clarissan letter and into all those copies, which each become a little "better" as they go through the transcription process. What happens to one who keeps making copy after written copy of one's own experience? Something rich and strange—even terrible, perhaps. One turns into a Pamela, or a Clarissa, or a Lovelace, or a Richardson. Depending on how seriously we take it, a letter diary *does* become another self, an externalized self to which one may go for confirmation and authorization of who one is—or was. Clarissa's constant preoccupation with reading, transcribing, collecting, and re-collecting her own book comes to exert a powerful influence on the self who does the writing.

Something similar happens to Lovelace. His constant preoccupation with writing and reading about his stratagems assists in entangling him ever more securely in his own devices. Clarissa and Lovelace are their own individual scribes. The very act of transcribing or copying something tends to validate and authorize it. We recall that Clarissa is physically unable to transcribe the letter from her sister conveying her father's curse, and even Lovelace is incapable of transcribing Clarissa's "mad" papers after he has had all the torn bits and pieces collected in an effort to put her back together for himself. In the authority with which it becomes endowed as the *true* record of her experience, the ever-expanding letter diary dictates to the mortal Clarissa. She believes what she has written. And in the reciprocal process of being written by her story as well as writing it—centered on the book of *Meditations*—Clarissa becomes what she has written.

Early in act 2 of the drama Clarissa had described to Anna Howe why it was necessary for her to keep on writing *even if she were not to send her letter to anyone*. She has found, she says, that writing down "everything of moment" that happens to her may be of "future use" to her, and that by writing things down she entered into a *"compact"* with herself, "having given it," she goes on, "under my own hand to *improve*, rather than to go *backward*, as I live longer" (2:128). She has made a written "compact" or covenant with her future self to improve herself. In the culminating third act of the drama, this "compact" has come to fruition. It replaces the "wretched composition" she once thought it might be necessary to arrange with Lovelace, a marriage of convenience to "save" her reputation, and she chooses a better salvation. Clarissa asks Belford to assemble her story because she shall be "too much discomposed by the retrospection . . . to proceed with the requisite temper in a task of still *greater* importance which I have before me" (4:74). This task is the new compact with God, a process of self-correction and restoration through writing, which we have traced in the book of her *Meditations* and its reliance on the Wisdom literature of the Bible. It is to the books of Job and Ecclesiasticus, not the Gospels, that Clarissa's Bible opens naturally in her harrowing stay at the Rowlands' debtors' prison (3:439). It would appear that the Wisdom literature of the Bible, not the New Testament, entered most deeply into Richardson's literary imagination in the composition of *Clarissa* partly, no doubt, because of its proverbial nature, partly because of its apocalyptic fervor (no less intriguing to Richardson), but most importantly, because these books—especially Job—spoke most directly to the willed preservation of the integrity of one's heart—in writing—in the experience of tragic suffering and loss.

John Belford, as Clarissa's future executor, editor, and virtual apostle, begins reading the Bible in earnest under the influence of Clarissa's example and her meditation of July 15. He collates the individual meditations he has access to with the original text, and the language he uses to characterize holy Scripture ("the clear, the pellucid fountainhead" of the Bible, "this all excelling collection of beauties" [4:7]) recalls the central image of the heart and is much like the language he uses to describe Clarissa and the style of her letters. In Belford's eyes, Clarissa is being fused with her meditations and the original scriptural text. She becomes for Belford Scripture personified, a "*bibliotheca Christi*" or "walking Bible," in Thomas Watson's words. For Belford and for Richardson's Christian readers, the chief impact of Clarissa as a suffering Job and Christ in one heroic female writing figure is that she translates herself into her own scripture, that she is the flesh made word.[56]

The developing divergence between Belford and Lovelace is nowhere more apparent than in their separate readings of the scriptural Clarissa. Lovelace responds to Belford's newfound edification with characteristic wit, reminiscent of Swift on Partridge. Lovelace is reminded of how scriptural enthusiasts will take the most far-fetched passages for "gospel," which seem to have any reference to the case at hand (here a person "in a heavy grief," recalling the "Deep Distress" noted on the title page of Clarissa's book of *Meditations*), so that "once, in a pulpit, I heard one . . . vehemently declare himself to be a *dead dog*; when every man, woman, and child, were convinced to the contrary by his howling" (4:33).[57]

In his very next letter, however, Lovelace becomes his own scriptural enthusiast in the case of Clarissa by assuming for himself, with a Lucretian twist, the patriarchal role of the Old Testament God who presides over female fertility. He interprets the lines from Clarissa's meditation, "For the arrows of the Almighty are within me; the poison whereof drinketh up my spirit. . . . For the thing which I greatly feared is come upon me!" as veiled indications of what Lovelace hopes for: "in plain English, that the dear creature is in the way to be a mamma" (4:38). He further declares that it would be the pride of his life "to prove, in this charming frost-piece, the triumph of nature over principle, and to have a young Lovelace by such an angel" (4:38). Lovelace epitomizes for Richardson the power of amoral, unregenerate nature in one exceptional man as Clarissa, with her affirmation to Anna Howe of the "ties of pure friendship" over the "ties of nature" (3:517), epitomizes—in her stress on principle—the exceptional woman. Lovelace finally realizes and accepts that, whether or not she is "in the way" he would have her be, she is going to die, and the final outcome of the history of Clarissa's responses to Lovelace's heart (as he and the reader both know) is now wholehearted rejection. To continue what amounts to his perverse parallel with the Hebrew God and woman, as Lovelace claimed Clarissa's womb, so will he now claim her heart, but his rhetoric of the heart has become more and more violent, parodic, literal, insane: "My heart is bent upon having her . . . though I marry her in the agonies of death. . . . I will overcome the creeping folly that has found its way into my heart, or I will tear it out in her presence, and throw it at hers, that she may see how much more tender than her own that organ is" (4:89–90).

Finally, after her death, Lovelace the natural man reveals to Belford the full state of his manic desperation in a way appropriately reminiscent of the behavior of Clarissa's mother in the early part of the novel ("The heart, Clary, is what I want" [1:90]), as well as defining himself as a demonic counterpart to Thomas Watson's depiction of Christ as "Heart-Searcher" and "surgeon": "I think it absolutely right that my ever-dear and beloved lady should be opened and embalmed. . . . Everything that can be done to preserve the charmer from decay shall also be done. . . . But her *heart*, to which I have such unquestionable pretensions, in which once I had so large a share, and which I will prize above my own, I *will* have" (4:375–76).

In his "Advertisement" to the *Meditations*, Richardson gives a poignant—almost wistful—further indication of his final intentions in *Clarissa* in a bald restatement of the "good heart/bad heart" doctrine: "The History of Clarissa must be owned to be carried into length. But the subject was pregnant. All bad nature was endeavoured to be set forth in the principal Men: All good in those of the two principal Women: so that the whole compass of human nature . . . was aimed to be taken into it."[58] Richardson's use of "compass" in this context may be set beside Jeremiah's by now familiar "for the Lord hath created a new thing in the earth, a woman shall compass a man" (31.22). We might remind ourselves at this point that no woman in Scripture is depicted as an important writer. This role is reserved exclusively for men, from Moses on through Ezekiel, Job, St. Paul, and the St. John of Revelation. Clarissa is represented in her own scripture (that is, virtually all of her own writing and the writing about her after the rape) in the traditional role of suffering female saint and martyr, but now as a female Job and Christ combined, and her creator's "new thing"—a more potent extension of his own role as searcher of the heart—is the woman hero with her own weapon—mightier than the proverbial sword, mightier even than all of Lovelace's phallocentric power—the crow-quill pen of a modern prophet aimed as an arrow to probe and prove the hearts of her family, of Lovelace, of herself, and finally of her reader. But Clarissa's ultimate role as prophet comprehends and enlarges her role as a "writer" whose life story inscribes the most comprehensive literary indictment of patriarchal and libertine authority in eighteenth-century literature.

All of her last "writings," diverse appeals to the head and the heart, work to justify Clarissa to a corrupt and inimical world and to an all-judging God, from the most literal expressions to the most figurative. There is a collection and collation of her "true story" drawn from her correspondence and Lovelace's, a task entrusted to Belford. There is her last will and testament (reminiscent of the traditional deathbed blessing in the Old Testament, as in Gen. 27), an extraordinary *aural* emblem meant to be read aloud (as it is by Colonel Morden) and her last letter heard in all its poignant nuances by her devastated family and friends of the family, of whom only Hickman and Morden saw her before her death: "my body . . . shall not be touched but by those of my own sex," nevertheless, "as I am nobody's," Lovelace may view *"her dead* whom he once before saw in a manner dead" (4:416). Such sentiments brought forth admiration, sighs, tears, then execrations from all assembled (4:429). This moving appeal to the ears of her assembled auditors will later be published for a second perusal by their weeping eyes.

There are her eleven posthumous letters to her family, friends, and Lovelace (eleven epistolary apostles to join Belford), which take seriously the injunction of Prov. 25.21–22, "If thine enemy be hungry, give him bread to eat; and if he be thirsty, give him water to drink: For thou shalt heap coals of fire upon his head, and the Lord shall reward thee," advice reiterated approvingly by the apostle Paul to the Romans in support of the Deuteronomic doctrine, "Vengeance is mine; I will repay, saith the Lord" (12.19–20). Since Clarissa, in these posthumous letters, believes she is now in the presence of the Lord, the enormous unspoken bitterness and implied reproach underlying her "forgiveness" in them seems to have the divine approval.[59] As so often happens in biblical narrative, the implied meaning takes precedence over the explicit: Clarissa *knows* that her parents are not going to be made happy by their two remaining children, that they will *not* forget their youngest child—that she was the very center of their life (4:361). To her brother she implies, despite "your rigorous heart, I know you are not such a monster that now I am dead you can refuse to forgive me; after all, what will it cost you? I hope when you have children there will not be one Clarissa among them" (4:361–63). Clarissa now believes herself to be beyond recrimination, and this is in a sense true, but the terrible energy released when her "best self" (3:321) was lost, destroyed, sacrificed, becomes transformed into an appropriation of divine condemnation. With such power, what is the most certain way of having them avenge her against Lovelace? By begging them not to. The posthumous letters are an expression of the nonhuman power of Clarissa's new divine self, and at the same time they are perfectly sincere in their forgiveness. Clarissa's *writing* self became progressively weaker: in these letters particularly we hear the full intensity of the *written* self, a power directed at those she has left behind. Clarissa in these letters has gone beyond the sphere of the most awesome of all satirists—the prophet with divine sanction—to the prophet deified.[60]

Counterbalancing the aural influence of her will is the sheer visual (and aural) impact of her coffin in the funeral procession, an extraordinary memorial emblem. The coffin-desk upon which Clarissa wrote her life out to the end has become the final "book" whose cover now shields her corpse. The coffin is an object charged with tremendous talismanic power (a counterpart in Clarissa's scripture to the ark of the covenant) as it comes, via the horse-drawn hearse with the solemn tolling of the church funeral bell in the distance, into the presence of the crowd of neighboring men, women, and children, and is then carried into the hall of her father's house by six maidens. Clarissa is no longer a person but her own religious force emanating from this terrific object, a power capable of "rewriting" her relationship to all of her family, including her inflexible brother, who stands—a final Richardsonian (and Lockean) impression—with "marks of stupefaction imprinted upon every feature" (4:396).

At the extreme limit of Clarissa's scripture is the nonverbal appeal of the Old Testament prophet's symbolic object, the linen girdle or potter's vessel of Jeremiah, the engraved brick of Ezekiel. The hieroglyphically inscribed coffin functions this way as a memorial sign of the martyr-prophet, but Clarissa is also careful to impress her waning but no less vivid physical presence itself as a memorial emblem, or a prophetic parable in action, upon the mind and heart of her auditor or reader when (of the many examples that could be cited) she writes to her mother on her knees for the last blessing that never comes (4:81), when she stitches a meditation to the bottom of her Uncle John's barbarous letter demanding to know if she thinks herself with child by Lovelace (4:101), when she drops to one knee, with clasped hands and uplifted eyes, imploring Anna Howe's Hickman to remember "that in this posture you see me, in the last moment of our parting, begging a blessing upon you both" (4:16). And over all of this hovers the powerful sense, in Clarissa's mind and gradually the reader's, that the biblical Lord God has intervened in her life to help write the new book of her heart as one of his elect, one of his specially called prophets; that by writing her "Book of Meditations" (virtually her "book of life"), she is writing her "name" in his book of the heart as well, for eternity. Put another way, by allowing Clarissa to write, like Jeremiah, her own "Book of Consolation" and vanquish her enemy Lovelace, God writes her, member by member, in his own.

Notes

Introduction: Writing the Heart from Plato to Hobbes

1. For Galen, each of the body's organs has its own special character or identity. The heart as the "Prince of all the Bowels" is found in Veslingus, *The Anatomy of the Body of Man* (1653), 39. Of recent work on gender, sex, "the humoral body," and the remaking of the sexual body discussed in the Preface, the Introduction, and elsewhere in this book, I am especially indebted to the articles of Randolph Trumbach, in particular "Sodomitical Subcultures, Sodomitical Roles, and the Gender Revolution of the Eighteenth Century: The Recent Historiography"; Thomas Laqueur, *Making Sex: Body and Gender from the Greeks to Freud*, chaps. 1–4; Gail Kern Paster, *The Body Embarrassed: Drama and the Disciplines of Shame in Early Modern England*, chaps. 1–2, 4. Concerning the behavior of heart transplant patients noted in the Preface, one recent study cites evidence that "some individuals seem to regard their heart as if it had a mind of its own," and "patients also worry that they have to take on the sexual behavior of the anonymous donor." They wonder if "the donor 'was promiscuous, oversexed, homo- or bisexual, excessively masculine or feminine, or afflicted with some sort of sexual dysfunction.'" Men were afraid of becoming effeminate after receiving a female heart, but no woman complained about having got a male heart (see B. Bunzel et al., "Does Changing the Heart Mean Changing Personality?" 252–55).

2. Plato, *The Collected Dialogues of Plato*, 1193–94.

3. *Galen on Respiration and the Arteries*, trans. David J. Furley and J. S. Wilkie, 3.

4. Galen, *On Semen*, trans. Phillip de Lacy, 71.

5. Galen, *On the Usefulness of the Parts of the Body*, trans. Margaret Tallmadge May, 631.

6. "Galen, who in the second century A.D. developed the most powerful and resilient model of the structural, though not spatial, identity of the male and female reproductive organs, demonstrated at length that women were essentially men in whom a lack of vital heat—of perfection—had resulted in the retention, inside, of structures that in the male are visible without. . . . In this world the vagina is imagined as an interior penis, the labia as foreskin, the uterus as scrotum, and the ovaries as testicles." Laqueur, *Making Sex*, 4. It should be remarked, however, that the Galenic anatomist Helkiah Crooke argued strenuously against Galen's one-sex model, noting (among other things) that women have no prostate and that the cavity of the penis is smaller than the neck of the womb (*Mikrokosmographia*, 249–50). See Laqueur, 90–91.

7. Galen, *On the Usefulness*, 626.
8. Galen, *On the Usefulness*, 382. See also May's excellent note 78 on male heat and female coldness.
9. *Hippocratic Writings*, ed. G. E. R. Lloyd, 351.
10. *Hippocratic Writings*, 347–49.
11. *Galen on Respiration*, 11–17.
12. Galen, *On the Usefulness*, 292; cf. Edward Mendelson on innate heat as "the single most important motive power in the animal system" (*Heat and Life*, 8).
13. *Galen on Respiration*, 19.
14. Owsei Temkin, *Galenism: Rise and Decline of a Medical Philosophy*, 54–55.
15. See May's commentary in Galen, *On the Usefulness*, 45.
16. We should note here also that Galen conceived "spirit" as an extremely subtle form of "body." The anatomist Helkiah Crooke says that Galen defines "spirite to bee *A certaine exhalation of benigne or wel-disposed blood . . . A subtle and thinne body always mooveable, engendered of blood and vapour . . .* It is therefor a body, but the finest and subtillest substance that is in this Little world [of the body]," *Mikrokosmographia*, 173–74.
17. See Peter Brain's commentary in *Galen on Bloodletting*, 7.
18. See May in Galen, *On the Usefulness*, 23, and Robert G. Richardson, *The Surgeon's Heart: A History of Cardiac Surgery*, 20.
19. I have yet to find an entirely satisfactory account of the flow of the blood in the Galenic system, and the difficulty may be owing more to Galen than to his interpreters. Some commentators argue for an "ebb and flow," some for a rudimentary form of circulation, most for a movement of the blood away from the heart (for the latter view see Peter Brain in *Galen on Bloodletting*, 6). The most detailed account is found in C. R. S. Harris, *The Heart and the Vascular System in Ancient Greek Medicine*, chap. 6. The clearest and most concise account is that of Gweneth Whitteridge, *William Harvey and the Circulation of the Blood*, 41–44. For the most part, I have followed May's description in her introduction to Galen, *On the Usefulness*, 47–54.
20. Robert G. Frank Jr., *Harvey and Oxford Physiologists*, 5.
21. See Harris, *The Heart and the Vascular System*, 327, 367.
22. May, introduction to Galen, *On the Usefulness*, 54; Harris, *The Heart and the Vascular System*, 329.
23. Frederick A. Willius and Thomas J. Dry, *A History of the Heart and the Circulation*, 17; cf. Geoffrey Keynes, *The Life of William Harvey*, 169–70. Keynes does not venture his own description of blood flow in Galen but relies on a summary by H. P. Bayon.
24. May, introduction to Galen, *On the Usefulness*, 47.
25. *Mikrokosmographia* (1615), 410. Hereafter all citations are to this edition and are indicated in the text.
26. See Brain's commentary in *Galen on Bloodletting*, 11.
27. Harris, *The Heart and the Vascular System*, 319.
28. Galen, *On the Usefulness*, 316.
29. Paster, *The Body Embarrassed*, 8.
30. "To most people who had the leisure to think about it in the seven-

teenth century, the unresolved problems about the motion of the heart and blood stemming from Harvey's publication were secondary—very secondary—to bigger problems about personal salvation, the correct interpretation of God's will, the coming millennium or the current wars. It is only with hindsight that we see Harvey's discovery as fundamental to a later 'biomedical science.' . . . I have been less concerned to show that the circulation was accepted because it was true than to show that it came to be seen as true because it was accepted." Roger French, *William Harvey's Natural Philosophy*, 2.

31. Thomas Vicary, *The Englishemans Treasvre*, 38.

32. The four "affections," rooted in the quadripartite heart, were joy, hope, dread, sorrow.

33. Galen, *On the Usefulness*, 293.

34. Galen, *On the Usefulness*, 294. Galen claims to have interviewed a number of women—the more "self-observant" ones—about whether they felt anything in the act of conception. Was conception different in a rational animal from an irrational one? "They said that they feel a certain movement in the uterus, crawling, as it were, and slowly contracting into itself, when they grasp the semen." He notes that some physicians write that the uterus "wraps itself around the semen and encloses it on all sides . . . often the men themselves could clearly perceive this very thing, the uterus drawing in the pudendum like a physician's suction pump" (*On Semen*, 67–69).

35. Thomas Watson, *God's Anatomy upon Man's Heart* (1649), 10.

36. Thomas Watson, *Heaven Taken by Storm*, 60.

37. In terms of the feminized discourse of the heart and the body, it is worth noting that the word "venter" is also a legal term for the uterus, used in designating maternal parentage (*Webster's New World Dictionary*).

38. "Ear": *OED* 2.7.1541 citation.

39. Thomas Watson, *How We May Read the Scriptures with Most Spiritual Profit*, 60.

40. Watson, *How We May Read the Scriptures*, 68.

41. Willius and Dry, *A History of the Heart and the Circulation*, 7.

42. Thomas Hobbes, *Leviathan*, 231.

43. Hobbes, *Leviathan*, 280–81.

44. John Bunyan, *Grace Abounding to the Chief of Sinners*, 35.

45. As quoted in Joseph E. Duncan, *Milton's Earthly Paradise*, 260.

46. John Bunyan, *Grace Abounding*, 14–15.

47. "It was my purpose at the beginning to inquire about the powers that govern us, whether they all have the heart as their only source, as Aristotle and Theophrastus supposed, or whether it is better to posit three sources for them, as Hippocrates and Plato believed" (Galen, *On the Doctrines of Hippocrates and Plato*, trans. Phillip de Lacy, 361).

48. Nathan Bailey, *Dictionarium Britannicum*, s.v. "nature": "NATURE . . . also the government of divine providence, directing all things by certain rules and laws."

49. See Carolyn Merchant, *The Death of Nature*, chaps. 4, 7–10.

50. The major exception is Richard W. F. Kroll's ample discussion of the

importance of Epicureanism in the early modern world in *The Material Word*, part 2. For the classical period, see Martha Nussbaum's discussion in *The Therapy of Desire*, chaps. 4–7.

51. *Lucretius His Six Books of Epicurean Philosophy*, trans. Thomas Creech, book 1, p. 15, hereafter cited in the text.

52. See Loeb edition, book 2, line 269.

53. *The Poetical Works of Dryden*, 188.

54. Samuel Richardson, *Clarissa*, Everyman ed., 3:250.

55. *Poetical Works of Dryden*, 189.

56. Hobbes, *Leviathan*, 1. The important seventeenth-century Epicurean-Lucretian natural scientist Walter Charleton goes far beyond Hobbes in his deployment of mechanistic images of the heart. He speaks of his admiration for "the skill of the Divine *Engineer* who contrived and made the *Machine* of the heart of so small a bulk, and yet so stupendous power and force" (*Three Anatomic Lectures*, 38).

57. Hobbes, *Leviathan*, 3.

58. Hobbes, *Leviathan*, 3.

59. Hobbes, *Leviathan*, 3–4.

60. John Locke, *An Essay Concerning Human Understanding*, 1:122.

Chapter 1. The Biblical Heart

1. I. Cohen, "The Heart in Biblical Psychology," 41.

2. Robert Alter, *The Art of Biblical Narrative*, 158.

3. On the meanings of "Puritan" and "Anglican" in the seventeenth and eighteenth centuries, see the discussion at the beginning of Chapter 5.

4. Stephen Charnock, "On the Existence and Attributes of God," *Complete Works*, 1:162–63.

5. Charnock, "The Sinfulness and Cure of Thoughts," in *Puritan Sermons*, 2:386–87.

6. Charnock, "The Sinfulness," 2:387.

7. Charnock, "The Sinfulness," 2:387–88.

8. This sense of Eve's preeminence to Adam was explored by seventeenth-century praisers of women, especially Cornelius Agrippa. See Robert A. Erickson, *Mother Midnight*, 25, 128.

9. See my review of Laqueur's *Making Sex* in *Eighteenth-Century Fiction* (1992).

10. Elaine Scarry's influential description of God's "making" activities would have had more particular force if she had focused on the motif of God's "making" as God's "writing" or "inscribing" (*The Body in Pain*, chap. 4).

11. *The Medieval Reader*, ed. Norman F. Cantor, 247.

12. Herbert N. Schneidau, *Sacred Discontent*, 30–31.

13. Watson, *Heaven Taken by Storm*, 23–24.

14. The New Revised Standard Version gives "common characters" for "a man's pen."

15. Scarry, *The Body in Pain*, 203–4.

16. Robert Boyle called Harvey "our English *Democritus*" (quoted in Robert G. Frank Jr., *Harvey and the Oxford Physiologists*, 146).

17. Watson, *Gods Anatomy upon Mans Heart*, 1–2, 15–18.

18. Watson, *Gods Anatomy*, 2–3.

19. Watson, *Gods Anatomy*, 2–3.

20. This is a pattern in prophetic writing seen most clearly in Jeremiah and Baruch, the pattern of God or the prophet dictating orally and the scribe writing.

21. John Bunyan, *The Pilgrim's Progress*, 235.

22. A similar dynamic occurs when King Jehoiakim burns the roll of Jeremiah's prophecy written by Baruch and the Lord commands Jeremiah to write another one (Jer. 36.20–32).

23. I discuss this psalm in *Mother Midnight*, 14–15.

24. Watson, *Gods Anatomy*, 3–4.

25. Watson, *Gods Anatomy*, 4–6, 10–11.

26. John Milton, *The Complete Prose Works*, 6:587.

27. The complex trope of the circumcised and uncircumcised heart occurs elsewhere in the Hebrew Bible in Lev. 26.41, Deut. 30.6, and Ezek. 44.7, 9. In Deut. 10.16 the circumcised heart will cause the Israelites to "be no more stiff-necked." There are also allusions to the uncircumcised ear (Jer. 6.10) and uncircumcised lips (Exod. 6.12, 30).

28. *Works of Richard Sibbes*, 5:69–70.

29. For a detailed exploration of women in the Quaker movement of the seventeenth century, see Phyllis Mack, *Visionary Women*, esp. chaps. 4 and 5.

30. Watson, *Gods Anatomy*, 14.

Chapter 2. The Phallic Heart

1. Geoffrey Keynes, *The Life of William Harvey*, 212–15.

2. In a poem of 1653, the physician Martin Llewellyn called Harvey the "*Circulator* of the *Lesser World*," comparing him to Drake. Llewellyn also invoked the "book of nature" trope in a novel way:

> From *Books* to *Nature* thy *Appeale* is made,
> Thy *Copies* by their *Archetype* are swayd.
> Though *High* and *Reverend* thy *Authors* sit,
> Yet the *Creation* is thy *Classick Writ*.

(Quoted in Robert G. Frank Jr., "The Image of Harvey in Commonwealth and Restoration England" in *William Harvey and His Age: The Professional and Social Context of the Discovery of the Circulation*, ed. Jerome J. Bylebyl.) Of recent scholarship on Harvey as anatomist and writer, I wish to note especially Peter N. Bradshaw, "The Idea of Anatomy in the Work of Seventeenth-Century Prose Writers," esp. chaps. 1 and 3; Robert G. Frank Jr., *Harvey and the Oxford Physiologists: Scientific Ideas and Social Interaction*; Walter Pagel, *William Harvey's Biological Ideas: Selected Aspects and Historical Background* and *New Light on William Harvey*.

3. See Gweneth Whitteridge, *William Harvey and the Circulation of the Blood*, 104–13. Cf. also Keynes, *The Life of William Harvey*, 93, 105–8.

4. On Harvey's relationship with Charles I, see the debate between Christopher Hill, "William Harvey and the Idea of Monarchy," and Gweneth Whitteridge, "William Harvey: A Royalist and No Parliamentarian," in *The Intellectual Revolution of the Seventeenth Century*, ed. Charles Webster, 160–96. As chief physician to his king, Harvey must have seen himself in the tradition of the anatomists Galen and Vesalius, who were each physicans to their respective emperors.

5. Another edition of this work appeared in 1673. The English version (translated anonymously) of Harvey's other great work, *Exercitationes de generatione animalium* (Anatomical exercitations on the generation of living creatures) (1651), hereafter referred to in the text as *De generatione*, was also first published in 1653.

6. John Aubrey, *Aubrey's Brief Lives*, ed. Oliver Lawson Dick, 131.

7. Marjorie Hope Nicolson, *The Breaking of the Circle: Studies in the Effect of the "New Science" Upon Seventeenth Century Poetry*, 113.

8. Charles Singer, *A Short History of Anatomy from the Greeks to Harvey*, 175.

9. William Harvey, *The Anatomical Exercises of Dr. William Harvey: "De Motu Cordis," 1628; "De Circulatione Sanguinis," 1649. The First English Text of 1653*, vii. All quotations from *The Motion of the Heart* and the two letters to Riolan (hereafter cited in the text) are to this edition and have been checked for accuracy against the original 1653 edition in the British Library and corrected where necessary. See also Roger French's comment on the 1653 translation in *William Harvey's Natural Philosophy*, 91 n. 40.

10. I am indebted to Jan V. Golinski's discussion of historicist methodology in "Robert Boyle: Scepticism and Authority in Seventeenth-Century Chemical Discourse," 59–60. For other discussions of Harvey's language, see Peter Jucovy, "Circle and Circulation: The Language and Imagery of William Harvey's Discovery," 92–107, and Peter Graham, "Harvey's *De Motu Cordis*: The Rhetoric of Science and Science of Rhetoric," 469–76. For a detailed study of *De motu cordis* as an example of the *exercitatio* form (and why it is not a "disputation"), see Roger French, *William Harvey's Natural Philosophy*, chap. 5.

11. Robert Burton, *The Anatomy of Melancholy*, ed. Holbrook Jackson, 1:150.

12. See the description and the two illustrations of this theater in Keynes, *William Harvey*, 25–26, plates 4 and 5.

13. Miguel Cervantes, *The History of Don Quixote of the Mancha*, trans. Thomas Shelton (1612), "The Authors Preface to the Reader," 5–7. Cf. "*I could not transgress the order of Nature, wherein every thing begets his like: which being so, what could my sterile and il-tild wit ingender, but the history of a dry tosted, and humorous son, full of various thoughts and conceits never before imagined of any other,*" 5.

14. "And if any man think that he knoweth any thing, he knoweth nothing yet as he ought to know" (1 Cor. 8.2).

15. See Frank, *Harvey and the Oxford Physiologists*, 16–17. Swift may have had the diminutive Harvey in mind when he imagined Gulliver in Brobdingnag doing battle with all manner of vermin.

16. See Carolyn Merchant, *The Death of Nature*, 181–82.

17. Quoted in Keynes, *William Harvey*, 158, 160.

18. Keynes, *William Harvey*, 93–94.

19. William Harvey, *Anatomical Exercitations, Concerning the Generation of Living Creatures: To which are added Particular Discourses, of Births, and of Conceptions, &c.* (London, 1653).

20. "I do indeed rejoice to see truly learned men everywhere illustrating the republic of letters, even in the present age" (Harvey's letter to John Nardi, Nov. 30, 1653, in *The Works of William Harvey, M.D.*, trans. Robert Willis (1847), 610. Cf. also Sir Charles Scarburgh's recollection of Harvey's allusion to "the Republick of Letters" in Keynes, *William Harvey*, 322. See also Devon Hodges, *Renaissance Fictions of Anatomy*, chap. 1, for further discussion of the scientific, spiritual, and literary meanings of "anatomy."

21. Abraham Cowley, *Selected Poetry and Prose*, ed. James G. Taaffe, 78–81. Cf. Jonathan Sawday's discussion of this poem in *The Body Emblazoned*, 239–41. Cf. also Evelyn Fox Keller's account of Bacon's aggressive/responsive portrayal of "the sons of knowledge" and their marital relationship to a coy feminine "Nature": "For you have but to follow and as it were hound nature in her wanderings, and you will be able, when you like, to lead and drive her afterwards to the same place again" (*Reflections on Gender and Science*, 36). Keller does not discuss Harvey. Also relevant in this context is the pioneering work of Carolyn Merchant, *The Death of Nature: Women, Ecology, and the Scientific Revolution* and Brian Easlea, *Witchhunting, Magic and the New Philosophy* and *Science and Sexual Repression: Patriarchy's Confrontation with Woman and Nature*. Harvey's own depiction of his relationship with Nature is closer in many ways to the seventeenth-century hermetical/alchemical model (seen particularly in Thomas Vaughan) of fruitful coition between male and female principles than it is to the aggressive Baconian model (see esp. Merchant, chap. 4, and Keller, chap. 3).

22. In his second letter to Riolan, Harvey describes three experiments that demonstrate how "the blood in the veins with a continuall and great flux runs continually towards the heart." The first experiment was made on "the internal jugular vein of a live Doe, which I laid open before a great part of the Nobility, and the King my Royal Master standing by," the second is one that Riolan (or the reader) can do by pressing out all the blood downward on any "visible long vein of your arm," and the third was performed on "a man's body, newly hang'd, two hours after his execution, before the rednesse of his face was gone, opening up his heart and Pericardium, the right ear of his heart and lungs much stuffed, and distended with blood; many witnesses standing by" (170–71). Here, the king as passive but potent witness, the nobility, the live doe, the reader, Aristotle, and an executed criminal are all brought into conjunction in the space of four brief paragraphs in order for Harvey, the master anatomist, to prove a crucial point in defense of his discovery.

23. See Erickson, *Mother Midnight*, 116–21.

24. Aubrey, *Brief Lives*, 129, 131.

25. In 1636, the Earl of Arundel chose Harvey as his personal physician to attend him on a diplomatic mission to Ratisbon. In a letter from Ratisbon, Arundel

reported that "Honest little Hervey is going a little start into Italy and I gave him some employment . . . about pictures for his Majesty" (Keynes, *William Harvey*, 245). Harvey was noted for his diminutive stature.

26. Pagel, *New Light on William Harvey*, 37. Walter Charleton, Harvey's contemporary, refers to Harvey's "invention" of the circulation of the blood and suggests that he came to the discovery "by assiduous Meditation, perhaps also by the secret Manduction of Fate, that had reserved the secret for his knowledge" (*Three Anatomic Lectures*, 23).

27. From the "Dramatis Personae," *Terence's Comedies: Made English. With His Life: and Some Remarks at the End. By Several Hands* (London, 1694).

28. Cf. the more empirical 1694 translation, with its stress on trial and experience: "Never did Man cast up the business of his Life so exactly; but still Experience, Years and Custom will bring in some new Particulars that he was not aware of; and shew his Ignorance of what he thought he knew, and after trial make him reject his former Opinions. This is plainly my case at present for since my Glass is almost out, I renounce this rigid Life I have always lead [*sic*]. But why so? Because Experience shews me there's nothing like gentleness and good nature." *Terence's Comedies*, 195.

29. Burton, *Anatomy of Melancholy*, 1:153.

30. Helkiah Crooke, *Mikrokosmographia*, 370.

31. Cf. Nicholas Venette on the link between the godlike penis and the heart: "It is observable, that the Ancients ranked the *Viril Member* among the number of their Gods . . . to intimate its Empire and Dominion. . . . 'tis the Father of human Kind. . . . The *Viril Member* has a notable Commerce with the whole Body; if you touch it sometimes never so rudely, the Heart at the same instant feels surprizing Faintness" (*The Pleasures of Conjugal Love Explain'd*, 1–2).

32. See Patricia K. Fumerton's detailed account of Charles's execution in *Cultural Aesthetics: Renaissance Literature and the Practice of Social Ornament*, chap. 1.

33. "When he had thus spoken, he spat on the ground, and made clay of the spittle, and he anointed the eyes of the blind man with the clay. . . . He went his way therefore, and washed, and came seeing" (John 9.6–7); "and [he] put his fingers into his ears, and he spit, and touched his tongue . . . and saith unto him . . . Be opened. And straightway his ears were opened, and the string of his tongue was loosed, and he spake plain" (Mark 7.33–35).

34. "Blood, according to Aristotle, in a more advanced stage becomes semen in the male who can thus concoct the *nourishment in its ultimate phase*. . . . Indeed the semen is the ultimate secretion of nutriment . . . and as such carried *to* all parts of the body—rather than coming *from* them" (Pagel, *William Harvey's Biological Ideas*, 258).

35. Aubrey, *Brief Lives*, 131. Keynes qualifies Aubrey's observation (*William Harvey*, 178).

36. Nicholas Venette, *Conjugal Love Reveal'd; In the Nightly Pleasures of the Marriage Bed*, 80–81.

37. Cf. Helkiah Crooke, Harvey's contemporary:

The habite [flesh] of a woman is fatter, looser and softer. . . . The flesh of men is more solide, their vesselles larger, their voyce baser: now it is heate which amplifieth and enlargeth, as cold straightneth and contracteth . . . *woemens food is more moyste*; and beside, they liue an idle and sedentarie life. . . . It is behoued therefore that man should be hotter, because his body was made to endure labour and travell, as also that his minde should bee stout and inuincible to vndergoe dangers, the onely hearing whereof will driue a woman as wee say out of her little wits. The woman was ordayned to receiue and conceiue the seede of the man, to beare and nourish the Infant, to gouerne and moderate the house at home, to delight and refresh her husband forswunke with labour and well-nigh exhausted and spent with care and travell; and therefore her body is soft, smooth and delicate, made especially for pleasure, so that whosoeuer vseth them for other doth almost abuse them. . . . It is therefore manifest, that the Chest and Paps, and the whole body of a woman is laxe & soft. . . . A mans body is ful; & like a cloath, thick and thight [sic] both to see to & to feele to, but a woman is rare, and laxe, and moyst, both to see to and to feele to . . . for women being of a shorter life then men, because they are colder, they sooner grow women and so also sooner grow old then men.

Mikrokosmographia, 274–76. Harvey's writings about women never betray this kind of antifeminist rhetoric.

38. Such wilt thou be to me, who must
   Like th' other foot, obliquely run;
   Thy firmness makes my circle just,
   And makes me end where I begun

(John Donne, "A Valediction: Forbidding Mourning")

39. Compare Don Quixote's "Balsamum of Fierebras" in Cervantes, *The History of Don Quixote*, Shelton trans., 143–44. Since in romance balsam is usually applied by a woman, it could conversely be considered a heroic "female" substance.

40. In *De generatione*, Harvey gives primacy to the blood over the heart as the originating principle of life.

41. Harvey, *De generatione*, 157–58. This passage is quoted in Keynes, *William Harvey*, 357.

42. Michael McKeon is one of the few critics to comment cogently and informatively (if briefly) on this issue in his discussion of Bakhtin and of "'Natural History' as a Narrative Model" in *The Origins of the English Novel, 1600–1740*, 11–14, 68–73. See also J. Paul Hunter, *Before Novels: The Cultural Contexts of Eighteenth-Century English Fiction*, esp. chap. 8, and Ilse Vickers, "The Influence of the New Sciences on Defoe," 200–218.

43. Mikhail Bakhtin, *The Dialogic Imagination: Four Essays*, ed. Michael Holquist, 24, 7, 15.

44. Keynes, *William Harvey*, 327.

45. Laurence Sterne, *Tristram Shandy*, ed. James A. Work, 176–77.

46. See Luke O. Wilson's stimulating but diffuse discussion of "anatomy" as "reconstitution" in "William Harvey's *Prelectiones*," 63, 75, 91.

47. For Harvey's comments on his own experiments, see *The Motion of the Heart*, 34, 46, 69, 75, and especially his careful analysis of the progress of his own bruise to the head: "I falling out of a Coach, and being somewhat hurt in my

forhead, there where the little branch of the *arterie* creeps out of the temples, I felt a swelling about the bigness of an egg in the space of twenty pulses, without either heat or much pain, *viz.* because of the nearness of the *arterie*, the blood was abundantly and more swiftly driven into the bruz'd place" (79). Defoe will carry over this carefully timed and detailed sort of description in Moll Flanders's analyses of her most proficient thefts.

Chapter 3. The Heart of Eve

1. Of the enormous outpouring of commentary on Milton's Eve since William Empson's groundbreaking *Milton's God* in 1965, I am most indebted to the following: Diane Kelsey McColley's *Milton's Eve* (1983) and *A Gust for Paradise* (1993), James Grantham Turner's *One Flesh: Paradisal Marriage and Sexual Relations in the Age of Milton* (1987), Joseph E. Duncan's *Milton's Earthly Paradise* (1972), John Halkett's *Milton and the Idea of Matrimony* (1970), Christopher Hill's *Milton and the English Revolution* (1977), Barbara K. Lewalski's *"Paradise Lost" and the Rhetoric of Literary Forms* (1985), William Kerrigan's *The Prophetic Milton* (1974) and *The Sacred Complex* (1983), Philip J. Gallagher's *Milton, the Bible, and Misogyny* (1990), Joseph Wittreich's *Feminist Milton* (1987). My starting point, to which I have returned again and again, is Empson.

2. For Milton's Cambridge curriculum, see Harris Francis Fletcher, *The Intellectual Development of John Milton*, 2:475. For Milton's conservative and traditional medical knowledge, see Kester Svendsen, *Milton and Science*, chap. 6, "The Human Body": "It would be strange . . . if Milton's abiding interest in medical matters failed to realize itself in images; and the prose teems with medical as the poetry with astronomical lore," 176. I will argue that the poetry, especially *Paradise Lost*, also teems with anatomical images.

3. *John Milton: Complete Poems and Major Prose*, ed. M. Y. Hughes, 635 n. 51.

4. *John Milton*, book 5, line 503; 10.1073; 11.565. All subsequent quotations from *Paradise Lost* are from the Hughes edition (unless otherwise noted) and are cited in the text.

5. Northrop Frye, *The Great Code*, 6.

6. For a suggestive and at times differing reading of Milton in relation to prophecy, see Kerrigan, *The Prophetic Milton*, introduction and chap. 1.

7. Milton, *The Christian Doctrine* in *The Complete Prose Works of John Milton*, 6:587.

8. *The Poems of John Milton*, ed. John Carey and Alastair Fowler, 459, note to lines 6–22. Further citations to this edition are in the text.

9. Cf. Fowler's note to "brooding . . . mad'st it pregnant" in lines 20–22: "Not a mixed metaphor, but a deliberate allusion to the Hermetic doctrine that God is both masculine and feminine"; he cites Nicolas Cusanus.

10. See Richard Brixton Onians, *The Origins of European Thought*, chaps. 1, 4.

11. Lancelot Andrewes, "The Fourth Sermon on the Nativity," in *Sermons*, 27.

12. Andrewes, "The Fourth Sermon on the Nativity," 47. Compare this sequence of inscribing Christ within the heart before his oral generation in the flesh with the writing and then speaking sequence of the creation of human beings discussed in Chapter 1. The writing in the heart precedes the voice.

13. Of the 205 uses of the "heart" in Milton's prose, 70 refer to the "hard" heart.

14. William Harvey, *The Motion of the Heart*, 35–36.

15. Crooke, *Mikrokosmographia* (1615), 41–42; all citations from Crooke are to this edition and are hereafter placed in the text. The unruly phallus is discussed in conjunction with the angry, wandering womb at the end of the *Timaeus* (*Collected Dialogues of Plato*, 1210).

16. "The Imperfect Enjoyment," *The Poems of John Wilmot, Earl of Rochester*, ed. Keith Walker, 31–32.

17. Galen, *On the Doctrines of Hippocrates and Plato*, 363–65. Galen distinguishes between *energeia*, the natural motion of the heart in pulsation, and *pathos*, the unnatural motion of the heart in palpitation. Anger and the other affections are runaway and immoderate motions. Galen's entire discussion of the autonomous heart, anger, and desire in this passage is relevant to Satan's opposition to God, his embrace of Hell, and his assault upon Adam and Eve.

18. I owe this connection to a reader of the prepublication manuscript.

19. Svendsen says, "Milton nowhere betrays any acquaintance with Harvey's discovery; his references to the blood and its functions and to the humors are traditional and almost always in a figurative context" (*Milton and Science*, 179). I suggest that if Milton was well aware of Galileo's astronomical discoveries, he almost certainly was aware of Harvey's anatomical ones.

20. This subtext is reinforced by the myth of Daphne, transformed by her father into one of the trees of her own sweet grove; Cham (or Ham), Noah's son, is linked to Ammon or Jove, the many-faceted father figure who, suspicious in this instance, hides his beautiful mistress and "florid," rosy-cheeked son Bacchus on an island, away from stepmother Rhea's eyes. And Ham of course returns as Noah's irreverent son whose own son is cursed because Ham saw his father naked (12.101).

21. The third aspect of the Galenic soul, the vegetative/nutritive faculty, whose seat is in the liver within the abdominal venter, is also more evident in Eve, who is associated with the green world of flowers and gardening, and who functions as provider of vegetarian food. The reader is referred to the discussion of male heat and female coldness, and to Galen's version of the human caloric economy in the Introduction.

22. Thomas Willis, *Two Discourses Concerning the Soul of Brutes* (1683), 38–39. This is a translation of *De anima brutorum quae hominis vitalis ac sensitiva est, exercitationes duae: prior physiologica* (London, 1672). For a good recent discussion of Willis on the soul, brain, and body in the context of emerging "neurocentrism," see Robert L. Martensen, "Alienation and the Production of Strangers: Western Medical Epistemology and the Architectonics of the Body," 143–61. Cf. also Walter Charleton on the "Sensitive" or "Corporeal Soul" and the "Rational Soul" in *Natural History of the Passions*, sig. A7–8, 14–79.

23. Willis, *Two Discourses*, 45–48.

24. When Milton reached sixty he may well have noted that he had now outlived—perhaps miraculously, considering his exposure to assassination and execution in 1660—the preceding great English poets, Chaucer, Spenser, Shakespeare. Michael Lieb's important recent study, *Milton and the Culture of Violence*, is relevant to my anatomical concerns in this chapter and the entire book, but Lieb does not discuss Satan's assault on Eve. He argues "that underlying Milton's sensibility is an anxiety about the body faced with the horrifying prospect of mutilation and dismemberment.... This is an anxiety deeply rooted in the Miltonic psyche, one intimately tied to Milton's sense of his own sexuality, his notion of gendered self, and the culture out of which his selfhood emerges" (9).

25. See "Posture 15" on p. 351 of Ellis's edition of Rochester's *Complete Works*.

26. Lewis, *A Preface to "Paradise Lost,"* 65. We may also recall at this point Lewis's less perceptive comment on the sex life of Milton's angels as noted by Gregory Bredbeck in *Sodomy and Interpretation*, 189–90, 192.

27. See Sara van den Berg, "Eve, Sin, and Witchcraft in *Paradise Lost*," and the influential essays on Eve and witchcraft by William B. Hunter Jr. and John M. Steadman.

28. R. David Freedman, "Woman, A Power Equal to Man," 56–58. My colleague, Professor Randall Garr, questions the root meaning of "be powerful" for *ezer*.

29. The Scottish physician James McMath, following Galen, notes in *The Expert Midwife* (1694) that in sexual intercourse the orifice of the womb "delightfully opens, and raveningly attracts the mans Seed (which is then sufficiently darted into the *Recesses* of the *Womb*)," 7. See Robert A. Erickson, "The Books of Generation," 81.

30. St. Paul says, in the context of fornication, "know ye not that your body is the temple of the Holy Ghost which is in you, which ye have of God, and ye are not your own?" (1 Cor. 6.19). And as we have seen, the activity of the Holy Spirit in the New Testament is intimately related to the human heart.

31. Or as Ajax says in *Troilus and Cressida*, "I do hate a proud man as I hate the engendering of toads" (2.3.58–59). The dynamic of Satan's engendering of pride in Eve seems to be modeled on Iago's engendering of jealousy in Othello.

32. See Erickson, *Mother Midnight*, 126, 156.

33. I have discussed this motif in some detail in *Mother Midnight*.

34. See Kroll, *The Material Word*, 223.

35. See [Geminus/Udall], *Compendiosa*, "Of the partes of Mannes bodye," sig. A1–6.

36. [Geminus/Udall], *Compendiosa*, sig. A4.

37. To my knowledge, the best discussion of unfallen and fallen sexuality in *Paradise Lost*—touching on angelic sex, Satan's sexual jealousy, and Satan's "rape" of Eve—is James Grantham Turner's *One Flesh*, esp. chap. 7.

38. John Milton, "Elegy I," translated in Hughes, *John Milton*, 91.

39. Satan's appropriation of Eve's image is a more subtle poetic version of the Eve-faced serpent coiled around the tree in Raphael's famous painting of the Fall.

40. Mary Wollstonecraft, *A Vindication of the Rights of Woman*, 52. Cf. Rilke's "Requiem": "Then from the night-warm soilbed of your heart / you dug the

seeds, still green from which your death / would sprout: your own, your perfect death, the one that was your whole life's perfect consummation." I owe this reference to Marisa Landa.

41. The *exercitatio* form employed by Harvey for his narrative of the heart, with its own proem, makes an interesting analogue to Milton's adaptation of the classical oration.

42. See, for example, John Cleland's *Fanny Hill*, 49.

43. Reinterpreting the tradition of the priority of the earth, Lucretius asserts that the gods did not create the world and are far removed from it (*On the Nature of the Universe*, 132–33), and that "the name mother has rightly been bestowed on the earth, since out of the earth everything is born. Even now multitudes of animals are formed out of the earth with the aid of showers and the sun's genial warmth" (149). Lucretius goes on, in language suggestive of Milton's maternal and fructifying Tree of Knowledge: "There was a great superfluity of heat and moisture in the soil. So . . . there grew up wombs, clinging to the earth by roots. These, when the time was ripe, were burst open by the maturation of the embryos. . . . Then nature directed towards that spot the pores of the earth, making it open its veins and exude a juice resembling milk, just as nowadays every female when she has given birth is filled with sweet milk because all the flow of nourishment within her is directed into the breasts. . . . Here then is further proof that the name of mother has rightly been bestowed on the earth, since it brought forth the human race and gave birth" to all beasts and birds (149).

44. Boehme defines the "tree of the knowledge of good and evil" as the "tree of self-knowledge of good and evil" (*Mysterium Magnum* in *Personal Christianity*, 193).

45. Concerning Adam's failure to save Eve, see John Leonard, *Naming in Paradise*, 217–22, 226–27.

46. Neither Diane Kelsey McColley in *Milton's Eve* nor James Grantham Turner in *One Flesh* discuss the implications of "thee . . . whose perfection far excell'd / Hers in all real dignity" (10.150–51).

47. See the two important articles on "patience" in Milton by Paul R. Baumgartner and William O. Harris.

48. One of Milton's most powerful expressions of this combined theme occurs in the autobiographical passage in his *Second Defense of the English People*: "There is, as the apostle has remarked, a way to strength through weakness. Let me then be the most feeble creature alive, as long as that feebleness serves to invigorate the energies of my rational and immortal spirit; as long as in that obscurity, in which I am enveloped, the light of the divine presence more clearly shines; then, in proportion as I am weak, I shall be invincibly strong, and in proportion as I am blind, I shall more clearly see. O! that I may thus be perfected by feebleness, and irradiated by obscurity!" (Hughes, *John Milton*, 826).

49. Willis, *Two Discourses*, 46.

50. Hobbes, *Leviathan*, 3.

51. Willis, *Two Discourses*, 46–47: "For indeed, the Blood containing Life as a most precious Jewel in it self, is not only heaped up more plentifully about the *Praecordia*, in all Fear and Danger, and is there lay'd up as it were for defence sake,

that it might better preserve its Flame: But further, in devout Affections, whil'st the Rational Soul orders the Spirits inhabiting the Brain into sacred Conceptions and Notions; by the Influence of the same Spirits, the Bosomes of the Heart are also so affected, that they cause the Blood to Centre, and to be more fully drawn into them, and there longer retain it . . . so as often as we Pray most earnestly, we endeavour nothing less, than that our Life with the Blood, be laid upon the Altar of the Heart. For truely, almost every body experiences in himself that in strong Prayer, the Blood is more and more heaped up in the Bosomes of the swelling Heart: wherefore, that the Vacuities of the Lungs might be supplied, we breath deeply, and so the Air being more fully drawn in, the Muscles of the Breast, and the *Diaphragma*, are detained almost in a continual *Systole* . . . for this end, that the Vital Blood, to be offered as it were a Sacrifice to God, should be there kept, nor suffer'd to go from thence, or to be inlarged, till as it were by a long immolation, together with Prayer, lieve may be had from the Godhead. Yea, 'tis to be observed, that those religiously affected, are apt at all times to call back the Blood towards the *Praecordia*, and to repress it from a more plentiful Excursion, which may give a loose to Delights or Mirth: Because 'tis just, that this Vital Humor should be Conserved, even Holy and Pure for God."

52. *The Reason of Church Government* in Hughes, *John Milton*, 668.

Chapter 4. The Generous Heart

1. *Lucretius His Six Books of Epicurean Philosophy* (1700), trans. Thomas Creech, 104.

2. Kroll, *The Material Word*, 95–96, 167–68.

3. *Lucretius His Six Books*, 1–2.

4. *The Works of Aphra Behn*, ed. Janet Todd, vol. 1: *Poetry*, 162; unless otherwise noted, all subsequent citations of Behn's poetry are to this edition and volume and are indicated by page numbers in the text.

5. Rochester translated *De rerum natura*, 1.1–5, 44–49 (Walker ed. of *The Poems of John Wilmot*, 50–51 and notes). See also the notes to Frank H. Ellis's recent edition of Rochester's *Complete Works*, 323 (and the allusions to Lucretius in Shadwell's *The Virtuoso*), 337, 338, 361, 373, 374.

6. *Lucretius His Six Books*, 118.

7. For Behn's biographical record I rely chiefly on Angeline Goreau's *Reconstructing Aphra: A Social Biography of Aphra Behn* (1980), and Maureen Duffy's *The Passionate Shepherdess: Aphra Behn, 1640–89* (1979).

8. See especially Duffy, *The Passionate Shepherdess*, on Prior (214, 221), and on Gould (219–20, 248, and 280–81 for the famous equation of "punk and poetess"). See also Catherine Gallagher, *Nobody's Story*, chap. 1.

9. *The Works of Aphra Behn*, ed. Montague Summers, vol. 6: *Poems of A. Behn*, 117, 119, 121. These dedicatory poems are not included in the Todd edition of Behn's poetry; all subsequent citations to the Summers edition are indicated in the text.

10. Goreau, *Reconstructing Aphra*, 10.

11. It is almost as if some male poets can accept Aphra Behn more easily as an androgyne than as a woman. Considering the influence of the androgynous *imago dei* in seventeenth-century hermetic thought, this could be construed as the ultimate male compliment to her, or it could be viewed more simply as another way of refusing to admit the unique power of feminine art and discourse.

12. Astraea was the Roman goddess of justice in the Age of Gold; she was driven to heaven by the wickedness and impiety of mankind to be constellated as Virgo.

13. Cf. Behn's possibly ironic praise of the "wondrous" erotic and political power of Gilbert Burnet's "Pen" in "A Pindaric Poem to the Reverend Doctor Burnet on the Honour he did me of Enquiring after me and my Muse," 308–9.

14. Duffy, *The Passionate Shepherdess*, 229.

15. Behn's Silvia compares herself to "the languishing abandon'd Mistress of the *Canticles*" in *Love Letters Between a Nobleman and His Sister* in *The Works of Aphra Behn*, ed. Janet Todd, 2:101–2.

16. Aphra Behn, *Oroonoko*, introd. Lore Metzger, 25. All subsequent citations from this edition are indicated by page number in the text.

17. Aphra Behn, *"Oroonoko," "The Rover" and Other Works*, ed. Janet Todd (1992), 160. For convenience, I have cited from this text and compared each citation with the best modern edition of the play, that by Frederick M. Link (1967). All subsequent citations to the Todd edition are indicated by page number in the text.

18. *"Oroonoko," "The Rover" and Other Works*, 147–48.

19. *"Oroonoko," "The Rover" and Other Works*, 30.

20. *"Oroonoko," "The Rover" and Other Works*, 33.

21. *The Works of Aphra Behn*, ed. Montague Summers, 1:130.

22. Locke, *An Essay Concerning Human Understanding*, 1:334.

23. Locke, *An Essay*, 1:334–36. See Ovid, *Metamorphoses*, 7.20–21.

24. Locke, *An Essay*, 1:338.

25. William Wycherley, *The Country Wife*, in *Restoration and Eighteenth-Century Comedy*, ed. Scott McMillin, 65.

26. See Catherine Gallagher, *Nobody's Story: The Vanishing Acts of Women Writers in the Marketplace, 1670–1820*, 22: "Aphra Behn managed to create the effect of a distinctively female integrity out of the very metaphor of prostitution," 22. Here Behn converts Willmore from "the gentleman" who would not "sell" himself (185) into a kind of male prostitute, similar to her Gayman in *The Lucky Chance*.

27. See Goreau, *Reconstructing Aphra*, 17. On the emergence of the female writer, cf. Goreau's chap. 9, "Literary Foremothers." See also Jacqueline Pearson, *The Prostituted Muse*, chaps. 1–4, and Catherine Gallagher, *Nobody's Story*.

28. Nathan Bailey, *Dictionarium*, s.v. "Woman." One of the features of Bailey's dictionary was the insertion of illustrative proverbs, including under this entry "*Women, Wealth, and Wine, have each two Qualities, a good and a bad. That is, they are either a blessing or a curse, according to the use we make of them,*" a definition that betrays the conventional view of woman as mere instrumentality, like language itself. In this view "woman" is shaped and defined by language as if she were a piece of woven stuff.

29. I have further explored the contrast between Lady Fulbank and Margery Pinchwife as "writers," and Behn's doctrine of virtuous female and male libertinism compared with Rochester's revisionist version of "right reason," in "Lady Fulbank and the Poet's Dream in Behn's *The Lucky Chance*," in *Broken Boundaries: Women and Feminism in Restoration Drama*, ed. Katherine M. Quinsey.

30. Of recent criticism (besides that cited elsewhere), I would like to note the following as the most pertinent to my concerns in this chapter: Katherine M. Rogers, "Fact and Fiction in Aphra Behn's *Oroonoko*," 1–15; Robert L. Chibka, "'Oh! Do Not Fear a Woman's Invention': Truth, Falsehood, and Fiction in Aphra Behn's *Oroonoko*," 510–37; Beverle Houston, "Usurpation and Dismemberment: Oedipal Tyranny in *Oroonoko*," 30–36; Martine Watson Brownley, "The Narrator in *Oroonoko*," 174–81; and Jacqueline Pearson, "Gender and Narrative in the Fiction of Aphra Behn," 40–56, 179–90, esp. pp. 184–90 for a sensitive account of the narrator's ambivalence.

31. For Behn's intellectual encounter with Scripture and French biblical criticism in her translation and publication, in early 1688, of Fontenelle's *Entretiens sur la pluralité des mondes* (accompanied by her "Essay on Translated Prose"), see Duffy, *The Passionate Shepherdess*, 270–74, and Robert Adams Day, "Aphra Behn and the Works of the Intellect," 374–80.

32. They are literally the first "African-American" protagonists in English fiction because they start out in Africa and die in South America.

33. I suggest that beginning in the second paragraph of *Oroonoko* ("the Hero . . . gave us the whole Transactions of his Youth" [1]), Behn, as "Mistress" of a special branch of "natural philosophy," is giving her own version of a "philosophical transaction" concerning a little known race and region of the world, a "curiosity" (though in the guise of a fiction) similar in topic and idiom to several communications in the pages of the *Philosophical Transactions* of the Royal Society in the first twenty years of its existence, including descriptions of exotic places (e.g., China [no. 180: 1686], the East and West Indies [no. 80: 1671/2], Jamaica [no. 36: 1668], the Antilles [no. 33: 1667/8], Barbados [no. 117: 1676]) and strange animals (e.g., the "Mexico Musk-Hog" [no. 153: 1683] and a variety of tropical birds). Concerning the use of "mistress," it is also noteworthy that Milton's Satan begins his final oratorical seduction of Eve—the one that wins her "heart"—with the appellation "sovran Mistress" (*Paradise Lost* 9.532), and that Defoe's original title for *Roxana* (1724) began with the words *The Fortunate Mistress*; the word "mistress" in that novel has many of the connotations noted here, as well as that of "mistress" to a single servant, the waiting maid Amy. "Mistress" could also connote a bawd (cp. *Othello* 4.2.89).

34. The epistle dedicatory is printed as an appendix to vol. 5 of *The Works of Aphra Behn*, ed. Montague Summers, 509–11.

35. Since the word "part" in reference to persons often had sexual overtones, Behn's identification of the "masculine Part in her" may be relevant to Laqueur's exposition (in *Making Sex*) of the "one-sex model" of sexual identity in medical discourse up into the eighteenth century. Cf. Defoe's Roxana: "I wou'd be a *Man-Woman*" (*Roxana*, 212).

36. Cf. *Paradise Lost*, 4.223–46.

37. Compare *Paradise Lost*, 4.736–47. Cf. also Claude Lévi-Strauss on nakedness and the fundamental role of the male-female couple among the Nambikwara: "Peoples who live entirely naked are not ignorant of what we call 'modesty': they simply have another frontier line. Among the Brazilian Indians . . . modesty has nothing to do with how much or how little of the body is exposed; tranquillity lies on one side of the frontier, agitation on the other" (*Tristes Tropiques*, 277–78). I have discussed the binary structure of the "island narrative" of *Robinson Crusoe* in "Starting Over with *Robinson Crusoe*," 51–73.

38. Especially relevant to Behn's *oeuvre* is the reevaluation of "Nature" as a highly complex seventeenth-century feminine construct in the recent work of Carolyn Merchant, Brian Easlea, Evelyn Fox Keller, Londa Schiebinger, Ludmilla Jordanova, and others. See also Erickson, *Mother Midnight*, xii, 14, 18, 211–16.

39. Cf. "Nature's Support, (without whose Aid / She can no Humane Being give) / It self now wants the Art to live" in the critical moment of impotence in Behn's poem "The Disappointment" (67). Cf. also Rochester's "The Imperfect Enjoyment," quoted in chap. 3, 101.

40. Cf. the "quite literal defacing of Imoinda, the lifting of her still-smiling face, as if it were a mask or portrait, off her body," in Gallagher, *Nobody's Story*, 83. This exceedingly delicate anatomical dissection recalls the even more delicate anatomical "defacing" of Eve by Satan discussed in the previous chapter; cf. Adam's silent reflection on the newly fallen Eve: "Defac't, deflow'r'd, and now to Death devote" (*Paradise Lost*, 9.901).

41. Guffey, "Aphra Behn's *Oroonoko*," 35–36; Duffy, *The Passionate Shepherdess*, 267; Brown, *Ends of Empire*, 58.

42. Cf. the complex rendering of the image of Arthegall that Britomart sees in Merlin's magic mirror and carries in her troubled dreams: "Tho gan she to renew her former smart, / And thinke of that faire visage, written in her heart" (*The Faerie Queene*, 3.2.260–61).

43. Cf. Behn's poem "To *Alexis* in Answer to His Poem Against Fruition. Ode":

Then, heedless Nymph, be rul'd by me
If e're your Swain the bliss desire;
Think like *Alexis* he may be
Whose wisht Possession damps his fire.
(273)

44. Janet Todd uses this term in her notes to the Burnet poem, *The Works of Aphra Behn*, 1:442.

45. In *The Works of Aphra Behn*, ed. Janet Todd, 1:443 n. 88. Cf. also Duffy, *The Passionate Shepherdess*, chap. 26.

46. *The Works of Aphra Behn*, ed. Janet Todd, 1:443–44. Cf. Carolyn Merchant, *The Death of Nature*, chap. 10: "The Management of Nature."

47. Cf. G. A. Starr: "In various ways, Behn tries to humanize Oroonoko without forfeiting his exoticism . . . her hero combines the best features of culture and of nature. Even more important is Oroonoko's attachment to Imoinda . . . [his] constancy is at least as important as his ardor . . . and [helps] to ally him . . . with

Behn's own voice as it emerges throughout this book" ("Aphra Behn and the Genealogy of the Man of Feeling," 367).

48. Duffy, *The Passionate Shepherdess*, 267.

Chapter 5. The Written Heart

1. Belford's allusion to Norris is found in the Everyman edition of *Clarissa; or, The History of a Young Lady*, 4:151. For convenience, all citations are from the Everyman edition, which "follows the 1751 text" of the third edition ("Editorial Note" following p. 582 of vol. 4). Citations from this edition of *Clarissa* were checked against the facsimile AMS edition for accuracy and are indicated hereafter in the text by volume and page number. There were no substantive variants in the citations between the two editions.

2. John Norris, *The Theory and Regulation of Love. A Moral Essay*, 17–20 (page numbers are cited hereafter in the text).

3. See the survey of responses in chap. 12, "The Reception of *Clarissa*: Richardson and Fielding," in T. C. Duncan Eaves and Ben D. Kimpel, *Samuel Richardson: A Biography*, 285–321. To Fielding's and Johnson's well-known appreciation of Richardson's knowledge of the human heart may be added this from the Marquis de Sade: "The example of Richardson, wrote Sade, teaches that one must explore the heart, not virtue, 'because virtue, however beautiful and necessary it may be, is still only one of the modes of this amazing heart, the profound study of which is so necessary to the novelist and which the novel, faithful mirror of the heart, must necessarily map out in all its windings'" (Jay Clayton, *Romantic Vision and the Novel*, 27; cf. also Eaves and Kimpel, 603). My ensuing comment on Richardson and the heart is based in part on his great letter to Sophia Westcomb [1746?] on "the converse of the pen . . . that makes distance, presence; and brings back to sweet remembrance all the delights of presence; which makes even presence but body, while absence becomes the soul" (*Selected Letters of Samuel Richardson*, ed. John Carroll, 64–67). Richardson's meditation on "presence" and "absence" in the epistolary process may owe something to St. Paul: "For I verily, as absent in body, but present in spirit, have judged already" (1 Cor. 5.3), and Richardson the writer's own diminutiveness may recall the words of Paul's opponents: "his letters . . . are weighty and powerful, but his bodily presence is weak, and his speech contemptible" (2 Cor. 10.10).

4. *Selected Letters*, to Hester Mulso, Aug. 15, 1755, 321.

5. Richardson was fond of referring in his correspondence to Clarissa as "my girl," and as her literary father he must have felt that after her demise he was suffering almost as much as her fictional father, whose own death from grief and remorse occurs shortly after Clarissa dies. In describing to a French acquaintance how busy he is with the third edition of the novel and with requests from a dozen ladies to give them a good man, he pauses: "But, Sir, my nervous infirmities you know—time mends them not—and Clarissa has almost killed me" (*Selected Letters*, to J. B. de Freval, Jan. 21, 1751, 174). A possible model for Clarissa is John Evelyn's daughter

Mary, who died at nineteen of smallpox. Evelyn praises her for the "extraordinary patience, and piety" with which she bore her sickness, and her "sanctified and blessed frame of mind. . . . the justness of her stature, person, comelinesse of her Countenance and gracefulnesse of motion . . . was one of the least, compar'd with the Ornaments of her mind, which was truely extraordinary. . . . Of early piety, and singularly Religious, so as spending a considerable part of every day in private devotion, Reading and other vertuous exercises, she had collected, and written out aboundance of the most usefull and judicious periods of the Books she read, in a kind of Commonplace." He mentions her command of history and the French language. "She had to all this an incomparable sweete Voice, to which she play'd a through-base on the Harpsichord. . . . She could not indure that which they call courtship, among the Gallants, abhorred flattery, and tho she had aboundance of witt, the raillery was . . . innocent and ingenuous. . . . No body living read prose, or Verse better and with more judgement, and as she read, so she writ not onely most correct orthography, but with that maturitie of judgement, and exactness of the periods, choice expressions, and familiarity of style, as that some letters of hers have astonish'd me." Then addressing her directly, he says "Thy Affection, duty and love to me was that of a friend, as well as of a Child, passing even the love of Women, the Affection of a Child." He notes that "Dr. Harvy somewhere writes, all young people should be let blood" around the age of nineteen, but Mary had an aversion to breathing a vein; all who beheld her thought she looked well, and "her extraordinary beauty was taken notice of, the last time she appeared at Church" (*The Diary of John Evelyn*, ed. John Bowle, 323–25). Cf. Anna Howe's long letter on Clarissa's accomplishments and virtues, especially "the correctness of her orthography," her grace in reading aloud, and her skill as a writer (4:494–95).

6. I have suggested in *Mother Midnight* that Clarissa's strongest feelings of affection are for women, and that her friend Anna Howe is the one love of her life (256, 128). The present commentary on Clarissa's heart suffering is meant to complement and extend my discussion of her spiritual progress, under the aspect of the metaphor of the "womb of fate," in *Mother Midnight*, 105–92. The source for Richardson's suggestive phrase "the womb of fate" (as it occurs in his preface and in the words of Clarissa's executor and literary editor, John Belford [4:81]) may be the opening lines of "The Advice" in John Norris, *A Collection of Miscellanies* (1687): "What's forming in the *Womb* of fate / Why art thou so *Concern'd* to know. Dost think 'twould be *advantage* to thy state / But *Wiser* heaven does not think it so" (33). Midway in the novel, Lovelace quotes the seventeenth-century poet Abraham Cowley's "Destinie" on the "unseen hand" that "makes all our moves" (2.397). Since Cowley's poetry figures importantly in one way or another with all four authors discussed in this book (especially Behn), and because he is a crucial link between *Mother Midnight* and this study, I wish to quote the lines describing his poetic muse following Lovelace's allusion: "Me from the *womb* the *Midwife Muse* did take: / She cut my *Navel, washt me,* and mine *Head* / With her own *Hands* she *Fashioned*; She did a *Covenant* with me make, / And *circumcis'ed* my tender *Soul.* . . . She spake, and all my years to come / Took their unlucky *Doom.* / Their several ways of *Life* let others *chuse,* / Their several pleasures let them use, / But I was born for *Love,* and for a *Muse*" (*Poems,* 193). In *Mother Midnight* I called *Clar-*

issa a "tragic prose epic" (109); although I still read the novel as a tragic representation of the womb of fate, I now think it at least equally relevant to refer to the novel as a "tragedy of the heart," or "tragic epic of the heart." (The phrase "tragedy of the heart" was used by T. McAlindon in a talk given at UCSB on *King Lear* in October, 1989.)

7. *Clarissa; or, The History of a Young Lady*, ed. Angus Ross (1985), a reprinting of the first edition (1747–48) with an excellent introduction and the first annotation of the complete text.

8. See Rosemary Bechler's discussion of Richardson and his "brethren" of the 1740s in "'Trial by What Is Contrary': Samuel Richardson and Christian Dialectic," 94–98. On Richardson's overtly religious views, see also Eaves and Kimpel, *Samuel Richardson*, 550–56.

9. In addition, for one so duty-bound as Richardson, at every stage of his life, the notion of "stealing in" suggests that which he most wishes to do. In the autobiographical letter to Stinstra he comments on how his "Thirst after Reading" led him to his arduous apprenticeship to a printer: "I stole from the Hours of Rest and Relaxation, my Reading Times for Improvement of my Mind" (*Selected Letters*, June 2, 1753, 229).

10. See Horton Davies, *Worship and Theology in England*, 1:40–56, 64–75, 255–324, 428–35; 2:117–32, 137–42, 161–84; 3:19–34, 94–113.

11. The word "trial" (which Richardson uses often in relation to Clarissa's experience) derives from the intensely physical verb *terere*, to rub, to thresh grain, the original gesture of rubbing the hands together to grind, sift, separate the wheat from the chaff. In heroic literature, the hands of the god or the Fate figure test the mettle of humankind through trial—"that which purifies us is trial, and trial is by what is contrary," in Milton's indelible phrase. Bailey, in his *Universal Etymological Dictionary*, guesses that trial is related to "tentatio," and to the notion of trial as "experiment" he adds the definition, "a temptation," recalling Satan's trial of Eve.

12. *Clarissa* has become almost the test-case text for a variety of contemporary critical approaches to the novel, of which the following citations form only a partial list. The brilliant but at times erratic poststructuralist studies of *Clarissa* (William B. Warner's *Reading "Clarissa": The Struggles of Interpretation*, Terry Castle's *Clarissa's Ciphers: Meaning and Disruption in Richardson's "Clarissa,"* and Terry Eagleton's *The Rape of Clarissa: Writing, Sexuality and Class Struggle in Samuel Richardson*) largely ignore the religious aspects of the novel while the important recent interpretations that do consider them, such as the early essay by John Dussinger (mentioned below, n.45), Cynthia Griffin Wolff's *Samuel Richardson and the Eighteenth-Century Puritan Character*, Mark Kinkead-Weekes's *Samuel Richardson: Dramatic Novelist*, Margaret Anne Doody's *A Natural Passion: A Study of the Novels of Samuel Richardson*, Jean H. Hagstrum's *Sex and Sensibility: Ideal and Erotic Love from Milton to Mozart*, chap. 8, Carol Houlihan Flynn's *Samuel Richardson: A Man of Letters*, Rita Goldberg's *Sex and Enlightenment: Women in Richardson and Diderot*, chap. 1, Linda S. Kauffman's *Discourses of Desire: Gender, Genre, and Epistolary Fictions*, chap. 4, Margaret Olofson Thickstun's *Fictions of the Feminine: Puritan Doctrine and the Representation of Women*, chap. 4, and especially Leopold Damrosch Jr.'s *God's Plot and Man's Stories: Studies in the Fic-*

tional Imagination from Milton to Fielding, chap. 6 (the best recent study of the Christian implications of *Clarissa*), do not pay enough attention to the specifically scriptural dimensions of the novel. Though Eagleton has some valuable things to say about "writing" in *Clarissa*, much poststructuralist criticism has overemphasized "reading" *Clarissa* at the expense of the powerful "writing" motif. A useful exception is Christina Marsden Gillis's finely honed exploration of "literal space" in *The Paradox of Privacy: Epistolary Form in "Clarissa."*

13. See Robert Alter (*The Art of Biblical Narrative*, 24–25) quoting Herbert Schneidau on the use and significance of the term "historicized fiction" in *Sacred Discontent*, 215.

14. Meir Sternberg, *The Poetics of Biblical Narrative*, 47.

15. William Sale, *Samuel Richardson: Master Printer*, 125.

16. "The number of hours in which he withdrew from [his business] to write, revise, and excise the text of his novels must have been extraordinary," Sale, *Master Printer*, 33.

17. For Richardson's own commentary on this phenomenon, see *Selected Letters*, 316, and Lovelace's "I love to write to the *moment*" (2:498). Cf. Eaves and Kimpel, *Samuel Richardson*, 597. On the possible connection between Richardson's practice here and its relation to biblical narrative practice, cf. Northrop Frye's comment on the word "*kairos*" ("a crucial moment in time") in the context of concrete "words of power" in *The Great Code*, 7, and Robert Alter's assertion that "biblical narrative characteristically catches its protagonists only at the critical and revealing points in their lives" (*The Art of Biblical Narrative*, 51). On the "critical moments" of birth, sex, and death in relation to eighteenth-century fiction, see Erickson, *Mother Midnight*, esp. 11, 40, 153, and 191.

18. On the relevance of "spiritual autobiographies" and "spiritual biographies" to early English fiction, especially Defoe's *Robinson Crusoe*, see the now standard studies of G. A. Starr, *Defoe and Spiritual Autobiography*, and J. Paul Hunter, *The Reluctant Pilgrim*. For a more detailed study of the subgenre itself, see Owen C. Watkins, *The Puritan Experience: Studies in Spiritual Autobiography*. There has been surprisingly little discussion of Richardson's reimagining of spiritual autobiography in *Pamela* and *Clarissa*. On the practice of copying passages from the Bible, cf. Richardson's observation to Stinstra that as a boy he "collected from ye Scripture Texts that made against" a certain backbiting widow (*Selected Letters*, 230).

19. *Puritan Sermons, 1659–1689*, 2:64, 58, 68. For a good discussion of English and American "preparationists" of the sixteenth and seventeenth centuries, see Norman Pettit, *The Heart Prepared: Grace and Conversion in Puritan Spiritual Life*, 1–21, 48–124.

20. In attempting to justify his representation of a good man some readers had found simply too good to be credible, Richardson quoted these words from Tillotson's sermon, "Of the Divine Perfections." See *The History of Sir Charles Grandison*, 3:466 and note.

21. *Puritan Sermons*, 2:284, 281. In discussing the duties of parents and children, Richard Adams points out, "we should take notice of those fair copies they have set us, and imitate whatsoever is good, commendable, and virtuous in our

parents," *Puritan Sermons*, 2:313. Cf. Damrosch's citation of Ames on parents' bearing the "image of God" in regard to their children (*God's Plot*, 234).

22. *Puritan Sermons*, 2:63, 68, 66, 70.

23. Sir Charles Grandison alludes indirectly to this passage when kindly admonishing his sister Charlotte for her unconsidered promise to Captain Anderson (*Sir Charles Grandison*, 1:408).

24. For all his gout-ridden debility, James Harlowe Sr. possesses one commanding attribute, "a terrible voice when he is angry" (1:30), a voice that will resonate in Clarissa's consciousness till the end. See Florian Stuber, "On Fathers and Authority in *Clarissa*," 560, and Damrosch's discussion of Clarissa's father "as a dreadful parody of the Augustinian God" (*God's Plot*, 234–36).

25. "Perhaps the gravest disappointment of Richardson's life was the death of four sons and one nephew by whom he hoped to see his press perpetuated.... In a desperate attempt to perpetuate the name of Samuel, [Richardson and his first wife, Martha] had named three of their infant boys after their father," Sale, *Master Printer*, 11. The fourth Samuel, by Richardson's second wife, Elizabeth, was baptized on April 26, 1739, and died less than a year later (Eaves and Kimpel, *Samuel Richardson*, 48–50).

26. The best and most comprehensive recent study is Lois A. Chaber's "'This Affecting Subject': An 'Interested' Reading of Childbearing in Two Novels by Samuel Richardson."

27. *Restoration and Eighteenth-Century Comedy*, ed. Scott McMillin, 234–35.

28. *Restoration and Eighteenth-Century Comedy*, 160.

29. *Restoration and Eighteenth-Century Comedy*, 239–40.

30. This is Dale Underwood's version, in *Etherege and the Seventeenth-Century Comedy of Manners*, 14, and it has not been substantially modified in the good recent studies by Weber and Chernaik.

31. *Aphra Behn: Five Plays*, ed. Maureen Duffy, 31.

32. *British Dramatists from Dryden to Sheridan*, ed. George H. Nettleton and Arthur E. Case, 412.

33. Terry Castle, *Clarissa's Ciphers*, 112. The tiny hands are replaced by asterisks in the Everyman edition.

34. Castle, *Clarissa's Ciphers*, 115.

35. Castle sees Mrs. Sinclair's "huge, quaggy carcase [as] ... a great summarizing image of Richardson's own problematic text," an assertion of the very real influence of Sinclair in the novel (*Clarissa's Ciphers*, 37; cf. Erickson, *Mother Midnight*, 138–47). Eagleton sees Richardson's novels "as *kits*, great unwieldy containers crammed with spare parts" (*The Rape of Clarissa*, 20). The two views are conveniently summed up in Angus Ross's sense of the "shifting quality" of the text (introduction to *Clarissa*, 16). Johnson and many other readers have been impressed with the massive "stillness" of the book. But the text is both stable and unstable, a living drama of voices within its houselike printer's frame. Cf. Gillis's discussion of Mrs. Sinclair's house (*Paradox of Privacy*, chap. 2).

36. On the nature of the "Puritan" family in relation to the Harlowes, see L. L. Schücking's still relevant *The Puritan Family: A Social Study from the Literary*

Sources, 56–95, 145–58, and Christopher Hill's "Clarissa Harlowe and Her Times," 102–23. The recent studies of the evolution of the family in the period 1500 to 1800 by Shorter and Trumbach have disappointingly little commentary on Puritan and religious elements in English family life, and even Stone's comprehensive work is not particularly illuminating for *Clarissa*.

37. The phrase "father's house" (like "father's curse") resonates throughout *Clarissa* and recalls the biblical repetition of the phrase in such passages as Deut. 22.21: "Then they shall bring out the damsel to the door of her father's house, and the men of her city shall stone her with stones that she die; because she hath wrought folly in Israel, to play the whore in her father's house. . . ."

38. *The Poetical Works of Dryden*, ed. George R. Noyes, 469, lines 375–80. With respect to mares, cf. the Galenic idiom of "let'em suck the seed with greedy force, / And close involve the vigor of the horse" (467, lines 222–23).

39. Cf. Geoffrey Keynes, *The Life of William Harvey*, 328n3.

40. *Puritan Sermons*, 2:321. In this connection, note Noah's curse on Canaan, the son of Noah's son Ham (Gen. 9.25).

41. Locke, *Essay Concerning Human Understanding*, 1:71; for clarity, I have omitted the square brackets in the text.

42. *Essay*, 1:121.

43. Cf. E. Talbot Donaldson on Griselda in *Chaucer's Poetry: An Anthology for the Modern Reader*, 920.

44. "By turning in her confusion to the written word, she [Clarissa] is clearly trying to reinstate order. In a sense, to go on writing is to go on living," H. Porter Abbott, *Diary Fiction: Writing as Action*, 92; "though raped and in one sense broken, Clarissa still writes. That is the important point. Writing sustains existence and affirms existence," Gillis, *Paradox of Privacy*, 53.

45. *Meditations Collected from the Sacred Books; And Adapted to the Different Stages of a Deep Distress*, viii. See also John A. Dussinger, "Conscience and the Pattern of Christian Perfection in *Clarissa*," 240–41, and Eaves and Kimpel, *Samuel Richardson*, 311–12. Cf. Robert A. Erickson, *Mother Midnight*, 180, 257, 282, and "'Written in the Heart': *Clarissa* and Scripture," 39–48; also, Tom Keymer, *Richardson's "Clarissa" and the Eighteenth-Century Reader*, 112, 212, 225.

46. Something similar happens to Robinson Crusoe in his spiritual ordeal on the island. The commencement of his serious reading of the Bible coincides with his three-day exploration of the interior of the "Island of Despair." Crusoe's panicked reaction to his discovery of the footprint also has interesting connections with Clarissa's immediate reaction to her realization of the rape. See Robert A. Erickson, "Starting Over With *Robinson Crusoe*," 61.

47. *Meditations*, 2. Cf. Michael Ragussis's discussion of how Clarissa's "pronominal transpositions displace the male from the center of language . . . and unname him" in *Acts of Naming: The Family Plot in Fiction*, 32–33; cf. Kauffman, *Discourses of Desire*, 155. See also John Norris, "The Third Chapter of Job Paraphrased" in *A Collection of Miscellanies* (20–22), and Richardson's friend Edward Young's "A Paraphrase on Part of the Book of Job" in *Edward Young: The Complete Works, Poetry and Prose*, ed. James Nichols, 1:245–59.

48. Preface to *Meditations*, vi. Clarissa's collecting and composing herself in this fashion brings to mind her creator's life work as an orderly "compositor," "collector" of extracts, and ultimately "composer" of fictions, and one wonders further just how much Richardson's "mystery" as master printer enters into the whole "mystery" of his particular kind of narrative creativity. See Eagleton's speculation on the ironies of the master printer (*The Rape of Clarissa*, 40–41). Robert Alter's discussion of "composite artistry" in *The Art of Biblical Narrative* (chap. 7) has interesting implications for Richardson's creative practice; Clarissa herself might be seen as engaging in a kind of *midrash*—or in Henry More's term, a "cabbala"—in the composition of her *Meditations*.

49. *Meditations*, 75–76.

50. Watson in *Puritan Sermons*, 5:464, 462; Robert South, *Sermons Preached upon Several Occasions*, 2:548 (Lovelace had supplied Clarissa's closet at Mrs. Sinclair's with copies of South's and Tillotson's sermons [2:194]). In a richly suggestive passage likening *"Mans nature to a Book, or law to itself"* in *The Resurrection of the Dead*, Bunyan discerns four books that will be opened at the last day: the Book of Creatures (the book of God's signs in nature), the Book of God's Remembrance (recording every good and every evil act ever performed), the Book of Law (the decalogue), and the Book of Life (containing the list of the names of the elect and their works, and a treatise on faith and love) (*"Christian Behavior," "The Holy City," "The Resurrection of the Dead,"* ed. J. Sears McGee, 252–85). Cf. also Warner on the relationship between the book of one's "works" and the book of the "saved" in *Reading "Clarissa,"* 71.

51. *Puritan Sermons*, 5:464–65. Cf. Starr, *Defoe and Spiritual Autobiography*, 6n. Clarissa's allegorical letter to Lovelace about embarking for her "father's house" might seem to qualify her sincerity, but see Damrosch's justification of the letter in the light of Baxter on the necessity of at times speaking "darkly" (*God's Plot*, 237). Cf. the Gospel precedent: "Jesus . . . said unto them, Destroy this temple, and in three days I will raise it up. Then said the Jews, Forty and six years was this temple in building, and wilt thou rear it up in three days? But he spake of the temple of his body" (John 2.18–21).

52. Thomas à Kempis, *The Christian's Pattern; or, A Treatise of the Imitation of Jesus Christ*, trans. George Stanhope, 104–5. When her sister Arabella asks Clarissa for her "Thomas à Kempis," Clarissa replies, "Here it is. You will find excellent things, Bella, in that little book" (1:367). One of the things Clarissa may have had in mind for her sister was the following: "We take a pleasure in being severe upon others, but cannot endure to hear of our own Faults" (27). Though Thomas seems to have a male reader in mind as the recipient of his advice, the book was expected to appeal to women readers because of its emphasis on the "feminine" (and "Christian") virtues of simplicity, sincerity, meekness, humility, modesty: "I had rather be affected with a true penitent Sorrow for Sin, than be able to resolve the most difficult Cases about it. Suppose you had all the Bible faithfully treasur'd up in your Memory, and a perfect Comprehension of all the Moral Philosophy in the World; To what purpose serves this mighty Stock of Rules, if not drawn out into Use by Charity, and seconded by Divine Grace?" (2). There were several translations of *The Imitation of Christ* in small duodecimo editions in the eighteenth century (see

Clarissa, ed. Ross, 1514), but Stanhope's translation, with its rich, dignified, periphrastic style, was the most popular and most influential, and the one that Richardson most likely had in mind.

53. Warner, *Reading "Clarissa,"* 71. Cf. Clarissa the day before her death on "the winding-up of our short story" (4:324).

54. South, *Sermons*, 2:548. Cf. Clarissa's impassioned plea to her mother, on her knees, for a last blessing *in writing*, "that I may hold it to my heart in my most trying struggles, and I shall think it a passport to Heaven" (4:84). It is not apparent that Clarissa would presume to be enumerated with the 144,000 martyr-witnesses in the first resurrection of Rev. 20.5.

55. Although she cannot "prove" that Richardson was steeped in Puritan devotional literature, Cynthia Griffin Wolff in *Samuel Richardson and the Eighteenth-Century Puritan Character*, 4–53, is certainly right in seeing Clarissa's close affinity to the writers of such works. Wolff notes that the seventeenth-century Puritan diarist represents himself in three primary roles, as self-examiner, as virtuous example, and as saint. Clarissa represents herself, and is represented by others, in all of these roles, and it is particularly interesting that "participation in the Community of the Elect in Heaven" is another way of becoming recorded in the "book of life," a connection that Wolff passes over. Cf. Gillis's pertinent comment (*The Paradox of Privacy*, 46) and Damrosch, *God's Plot*, 220.

56. If we were to take Richardson's transformation of the New Testament into fiction in its broadest sense and were to see the Gospels as four narratives of the same Christ-event (i.e., as the first "novel" [a new thing, good news] incorporating multiple points of view) and the letters of Paul as the first epistolary "novel," it could be said that *Clarissa* combines both narrative techniques to extraordinarily complicated effect in representing the Clarissa-event.

57. Cf. Bickerstaff on the gentlemen who bought Partridge's almanacs: "at every Line they read, they would lift up their Eyes and cry out, betwixt Rage and Laughter, *They were sure no Man* alive *ever writ such damned Stuff as this*," "A Vindication of Isaac Bickerstaff, Esq." in *The Writings of Jonathan Swift*, ed. Greenberg and Piper, 439.

58. *Meditations*, iii.

59. Cf. Flynn on Clarissa's "infernal forgiveness" in *Samuel Richardson: A Man of Letters*, 42–45.

60. As Richardson was composing *Clarissa*, the great age of English satire—according to traditional literary history—had come to an end with the deaths of Pope and Swift. Fielding is usually thought of as the heir to the satirical tradition. But Richardson was not immune to the influence of the Tory satirists in verse or prose, nor to the satirical *zeitgeist*. *Clarissa* in its protracted and massive social sweep is at least as powerful a condemnation of the errors of midcentury English culture as is *The Dunciad*.

Works Cited

Abbott, H. Porter. *Diary Fiction: Writing as Action*. Ithaca, N.Y.: Cornell University Press, 1984.
Alter, Robert. *The Art of Biblical Narrative*. New York: HarperCollins, 1981.
Adams, Richard. "What Are the Duties of Parents and Children, and How Are They to be Managed According to Scripture?" In *Puritan Sermons* 2:303–58.
Andrewes, Lancelot. *Sermons By the Right Honorable and Reverend Father in God, Lancelot Andrewes, Late Lord Bishop of Winchester*. London, 1629.
Aubrey, John. *Aubrey's Brief Lives*. Ed. Oliver Lawson Dick. London: Secker and Warburg, 1958.
Bailey, Nathan. *Dictionnarium Britannicum; or, A more Compleat Universal Etymological English Dictionary than Any Extant.* . . . 2d ed. London, 1736.
Bakhtin, Mikhail. *The Dialogic Imagination: Four Essays*. Ed. Michael Holquist, trans. Caryl Emerson and Michael Holquist. Austin: University of Texas Press, 1981.
Baumgartner, Paul R. "Milton and Patience." *Studies in Philology* 44 (1963): 203–13.
Bechler, Rosemary. "'Trial by What is Contrary': Samuel Richardson and Christian Dialectic." In *Samuel Richardson: Passion and Prudence*, ed. Valerie Grosvenor Myer. London: Vision, 1986.
Behn, Aphra. *Aphra Behn: Five Plays*, Introd. Maureen Duffy. London: Methuen, 1990.
———. *"Oroonoko," "The Rover" and Other Works*. Ed. Janet Todd. London: Penguin, 1992.
———. *Oroonoko: or, The Royal Slave*. Introd. Lore Metzger. New York: W. W. Norton, 1973.
———. *The Rover*. Ed. Frederick M. Link. Lincoln: University of Nebraska Press, 1967.
———. *The Rover, or The Banished Cavaliers*. Ed. Anne Russell. Peterborough: Broadview, 1994.
———. *The Works of Aphra Behn*. Ed. Montague Summers. 6 vols. London, 1915. Repr., New York: Benjamin Blom, 1967.
———. *The Works of Aphra Behn*. Ed. Janet Todd. Vols. 1–4. Athens: Ohio State University Press, 1992–93.
Boehme, Jacob. *Personal Christianity: The Doctrines of Jacob Boehme*. Ed. Franz Hartmann. New York: Frederick Ungar, n.d.
Bradshaw, Peter N. "The Idea of Anatomy in the Work of Seventeenth-Century Prose Writers." Cambridge University Ph.D. diss., 1989.

Bredbeck, Gregory. *Sodomy and Interpretation*. Ithaca, N.Y.: Cornell University Press, 1991.
British Dramatists from Dryden to Sheridan. Ed. George H. Nettleton and Arthur E. Case. Boston: Houghton Mifflin, 1939.
Brown, Laura. *Ends of Empire: Women and Ideology in Early Eighteenth-Century English Literature*. Ithaca, N.Y.: Cornell University Press, 1993.
Brownley, Martine Watson. "The Narrator in *Oroonoko*." *Essays in Literature* 4 (1977): 174–81.
Bunyan, John. *"Christian Behavior," "The Holy City," "The Resurrection of the Dead."* Ed. J. Sears McGee. Oxford: Clarendon, 1987.
———. *Grace Abounding to the Chief of Sinners*. Ed. W. R. Owens. New York: Penguin, 1987.
———. *The Pilgrim's Progress*. Ed. Roger Sharrock. New York: Penguin, rev. ed., 1987.
Bunzel, B., B. Schmidi-Mohl, A. Grundböck, G. Wollenek. "Does Changing the Heart Mean Changing Personality? A Retrospective Inquiry on 47 Heart Transplant Patients." *Quality of Life Research* 1 (1992): 251–56.
Burton, Robert. *The Anatomy of Melancholy*. Ed. Holbrook Jackson. 3 vols. London: J. M. Dent, 1932.
Castle, Terry. *Clarissa's Ciphers: Meaning and Disruption in Richardson's "Clarissa."* Ithaca, N.Y.: Cornell University Press, 1982.
Cervantes, Miguel. *The Historie of Don Quixote of the Mancha*. Trans. Thomas Shelton. 1612. Repr., New York: AMS Press, 1967.
Chaber, Lois A. "'This Affecting Subject': An 'Interested' Reading of Childbearing in Two Novels by Samuel Richardson." *Eighteenth-Century Fiction* 8 (1996): 193–250.
Charleton, Walter. *Natural History of the Passions*. London, 1674.
———. *Three Anatomic Lectures, Concerning 1. The Motion of the Blood through the Veins and Arteries; 2. The Organic Structure of the Heart; 3. The Efficient Causes of the Pulsation*. London, 1683.
Charnock, Stephen. *The Complete Works of Stephen Charnock, B. D. (1681–82)*. 5 vols. Edinburgh, 1864.
———. "The Sinfulness and Cure of Thoughts." In *Puritan Sermons* 2: 386–420.
Chaucer, Geoffrey. *Chaucer's Poetry: An Anthology for the Modern Reader*. Ed. E. Talbot Donaldson. New York: Ronald, 1958.
Chernaik, Warren. *Sexual Freedom in Restoration Literature*. Cambridge: Cambridge University Press, 1995.
Chibka, Robert L. "'Oh! Do Not Fear a Woman's Invention': Truth, Falsehood, and Fiction in Aphra Behn's *Oroonoko*." *TSLL* 30 (1988): 510–37.
Cibber, Colley. *The Careless Husband*. In *British Dramatists from Dryden to Sheridan*.
Clayton, Jay. *Romantic Vision and the Novel*. Cambridge: Cambridge University Press, 1987.
Cleland, John. *Fanny Hill, or Memoirs of a Woman of Pleasure*. Ed. Peter Wagner. Harmondsworth: Penguin, 1985.

Cohen, I. "The Heart in Biblical Psychology." In *Essays Presented to Israel Brodie*, ed. H. J. Zimmels, J. Rabbinnowitz, and I. Finestein. London: Soncino, 1967.

Congreve, William. *The Way of the World*. In *Restoration and Eighteenth-Century Comedy*.

Cowley, Abraham. *Poems*. Ed. A. R. Waller. Cambridge: Cambridge University Press, 1905.

———. *Selected Poetry and Prose*. Ed. James G. Taaffe, New York: Meredith, 1970.

Crooke, Helkiah. *Mikrokosmographia: A Description of the Body of Man, Collected and Translated out of All the Best Authors of Antiquity*. London, 1615.

Damrosch, Leopold, Jr. *God's Plot and Man's Stories: Studies in the Fictional Imagination from Milton to Fielding*. Chicago: University of Chicago Press, 1985.

Davies, Horton. *Worship and Theology in England*. 5 vols. Princeton, N.J.: Princeton University Press, 1961–1975.

Day, Robert Adams. "Aphra Behn and the Works of the Intellect." In *Fetter'd or Free: British Women Novelists, 1670–1815*, ed. Mary Anne Schofield and Cecilia Macheski. Athens: Ohio University Press, 1989.

Defoe, Daniel. *Roxana*. Ed. David Blewett. New York: Penguin, 1982.

Derrida, Jacques. *Writing and Difference*. Chicago: University of Chicago Press, 1978.

Doody, Margaret Anne. *A Natural Passion: A Study of the Novels of Samuel Richardson*. Oxford: Clarendon, 1974.

Dryden, John. *The Poetical Works of Dryden*. Ed. George R. Noyes. Boston: Houghton Mifflin, 2d ed., 1950.

Duffy, Maureen. *The Passionate Shepherdess: Aphra Behn, 1640–89*. London: Jonathan Cape, 1979.

Duncan, Joseph E. *Milton's Earthly Paradise: A Historical Study of Eden*. Minneapolis: University of Minnesota Press, 1972.

Dussinger, John A. "Conscience and the Pattern of Christian Perfection in *Clarissa*." PMLA 81 (1966): 236–45.

Eagleton, Terry. *The Rape of Clarissa: Writing, Sexuality and Class Struggle in Samuel Richardson*. Oxford: Blackwell, 1982.

Easlea, Brian. *Science and Sexual Repression: Patriarchy's Confrontation with Woman and Nature*. London: Weidenfeld and Nicolson, 1981.

———. *Witchhunting, Magic and the New Philosophy*. Brighton: Harvester Press, 1980.

Eaves, T. C. Duncan, and Ben D. Kimpel. *Samuel Richardson: A Biography*. Oxford: Clarendon, 1971.

Empson, William. *Milton's God*. London: Chatto and Windus, rev. ed., 1965.

Erickson, Robert A. "'The Books of Generation': Some Observations on the Style of the English Midwife Books, 1671–1764." In *Sexuality in Eighteenth-Century Britain*, ed. Paul-Gabriel Boucé, 74–94. Manchester: Manchester University Press, 1982.

———. "Lady Fulbank and the Poet's Dream in Behn's *The Lucky Chance*." In *Broken Boundaries: Women and Feminism in Restoration Drama*, ed. Katherine Quinsey. Lexington: University of Kentucky Press, 1996.

———. *Mother Midnight: Birth, Sex, and Fate in Eighteenth-Century Fiction (Defoe, Richardson, and Sterne)*. New York: AMS Press, 1986.

———. Review of Thomas Laqueur, *Making Sex: Body and Gender from the Greeks to Freud*. *Eighteenth-Century Fiction* 4 (1992): 270–71.

———. "Situations of Identity in the *Memoirs of Martinus Scriblerus*." *Modern Language Quarterly* 26 (1965): 388–400.

———. "Starting Over with *Robinson Crusoe*." In *Daniel Defoe: The Making of His Prose Fiction*, ed. Malinda Snow, *Studies in the Literary Imagination* 15 (1982): 51–73.

———. "'Written in the Heart': *Clarissa* and Scripture." *Eighteenth-Century Fiction* 2 (1989): 17–54.

Etherege, George. *The Man of Mode or, Sir Fopling Flutter*. In *Restoration and Eighteenth-Century Comedy*.

Evelyn, John. *The Diary of John Evelyn*. Ed. John Bowle. Oxford University Press, 1985.

Fletcher, Harris Francis. *The Intellectual Development of John Milton*. 2 vols. Urbana: University of Illinois Press, 1961.

Flynn, Carol Houlihan. *Samuel Richardson: A Man of Letters*. Princeton, N.J.: Princeton University Press, 1982.

Foucault, Michel. *The Order of Things: An Archaeology of the Human Sciences*. New York: Random House, 1970.

Frank, Robert G., Jr. *Harvey and the Oxford Physiologists: Scientific Ideas and Social Interaction*. Berkeley: University of California Press, 1980.

Freedman, R. David. "Woman, A Power Equal to Man." *Biblical Archaeology Review* 9 (1983): 56–58.

French, Roger. *William Harvey's Natural Philosophy*. Cambridge: Cambridge University Press, 1994.

Frye, Northrop. *The Great Code: The Bible and Literature*. New York: Harcourt Brace Jovanovich, 1982.

Fumerton, Patricia K. *Cultural Aesthetics: Renaissance Literature and the Practice of Social Ornament*. Chicago: University of Chicago Press, 1991.

Galen, *On the Doctrines of Hippocrates and Plato*. Trans. Phillip de Lacy. Berlin: Akademie-Verlag, 1984.

———. *On the Natural Faculties*. Trans. Arthur H. Brock. Cambridge, Mass.: Harvard University Press, 1916.

———. *On Semen*. Trans. Phillip de Lacy. Berlin: Akademie-Verlag, 1992.

———. *On the Usefulness of the Parts of the Body*. Trans. Margaret Tallmadge May. 2 vols. Ithaca, N.Y.: Cornell University Press, 1968.

Galen on Bloodletting: A Study of the Origins, Development and Validity of his Opinions, with a Translation of the Three Works. Trans. Peter Brain. Cambridge: Cambridge University Press, 1986.

Galen on Respiration and the Arteries. Trans. David J. Furley and J. S. Wilkie. Princeton, N.J.: Princeton University Press, 1984.

Gallagher, Catherine. *Nobody's Story: The Vanishing Acts of Women Writers in the Marketplace, 1670–1820*. Berkeley: University of California Press, 1994.

Gallagher, Philip J. *Milton, the Bible, and Misogyny.* Ed. Eugene R. Cunnar and Gail L. Mortimer. Columbia: University of Missouri Press, 1990.
[Geminus/Udall]. *Compendiosa totius Anatomie delineatio, and re exarata: per Thomam Geminum.* . . . [Trans. Nicholas Udall.] London, 1553.
Gillis, Christina Marsden. *The Paradox of Privacy: Epistolary Form in Clarissa.* Gainesville: University of Florida Press, 1984.
Goldberg, Rita. *Sex and Enlightenment: Women in Richardson and Diderot.* Cambridge: Cambridge University Press, 1984.
Golinski, Jan V. "Robert Boyle: Scepticism and Authority in Seventeenth-Century Chemical Discourse." In *The Figural and the Literal: Problems of Language in the History of Science and Philosophy, 1630–1800*, ed. Andrew E. Benjamin, Geoffrey N. Cantor, and John R. R. Christie. Manchester: Manchester University Press, 1987.
Goreau, Angeline. *Reconstructing Aphra: A Social Biography of Aphra Behn.* New York: Dial, 1980.
Graham, Peter. "Harvey's *De Motu Cordis*: The Rhetoric of Science and Science of Rhetoric." *Journal of the History of Medicine* 33 (1978): 469–76.
Guffey, George. "Aphra Behn's *Oroonoko*: Occasion and Accomplishment." In George Guffey and Andrew Wright, *Two English Novelists: Aphra Behn and Anthony Trollope.* Los Angeles: William Andrews Clark Memorial Library, 1975.
Hagstrum, Jean H. *Sex and Sensibility: Ideal and Erotic Love from Milton to Mozart.* Chicago: University of Chicago Press, 1980.
Halkett, John. *Milton and the Idea of Matrimony.* New Haven, Conn.: Yale University Press, 1970.
Harris, C. R. S. *The Heart and the Vascular System in Ancient Greek Medicine.* Oxford: Clarendon, 1973.
Harris, William O. "Despair and 'Patience as the Truest Fortitude' in *Samson Agonistes*." *ELH* 30 (1963): 107–20.
Harvey, Christopher. *Schola Cordis, or The Heart of it Selfe gone away from God; brought back againe to him & instructed by him. in 47 Emblems.* London, 1647.
Harvey, E. Ruth. *The Inward Wits: Psychological Theory in the Middle Ages and the Renaissance.* London: Warburg Institute, 1975.
Harvey, William. *The Anatomical Exercises of Dr. William Harvey: "De Motu Cordis," 1628; "De Circulatione Sanguinis," 1649. The First English Text of 1653 Now Newly Edited by Geoffrey Keynes.* London: Nonesuch, 1928.
———. *Exercitatio anatomica de motu cordis et sanguinis in animalibus.* Frankfurt, 1628.
———. *Exercitationes de generatione animalium.* London, 1651. (*Anatomical Exercitations, Concerning the Generation of Living Creatures: To which are added Particular Discourses, of Births, and of Conceptions, &c.* London, 1653.)
———. *The Works of William Harvey, M.D.* Trans. Robert Willis. 1847. Repr., New York: Johnson Reprint, 1965.
Hill, Christopher. "Clarissa Harlowe and Her Times." *Essays in Criticism* 5 (1955): 315–40.

———. *Milton and the English Revolution*. London: Faber and Faber, 1977.
Hippocratic Writings. Ed. G. E. R. Lloyd. New York: Penguin, 1978.
Hobbes, Thomas. *Leviathan*. London: J. M. Dent, 1914.
Hodges, Devon. *Renaissance Fictions of Anatomy*. Amherst: University of Massachusetts Press, 1985.
Houston, Beverle. "Usurpation and Dismemberment: Oedipal Tyranny in *Oroonoko*." *Literature and Psychology* 32 (1985): 30–36.
Hunter, J. Paul. *Before Novels: The Cultural Contexts of Eighteenth-Century English Fiction*. New York: Norton, 1990.
———. *The Reluctant Pilgrim: Defoe's Emblematic Method and Quest for Form in "Robinson Crusoe."* Baltimore: Johns Hopkins University Press, 1966.
Hunter, William B. "Eve's Demonic Dream." *ELH* 13 (1946): 255–65.
The Intellectual Revolution of the Seventeenth Century. Ed. Charles Webster. London: Routledge and Kegan Paul, 1974.
Johnson, Samuel. *A Dictionary of the English Language*. London, 1755.
Jordanova, Ludmilla. *Sexual Visions: Images of Gender in Science and Medicine between the Eighteenth and Twentieth Centuries*. New York: Harvester Wheatsheaf, 1989.
Jucovy, Peter. "Circle and Circulation: The Language and Imagery of William Harvey's Discovery." *Perspectives in Biology and Medicine* 20 (1976): 92–107.
Kauffman, Linda S. *Discourses of Desire: Gender, Genre, and Epistolary Fictions*. Ithaca, N.Y.: Cornell University Press, 1986.
Keller, Evelyn Fox. *Reflections on Gender and Science*. New Haven, Conn.: Yale University Press, 1985.
Kempis, Thomas à. *The Christian's Pattern; or A Treatise of the Imitation of Jesus Christ.* . . . Trans. George Stanhope. 11th ed. London, 1727.
Kerrigan, William. *The Prophetic Milton*. Charlottesville: University Press of Virginia, 1974.
———. *The Sacred Complex: On the Psychogenesis of "Paradise Lost."* Cambridge, Mass.: Harvard University Press, 1983.
Keuls, Eva C. *The Reign of the Phallus: Sexual Politics in Ancient Athens*. New York: Harper and Row, 1985.
Keymer, Tom. *Richardson's "Clarissa" and the Eighteenth-Century Reader*. Cambridge: Cambridge University Press, 1992.
Keynes, Geoffrey. *The Life of William Harvey*. Oxford: Clarendon, 1966.
Kinkead-Weekes, Mark. *Samuel Richardson: Dramatic Novelist*. Ithaca, N.Y.: Cornell University Press, 1973.
Kroll, Richard W. F. *The Material Word: Literate Culture in the Restoration and Early Eighteenth Century*. Baltimore: Johns Hopkins University Press, 1991.
Laqueur, Thomas. *Making Sex: Body and Gender from the Greeks to Freud*. Cambridge, Mass.: Harvard University Press, 1990.
Leonard, John. *Naming in Paradise: Milton and the Language of Adam and Eve*. Oxford: Clarendon, 1990.
Lévi-Strauss, Claude. *Tristes Tropiques*. Trans. John Russell. New York: Atheneum, 1972.

Lewalski, Barbara K. *"Paradise Lost" and the Rhetoric of Literary Forms*. Princeton, N.J.: Princeton University Press, 1985.

Lewis, C. S. *A Preface to "Paradise Lost."* New York: Oxford University Press, 1961.

Lieb, Michael. *Milton and the Culture of Violence*. Ithaca, N.Y.: Cornell University Press, 1994.

Locke, John. *An Essay Concerning Human Understanding*. Ed. Alexander Campbell Fraser. [1894.] 2 vols. New York: Dover, 1959.

Lucretius. *De rerum natura (On the Nature of Things)*. Trans. W. H. D. Rouse. Cambridge, Mass.: Harvard University Press, 1937.

———. *On the Nature of the Universe*. Trans. R. E. Latham. London: Penguin, 1994.

———. *Lucretius His Six Books of Epicurean Philosophy....* Trans. Thomas Creech. London, 1700.

Mack, Phyllis. *Visionary Women: Ecstatic Prophecy in Seventeenth-Century England*. Berkeley: University of California Press, 1992.

Martensen, Robert L. "Alienation and the Production of Strangers: Western Medical Epistemology and the Architectonics of the Body. An Historical Perspective." *Culture, Medicine and Psychiatry* 19 (1995): 141–82.

McColley, Diane Kelsey. *A Gust for Paradise: Milton's Eden and the Visual Arts*. Urbana: University of Illinois Press, 1993.

———. *Milton's Eve*. Urbana: University of Illinois Press, 1983.

McKeon, Michael. *The Origins of the English Novel, 1600–1740*. Baltimore: Johns Hopkins University Press, 1987.

McMath, James. *The Expert Mid-wife*. London, 1694.

The Medieval Reader. Ed. Norman F. Cantor. New York: HarperCollins, 1994.

Mendelson, Everett. *Heat and Life: The Development of the Theory of Animal Heat*. Cambridge, Mass.: Harvard University Press, 1964.

Merchant, Carolyn. *The Death of Nature: Women, Ecology, and the Scientific Revolution*. New York: Harper and Row, 1980.

Milton, John. *The Complete Prose Works of John Milton*. 8 vols. Ed. Don M. Wolfe. New Haven: Yale University Press, 1953–82.

———. *John Milton: Complete Poems and Major Prose*. Ed. Merritt Y. Hughes. New York: Odyssey Press, 1957.

———. *The Poems of John Milton*. Ed. John Carey and Alastair Fowler. London: Longman, 1968.

Nicolson, Marjorie Hope. *The Breaking of the Circle: Studies in the Effect of the "New Science" upon Seventeenth-Century Poetry*. Evanston, Ill.: Northwestern University Press, 1950.

Norris, John. *A Collection of Miscellanies*. 1687. Repr., New York: Garland, 1978.

———. *The Theory and Regulation of Love. A Moral Essay. In Two Parts. To Which Are Added Letters Philosophical and Moral between the Author and Dr Henry More*. London, 1688.

Nussbaum, Martha. *The Therapy of Desire: Theory and Practice in Hellenistic Ethics*. Princeton, N.J.: Princeton University Press, 1994.

Onians, Richard Brixton. *The Origins of European Thought About the Body, the*

Mind, the Soul, the World, Time and Fate. Cambridge: Cambridge University Press, 1951.

Otway, Thomas. *Venice Preserved.* In *British Dramatists from Dryden to Sheridan.*

Ovid. *Metamorphoses.* Trans. Frank Justus Miller. 2 vols. Cambridge, Mass.: Harvard University Press, 1921.

Pagel, Walter. *New Light on William Harvey.* Basel and New York: S. Karger, 1976.

———. *William Harvey's Biological Ideas: Selected Aspects and Historical Background.* Basel and New York: S. Karger, 1967.

Paster, Gail Kern. *The Body Embarrassed: Drama and the Disciplines of Shame in Early Modern England.* Ithaca, N.Y.: Cornell University Press, 1993.

Jacqueline Pearson. "Gender and Narrative in the Fiction of Aphra Behn." *RES* 5 (1991): 40–56 and 5 (1991): 179–90.

———. *The Prostituted Muse: Images of Women and Women Dramatists, 1642–1737.* New York: St. Martin's Press, 1988.

Pettit, Norman. *The Heart Prepared: Grace and Conversion in Puritan Spiritual Life.* New Haven: Yale University Press, 1966.

Philosophical Transactions: Giving Some Accompt of the Present Undertakings, Studies, and Labours of the Ingenious in Many Considerable Parts of the World. London, 1666–87.

Pico della Mirandola, Giovanni. *Oration of the Dignity of Man.* In *The Renaissance Philosophy of Man,* ed. Ernst Cassirer, Paul Oskar Kristeller, and John Herman Randall, Jr. Chicago: University of Chicago Press, 1948.

Plato. *The Collected Dialogues of Plato.* Ed. Edith Hamilton and Huntington Cairns. New York: Pantheon, 1961.

Poulet, Georges. *Studies in Human Time.* Trans. Elliott Coleman. New York: Harper and Brothers, 1956.

Puritan Sermons, 1659–1689. Ed. James Nichols. 1844. 5 vols. Repr., Richard Owen Roberts, Wheaton, Ill., 1981.

Ragussis, Michael. *Acts of Naming: The Family Plot in Fiction.* New York: Oxford University Press, 1986.

Restoration and Eighteenth-Century Comedy. Ed. Scott McMillin. New York: W. W. Norton, 1973.

Richardson, Robert G. *The Surgeon's Heart: A History of Cardiac Surgery.* London: Heinemann, 1969.

Richardson, Samuel. *Clarissa; or, The History of a Young Lady.* Everyman Library. 4 vols. London: Dent, 1967.

———. *Clarissa; or, The History of a Young Lady.* Ed. Angus Ross. Harmondsworth: Penguin, 1985.

———. *Clarissa; or, The History of a Young Lady.* 8 vols. New York: AMS Press, 1990.

———. *The History of Sir Charles Grandison.* Ed. Jocelyn Harris. London: Oxford University Press, 1972.

———. *Meditations Collected from the Sacred Books; And Adapted to the Different Stages of a Deep Distress; Gloriously surmounted by Patience, Piety, and Resignation. Being those mentioned in the History of Clarissa as drawn up by her for her own use. . . .* 1750. Repr., London: Garland, 1976.

———. *Selected Letters of Samuel Richardson*. Ed. John Carroll. Oxford: Clarendon Press, 1964.
Rogers, Katharine M. "Fact and Fiction in Aphra Behn's *Oroonoko*." *Studies in the Novel*, 20 (1988): 1–15.
Sale, William. *Samuel Richardson: Master Printer*. Ithaca, N.Y.: Cornell University Press, 1950.
Samuel Richardson: A Collection of Critical Essays. Ed. John Carroll. Englewood Cliffs, N.J.: Prentice-Hall, 1969.
Sawday, Jonathan. *The Body Emblazoned: Dissection and the Human Body in Renaissance Culture*. London: Routledge, 1995.
Scarry, Elaine. *The Body in Pain: The Making and Unmaking of the World*. New York: Oxford University Press, 1985.
Schiebinger, Londa. *The Mind Has No Sex? Women in the Origins of Modern Science*. Cambridge, Mass.: Harvard University Press, 1989.
Schneidau, Herbert. *Sacred Discontent: The Bible and Western Tradition*. Berkeley: University of California Press, 1976.
Schücking, L. L. *The Puritan Family: A Social Study from the Literary Sources*. 1929. Repr., New York: Schocken Books, 1970.
Sibbes, Richard. *Works of Richard Sibbes*. Ed. Alexander B. Grosart. 7 vols. London, 1862–64.
Singer, Charles. *A Short History of Anatomy from the Greeks to Harvey*. 2d. ed. New York: Dover, 1957.
South, Robert. *Sermons Preached upon Several Occasions*. London, 1845.
Spengemann, William C. "The Earliest American Novel: Aphra Behn's *Oroonoko*." *Nineteenth-Century Fiction* 38 (1984): 384–414.
Starr, G. A. "Aphra Behn and the Genealogy of the Man of Feeling." *Modern Philology* 87 (1990): 362–72.
———. *Defoe and Spiritual Autobiography*. Princeton, N.J.: Princeton University Press, 1965.
Steadman, John M. "Eve's Dream and the Conventions of Witchcraft." *Journal of the History of Ideas* 26 (1965): 567–74.
Steele, Richard. "What Are the Duties of Husbands and Wives Towards Each Other?" In *Puritan Sermons* 2:272–303.
Steele, Sir Richard. *The Conscious Lovers*. In *Restoration and Eighteenth-Century Comedy*.
Sternberg, Meir. *The Poetics of Biblical Narrative: Ideological Literature and the Drama of Reading*. Bloomington: Indiana University Press, 1985.
Sterne, Laurence. *Tristram Shandy*. Ed. James A. Work. New York: Odyssey, 1940.
Stuber, Florian. "On Fathers and Authority in *Clarissa*." *Studies in English Literature* 25 (1985): 557–74.
Svendsen, Kester. *Milton and Science*. Cambridge, Mass.: Harvard University Press, 1956.
Swift, Jonathan. *The Writings of Jonathan Swift*. Ed. Robert A. Greenberg and William B. Piper. New York: Norton Critical Edition, 1973.
Temkin, Owsei. *Galenism: Rise and Decline of a Medical Philosophy*. Ithaca, N.Y.: Cornell University Press, 1973.

Terence. *Terence's Comedies: Made English. With His Life: and Some Remarks at the End. By Several Hands.* London, 1694.
Thickstun, Margaret Olofson. *Fictions of the Feminine: Puritan Doctrine and the Representation of Women.* Ithaca, N.Y.: Cornell University Press, 1988.
Trumbach, Randolph. *The Rise of the Egalitarian Family: Aristocratic Kinship and Domestic Relations in Eighteenth-Century England.* New York: Academic Press, 1978.
———. "Sodomitical Subcultures, Sodomitical Roles, and the Gender Revolution of the Eighteenth Century: The Recent Historiography." In *'Tis Nature's Fault: Unauthorized Sexuality during the Enlightenment*, ed. Robert Purks Maccubbin. Cambridge: Cambridge University Press, 1987.
Turner, James Grantham. *One Flesh: Paradisal Marriage and Sexual Relations in the Age of Milton.* Oxford: Clarendon, 1987.
Underwood, Dale. *Etherege and the Seventeenth-Century Comedy of Manners.* New Haven, Conn.: Yale University Press, 1957.
Van den Berg, Sara. "Eve, Sin, and Witchcraft in *Paradise Lost.*" *Modern Language Quarterly* 47 (1986): 347–65.
Venette, Nicholas. *Conjugal Love Reveal'd; In the Nightly Pleasures of the Marriage Bed, and the Advantages of that Happy State. In an Essay Concerning Humane Generation. Done from the French of Monsieur Venette By a Physician.* 7th ed. London, n.d. [c. 1700]
———. *The Pleasures of Conjugal Love Explain'd in an Essay concerning Human Generation.* London, n.d. [c. 1730].
Veslingus, Johann. *The Anatomy of the Body of Man: Wherein is exactly described every Part thereof, in the same Manner as it is Commonly shewed in Publick Anatomies....* London, 1653.
Vicary, Thomas. *The Englishmans Treasvre . . . With the true Anatomye of Mans body....* London, 1586.
Vickers, Ilse. "The Influence of the New Sciences on Defoe." *Literature and History* 13 (1990): 200–218.
Warner, William B. *Reading Clarissa: The Struggles of Interpretation.* New Haven, Conn.: Yale University Press, 1979.
Watkins, Owen C. *The Puritan Experience: Studies in Spiritual Autobiography.* New York: Schocken Books, 1972.
Watson, Thomas. *Gods Anatomy upon Mans Heart....* London, 1649.
———. *Heaven Taken by Storm; or, The Holy Violence a Christian is to Put Forth in the Pursuit after Glory....* London, 1669.
———. "How We May Read the Scriptures with Most Spiritual Profit." In *Puritan Sermons*, 2:57–71.
———. "The Day of Judgment Asserted." In *Puritan Sermons*, 5: 459–70.
Weber, Harold. *The Restoration Rake-Hero: Transformations in Sexual Understanding in Seventeenth-Century England.* Madison: University of Wisconsin Press, 1986.
Whitteridge, Gweneth. *William Harvey and the Circulation of the Blood.* New York: American Elsevier, 1971.

William Harvey and His Age: The Professional and Social Context of the Discovery of the Circulation. Ed. Jerome J. Bylebyl. Baltimore: Johns Hopkins University Press, 1979.
Willis, Thomas. *De anima brutorum quae hominis vitalis ac sensitiva est, exercitationes duae: prior physiologica*. London, 1672. (*Two Discourses Concerning the Soul of Brutes*. London, 1683.)
Willius, Frederick A., and Thomas J. Dry. *A History of the Heart and the Circulation*. Philadelphia: Saunders, 1948.
Wilmot, John, Earl of Rochester. *The Complete Works*. Ed. Frank H. Ellis. London: Penguin, 1994.
———. *The Poems of John Wilmot, Earl of Rochester*. Ed. Keith Walker. Oxford: Blackwell, 1984.
Wilson, Luke O. "William Harvey's *Prelectiones*: The Performance of the Body in the Renaissance Theater of Anatomy." *Representations* 17 (1987): 62–95.
Wither, George. *A Collection of Emblems, 1635*. Ed. John Horden. London: Scolar Press, 1968.
Wittreich, Joseph. *Feminist Milton*. Ithaca, N.Y.: Cornell University Press, 1987.
Wolff, Cynthia Griffin. *Samuel Richardson and the Eighteenth-Century Puritan Character*. Hamden, Conn.: Archon Books, 1972.
Wollstonecraft, Mary. *A Vindication of the Rights of Woman*. Ed. Carol H. Poston, 2d ed. New York: W. W. Norton, 1988.
Wycherley, William. *The Country Wife*. In *Restoration and Eighteenth-Century Comedy*.
Young, Edward. *Edward Young: The Complete Works Poetry and Prose*. Ed. James Nichols. 1854. 2 vols. Repr., Hildesheim: Georg Olms, 1968.

Index

Abel, 30–31
Adam, xviii, 166; in Bible, 29–30, 35, 70, 182. *See also* Milton, *Paradise Lost*
Adams, Richard, 213
Addison, Joseph, 198
Adelphi (Terence), 74
Aeneid (Virgil), 182
Alter, Robert, 26, 192
Anastomosis, 76
Anatomical theater, in Padua, 66
Anatomists, 77–78, 158
Anatomy and anatomical discourse, xi, xv, xvii–xviii, 40, 64–74; early modern, 70, 89–90, 101–2, 103–5, 119, 125, 193, 216. *See also* Harvey, William; Crooke, Helkiah
Andrews, Lancelot, 98
Anglicans, 38, 52, 67, 82, 98, 189–92, 195–96, 211
Animal spirits. *See* Spirits
Apollo, 178
Arbuthnot, John, xiv, 192
Árgent, John, 66–67, 72, 74, 79
Aristotle, xv, 70, 112; on heart and blood flow, 2–5, 11, 16, 23, 77, 112, 186, 199–200; *Physics*, 19–20
Astraea, 152, 157
Atomism, 19
Aubrey, John, 68, 73, 79
Augustine, 63, 113, 185

Bacon, Francis, 19, 68
Bailey, Nathan, 18, 162
Bakhtin, Mikhail, xiv, 84–85
Banister, John, 172
Barry, Elizabeth, 139
Behn, Aphra, xvi, xvii, xviii, 3, 19, 85–86, 91, 122, 136, 190, 200–201; and the gendered heart, 15, 147–85, 193, 197, 198, 200–201, 207 *passim*; as woman writer, 161–62; as androgyne, 151–53; as prophet, 152–53, 172–79; as "Great Mistress," 164–65, 169; self-inscription as poet, 175, 182; Works: *The Lucky Chance*, xvii, 147, 161–62, 201; *Oroonoko*, xi, xvii, 151, 153–54, 161, 162–72, 174, 176, 179, 183–84, 191, 216; heart rhetoric in, 151–84; narrative structure of, 168–69; narrator of, 163–64; *The Rover*, xvii, 155–61, 200, 207; *The Rover, Part 2*, 158; *The Fair Jilt*, 158; *Love Letters to a Gentleman*, 156–57; *Poems on Several Occasions*, 151; "Congratulatory Poem . . . on the Happy Birth of the Prince of Wales," 175–76; "Congratulatory Poem to Her Sacred Majesty Queen Mary," 175–76; "Congratulatory Poem to Her Most Sacred Majesty," 175; "Coronation" poem 1685, 174–75; "The Golden Age," 166; "The Juniper Tree," 178; "Lycidus," 152, 198; "On Desire," 157–58; "A Pastoral Pindarick . . . ," 159; "A Pindaric Poem to the Reverend Doctor Burnett," 176–77; "A Pindarick on the Death of Our Late Sovereign," 172; "Poem Humbly Dedicated to . . . Catherin Queen Dowager," 172–73; "Selinda and Chloris," 89; "To Lysander at the Musick Meeting," 147, 156, 180
Bible, xv, xviii, xix, 7, 16, 20, 211; and the gendered heart, 31–35, 37, 40–44, 52–60, 200; hardness of heart in, 40; circumcision of heart in, xv, 37, 51–52, 55; ambivalence of heart in, 28; evil of heart in, 27, 36; testing/searching motif of heart in, 50, 54; and women readers, 38–39, 52, 118; and writing motif in, 37–41, 47–48, 52–53; Authorized Version of, xi, 25–27, 33, 63, 86, 92; blessing motif in, 30, 38, 57, 208, 226; cursing motif in, 32–33, 36, 38, 210, 213; covenant in, 53–54; Wisdom books, 192, 223; Apoc-

Bible (*continued*)
   rypha: Ecclesiasticus, 192, 197, 210, 218, 223; Gospels, xvi, 17, 35, 47–48, 55, 67, 167, 224; Books of: Genesis, 27, 30, 135, 192, 206; Leviticus, 31; Numbers, 196; Deuteronomy, 29, 36; Joshua, 41, 173; Esther, 39; Job, 96, 141, 168, 218, 223, 216, 226; Psalms, xv, 45–51; Song of Solomon, 120, 154; Isaiah, 38–39, 47; Jeremiah, xii, xv, 19, 25, 39, 49, 51–55, 191, 206–7, 215, 225–28; Ezekiel, 39, 47, 53–54, 226–27; Daniel, 58; Matthew, 58; Luke, 34, 89, 165; John, 89, 142, 166; 1 & 2 Corinthians, 55, 89, 191; Galatians, 17, 55; Ephesians, 15–16; Philippians, 52; James, 175; 1 & 2 Peter, 15, 55, 165; Revelation, 47–48, 115, 192, 226. *See also* individual names, e.g. Moses
Birth studies, xiv
Blake, William, 191
Blazon, 110
Blood, xv, 4, 26; in Bible, 31; blood flow (Galenic), 5–8; circulation of, 8–10, 14, 63, 66–67, 69–70, 95, 100; pulmonary, 79; systemic, 79
Bloodletting, 7, 18
"Blossom, The" (Donne), 11
Bloody Assizes, 182
Body, xiii, xvi, 1, 7; Galenic/humoral model of, 7, 10, 14, 18, 22, 154; Harveian model of, 10; Hobbesian model of, 23–24; male biblical representations of, 35–39; female biblical representations of, 28–35; official members of, 12. *See also* Anatomy; Gender; Heart
Boehme, Jacob, 139
"Book of life," biblical trope of, xv, xix, 16, 44–50, 188, 228
Bowels, 1
Brain, 4, 12, 18, 20
Breasts, 12, 30
Bruno, Giordano, 73–74
Buchanan, George, 178
Bunyan, John, 15, 17–18, 44, 207
Burnet, Gilbert, 176
Burney, Francis, 87
Burton, Robert (*Anatomy of Melancholy*), 64; on the heart, 75
Byam, William, 172

Cabal, the, 163
Cain, 30–32, 35–36
Campbell, Archibald, Earl of Argyle, 182
Campbell, Lady Agnes, 182. *See* Maitland, Richard
Cardiocentrism, xii
Careless Husband, The (Cibber), 201
Carew, Thomas, 154
Castle, Terry, 205
Catherine of Braganza, 172–73
Ceres, 122
Charles I, 61–65, 71, 77, 80, 171, 179, 181
Charles II, 172–73, 177–79
Charleton, Walter, 123, 186
Charnock, Stephen, 27, 29, 38, 189, 206
Chaucer, Geoffrey, xiv, 86, 194, 216
Childbearing, 30, 32, 197–98
Cibber, Colley, 201
Circumcision, 36–37, 51, 54–55, 200; circumcision of the heart, xv, 37, 51–52, 55, 200
Civil War, English, 41
Clerk's Tale, The (Chaucer), 216
Colonialism, xviii
Congreve, William, 198
Conscious Lovers, The (Steele), 198
Cooper, John, 151
Country Wife, The (Wycherley), 155–56, 161
Cowley, Abraham, 71, 177–78, 200
Creech, Thomas, xvii, 19, 91, 147–49, 153–54, 164
Cromwell, Oliver, 63
Crooke, Helkiah, 7, 8, 11, 12, 13, 22, 66, 81–82, 100, 102, 104–5, 118–19, 193, 200
Cultural studies, xiii, 1
Cupid (cupido), 22, 50, 153

Daphne, 177
David, in Bible, 32, 45–46, 49–50, 151
Davies, Horton, 190
De corde ("Hippocrates"), 3, 20, 199, 206
De generatione animalium (Harvey), 69–70, 71, 79, 82, 86
De motu cordis. *See* Harvey, William
De rerum natura (Lucretius), 11, 19–22, 91, 111, 147–50, 154
De semine (Galen), 81–82
Defoe, Daniel, xvi, 84–85, 122, 190
Delilah, in Bible, 33–34
Democritus, 41

Derrida, Jacques, xiv
Dialogic Imagination, The (Bakhtin), 84–85
Don Quixote (Cervantes), 87
Donne, John, 11, 42
Drake, Francis, 63
Dryden, John, 19, 111, 200, 211
Duffy, Maureen, 153, 172, 181
Dürer, Albrecht, 110
Dutch nation, 168
Dyscrasia. *See* Humors, theory of

Eagleton, Terry, 191
Earth, in *Paradise Lost*, 95, 121, 126–27, 185
Earth, Mother, 138
Eclogues (Virgil), 69
Elijah, 56–57, 68
Elisabeth, in Bible, xvi, 34, 56, 207
Empedocles, 2
Empiricism, early English, xv, 19
Empson, William, 115
Enoch, in Bible, 220–21
Epicureanism. *See* Lucretius
Epistolary novel, 195–96
Erasistratus, 5
Esau, 31–33
Essay Concerning Human Understanding, An (Locke), 159–60, 214–15
Etherege, George (*The Man of Mode*), 155–57
Eucrasia. *See* Humors, theory of
Eve, in Bible, xv, xviii, 27–31, 39, 70, 166, 182, 216. *See also* Milton, *Paradise Lost*
Evelina (Burney), 87
Evelyn, John, 148, 177, 211
Evelyn, Mary, 148, 211
Exercitatio anatomica de motu cordis et sanguinis in animalibus. *See* Harvey, William
Ezer kenegdo, 115

Fabrica (Vesalius), 71
Fabricius ab Aquapendente, 63, 70, 72
Fair Jilt, The (Behn), 158
Fate (and the Fates), xix, 72–74, 173
Feminist theory, xiv
Fielding, Henry, 84
"Flower, The" (Herbert), 17
Foucault, Michel, xiv
Fowler, Alastair, 96, 103, 144
Fracastoro, Girolamo, 72

Frank, Robert G., 68
Frankfurt-am-Main, 63
Freedman, R. David, 115
Freud, Sigmund, xiv
Frye, Northrop, xiv, 95

Galen, xv, 2–12, 16, 18, 20, 22, 31, 51, 68, 70, 78, 80–82, 87, 100, 102, 107, 119, 123, 130, 154, 156–58, 160–61, 186–87, 200, 202; *De semine*, 81–82. *See also* Body; Anatomy; Heart
Gall bladder, 1
Gender, xi, xii, xiii, 18, 26. *See also* Body; Heart; Writing
Generation, literature of, 44–45
Georgics (Virgil), 211
Gildon, Charles, 151
God, in Bible, xv, xvi, xix, 26–58 *passim*; as anatomist, 30, 32, 215–16; as writer/author, 37–41, 43–44, 69; heart of, 26–27; seminal, 28–35; semiotic, 35–44, 78; and "book of life," 44–50. *See also* Milton, John
Gods Anatomy Upon Man's Heart (Watson), 65
Gold Coast, 167
Golden Age, 148
"Golden Age, The" (Behn), 166
Goreau, Angeline, 162
Gould, Robert, 151
Greek medicine and physiology, ancient, 1–11, 18, 20, 36, 52, 100, 199–200, 206
Guffey, George, 171

Hades, 14
Hannah, in Bible, xv, 34–35, 57, 184, 206
Harvey, Christopher, xiv
Harvey, William, xi, xvi, xvii, 8–11, 14, 15, 19, 61–88, 91–92, 95, 99, 106, 111, 119, 147, 177, 187, 192, 200, 206; and the "republick of Literature," 74; as author, 64–71; as anatomist, 63–64, 69–70, 72–73, 77–78; as fate figure, 72–74, 86; as "vitalist," 84; and Aristotle, 70–71; and Galen, 70, 81–82; and "Mistris Antiquity," 70, 73; and witchcraft, 61–63; and the circulation of the blood, 78–82; on book as offspring motif, 66–67, 71; and the novel, 84–88; and ejaculatory na-

270 Index

Harvey, William (*continued*) ture of the heart, 76–78; and erotics of blood circulation, 86; and "nature," 68–71; Works: *De motu cordis*, xvi, 61–88, 98, 100, 181, 191; *De generatione animalium*, 69–70, 71, 79, 82, 86; *Prelectiones*, 66, 68–69

Heart, xi, xii, xiii, 2, 11, 12, 14, 18; and gender/sexuality, xi, xv, xix, 2–11, 12, 13, 15, 21–22, 26, 31–35, 37, 52–60, 71, 73–78, 97–98, 99–103, 113–14, 126, 128, 130–39, 150, 155, 156–59, 170–71, 173–75, 179, 199–216, 224–25; bisexual heart, 11; male heart function, 199–200; female heart function, 206–7; ancient Greek view of, xv, 1–11, 12, 16, 18, 20, 52, 199–200, 206; Platonic model of, 1–2; Aristotelian model of, 2, 3–4; "Hippocratic" model of, 3; Galenic "attractive" model of, 4–11, 15–16, 27, 103, 202; biblical view of (*see* Bible); Lucretian model of, 20–21; Harveian "ejaculatory" model of, 8–11; Hobbesian model of (and recoil effect), 22–24; early modern meanings of, 11; "naked thinking heart," trope of, 11; and heat, 12, 13, 16, 52, 186; and memory, 17; and music, 16; and religion, 16; preparation of, 16; and book/writing motif, xiii, 16–18, 35–52, 64–71, 93–94, 164–65, 172–74, 187–99, 217–28; as *primum sensorium*, 12; as microcosm of body, 14; as fountain, 14–15, 28, 76, 106, 119, 127, 186; as house, 15–16; as ground, 17–18; as king, 65; aural dimension of, 13; quadripartite structure of, 14–16; bipartite structure of, 16–17; caul of, 44; ears of, 41, 77; intelligence in, 3–4, 11–12, 20, 42–43; story of heart motif, 151. *See also* Body; Gender; Bible; and *entries under individual authors*

Heartbeat, 13–14
Heart studies, xiv
Heat, innate, 2, 3, 4, 80–82; heat of God's anger, 54. *See also* Gender
Hedda Gabler (Ibsen), 185
Helen of Troy, 157
Helicon, 96
Hell. *See* Milton, John
Herbert, George, 17

Herophilus, 5
"Hippocrates," 3–5, 7, 14, 20, 199, 206
"Historicized prose fiction," 192
Hobbes, Thomas, 16–17, 22–25, 27–28, 63, 145, 185–86, 188, 200
Hogarth, William, 195
Holy Spirit (Ghost), as writer in the heart, 55–57
Homer, 94
Horace, 66
Howard, Edward, 152
Hoyle, John, 149
Hughes, Merritt, 115
Humoral body. *See* Body
Humors, theory of, 4, 7, 10, 14, 18
Hutchinson, Lucy, 148

Ibsen, Henrik, 185
"Il Penseroso" (Milton), 154
Imago dei, 97, 105, 214
Indians, in *Oroonoko*, 166–68, 179, 182

Jacob/Israel, 30, 32–33, 47, 96, 159
Jael, in Bible, 39
James I, 63
James II, 163, 171–72, 174, 176, 182
Jeffreys, Judge, 182
Jerusalem, 96
Jesus Christ, 15, 24, 52–60, 83, 142–45, 173, 216, 220
Jezebel, in Bible, 15, 39
Johnson, Samuel (*Dictionary*), 165, 190
Jonson, Ben, 140
Jove, 174
Jung, Carl, xiv
"Juniper Tree, The" (Behn), 178

Kardiognostes, 47, 220
Kempis, Thomas à, xix, 221
Kendrick, Daniel, 151
Keuls, Eva, 201
Keynes, Sir Geoffrey, 64
Kidneys, 1
King Lear (Shakespeare), 15, 211
Kroll, Richard, 148

Lacan, Jacques, xiv
Laqueur, Thomas, xiii
Lauderdale, John Maitland, duke of, 163
Law, William, 189, 191
Leviathan (Hobbes), 22, 25

Levite's concubine, in Bible, 39, 181
Lewis, C. S., 103, 113
Libertinism, xvi, xvii, 100–101, 149; characteristics of, 201
Liver (organ), 1, 5, 12, 18
Locke, John, 19, 24, 33, 167, 188, 207, 214–15, 227
Love Letters to a Gentleman (Behn), 156–57
Lovelace, Richard, 200
Lucretius, xii, xvii, 3, 19–23, 25, 28–29, 50–51, 91–92, 101, 116, 135, 147–51, 154–55, 157–58, 161, 164, 166, 167, 180, 184, 199–200, 210
Lungs, 1–3, 12–13, 206
Luther, Martin, 17
"Lycidas" (Milton), 123
"L'Allegro" (Milton), 107, 154

Macbeth (Shakespeare), 121, 132
Magic, 61–63, 95
Maitland, Richard, fourth earl of Lauderdale, 163–64, 172, 182–83
"Marriage of Heaven and Hell, The" (Blake), 191
Martin, George, 172, 179
Mary II (of England), 176
Mary Magdalene, 59–60
Mary of Modena, 172, 174–75
Mary, Virgin, xvi, 56–59, 173–74, 176, 184, 207
Meditations (Richardson), 216–17, 219–20, 223–25, 228
Memoirs of Martinus Scriblerus (Arbuthnot and Pope), xiv
Middle Ages, xiv
Midwife, 73
Midwife books, 118, 125
Mikrokosmographia. *See* Crooke, Helkiah
"Miller's Tale, The" (Chaucer), 11
Milton, John, xvi, xviii, 11, 15, 19, 32, 56, 109, 147–49, 151, 153, 167, 175, 178, 184–85, 191, 194, 203–4, 206, 214–16; on double scripture, 48; and unfallen language, 94; blindness of, 109; and Muse, 93–96, 129; Eve in *Paradise Lost*: xv, xvii, xviii, 3, 13, 39, 63, 75, 89–146 *passim*, 167, 184, 187, 221; creation of, 127–28; as artist, 123–30; as *ezer kenegdo*, 115; heart rhetoric and, xvi–xvii, 89, 93, 99, 117, 127–43; Bower of, 117–20; Nursery of, 120–30; patience of, 144; softness of, 109; and sense of identity, 115–16; and rose symbolism, 125; Adam in *Paradise Lost*: xvii, 75, 89–146 *passim*, 167; heart rhetoric and, 126–27; God in *Paradise Lost*: 69, 90–146 *passim*, 200; sexuality of, 97; heart/bosom of, 141–42; Satan in *Paradise Lost*, xii, xvi, xvii, xix, 4, 23, 63, 71, 76, 89–146 *passim*, 158, 184, 186; as anatomist, 103–4, 119; body of, 101; heart of, 99; and Hell, 113–14; sexuality/phallicism of, 110–13; and gaze upon Eve, 110–17; and classical oration, 132–39; Works: *Paradise Lost*, xi, xviii, 45, 50, 75, 89–146, 147, 159, 174, 191, 218–19; paradise in, 103–10; visual motif in, 91–92, 107; nature in, 106; "L'Allegro," 107, 154; "Il Penseroso," 154; "Lycidas," 123; *Samson Agonistes*, 35
Mirandola, Pico della ("The Dignity of Man"), 19
Miscellanies (Norris), 212
"Mistress Antiquity," 70, 73, 79–80
Moll Flanders (Defoe), 84, 86–87, 163
Monmouth, James Scott, Duke of, 182
Moses, xv, 17, 32, 36, 40–41, 43–44, 52, 68, 173, 176, 197, 212, 226
Mother Midnight, 70
Mother Midnight (Erickson), xii, xiv, 70, 86, 173, 197
Motion, Greek representation of, 2
Mount Horeb, 95
Mount Sinai, 95
Mount Zion, 96
Muses, the, 96

Narrative, as discourse of motion, 85
Natura, 148
Natural philosophy, 19
Nature, xiii, xvi, xviii, 20, 63, 69–71, 73, 80, 126, 148–49, 155, 166, 168, 173, 177; feminized, 2, 4; as machine, 18; Galenic, 30, 68; book of, 69
Neo-Platonism, xviii
Neurocentrism, xii
New Atlantis (Bacon), 68
New Criticism, xiv
New Historicism, xiv
Newton, Sir Isaac, 185–86
Nicolson, Marjorie Hope, 63–64

Norris, John, xviii, 185–87, 211–12, 220–21
Novel, xvi, 84–88, 163
Nymphs, 104–5

"Ode: Upon Dr. Harvey" (Cowley), 71, 177
"On Desire" (Behn), 154, 157–58
Orpheus, 95, 154
Othello (Shakespeare), 119, 211
Otway, Thomas, 211
Ovid, 160

Padua, 63, 66, 74
Pagel, Walter, 73–74
Pamela (Richardson), 87, 122, 167, 197, 223
Passions, the, 12
Pastor, Gail Kern, 10
"Pastoral Pindarick . . . Between Damon and Aminta, A" (Behn), 159
Paul, xvi, 16, 35, 48–49, 67, 94, 129, 160, 191, 226
Penis, 13; Jewish circumcision vs. Christian uncircumcision, 37
Pergamon, 5
Pericardium, 1
Pharoah, in Bible, 40, 51, 53
Philips, Katherine (Orinda), 178
Phillips, Edward, 91
Philosophical Transactions of the Royal Society, 85
Phlebotomy, 7, 18
Picard, Jeremy, 94
Pilgrim's Progress, The (Bunyan), 44, 207
Plantarum (Cowley), 177–78
Plato, 1–2, 12, 15, 20, 186, 199, 206; doctrine of three souls, 4; *Timaeus*, 1, 100
Pneuma, 3, 5, 7, 55, 119
Poe, Edgar Allan, 13
"Poem Humbly Dedicated to . . . Catherine Queen Dowager, A" (Behn), 172–73
Poems on Several Occasions (Behn), 151
Polygamy, 171, 192
Pomona, 122
Pope, Alexander, xiv
Popish Plot, the, 182
Poulet, Georges, xiv
Praecordia, 108, 145, 207
Preface to Paradise Lost, A (Lewis), 103
Prelectiones (Harvey), 66, 68–69
Primum sensorium, 12, 207
Prior, Matthew, 151

Proserpine, 122
Protestantism, xviii, 189, 191
Puritans, xix, xv, 11, 16–17, 27–28, 38, 43–44, 52, 189–92, 193, 195–96, 207–9, 213

Rachel, in Bible, xv, 33, 39, 159, 184
"Ramble in St. James Park, A" (Rochester), 156
Rebekah, in Bible, 32–33, 39, 184
Reign of the Phallus, The (Keuls), 201
Renaissance, the, 19, 63, 86
Republic of literature, 67
Restoration, the, 10–11, 86, 139, 201
Richardson, Samuel, xvi, xix, 15, 22, 32, 56, 84–85, 92, 184, 185–238; and the Bible, 192, 195–97; as Anglican/Puritan, 190–92; as *kardiognostes*, 187–99; Works: *Clarissa*, xi, xvi, xviii, xix, 11, 15, 22, 29, 32, 39, 40, 61, 71, 84, 87, 117, 122, 167, 185–238; and the Bible, 192–93; as representation of Christianity, 189; parental curse motif in, 210–11; allusions to Bible in, 218; gendered heart in, 199–238 *passim*; Lovelace, xix, 22, 32, 40, 190, 192, 223–28; the male heart in, 199–205; the female heart in, 205–28 *passim*; the good heart in, 188, 199, 213–22; rape of Clarissa, 204–5; writing motif in, 215–28; *Pamela*, 87, 122, 167, 197, 223
Riolan, Jean, 63
Robinson Crusoe (Defoe), 84, 86, 166
Rochester, Earl of. *See* Wilmot, John
Roman Catholicism, 182
Romano, Giulio, 111–12
Romantic poets, the, xiv
Rome, 5
Royal College of Physicians, the, 66
Royal Society, the, 85
Rye House Plot, the, 182

Sale, William, 193
Samson Agonistes (Milton), 34
Samson, xv, 33–34, 56–57, 206
Samson's mother, 33, 206
Sappho, 178
Sarai/Sarah, in Bible, xv, 31–32, 39, 47, 184
Satyr Against Mankind, A (Rochester), 214
Sawday, Jonathan, xi
Scarry, Elaine, 40

self, as narrative, 18
"Selinda and Cloris" (Behn), 89
Semele, 174
Sexuality. *See* Body; Gender; Heart
Shakespeare, William, xiv, 15, 17, 106, 113, 119, 121, 132, 157, 163, 211
Sheridan, Richard Brinsley, 140
Sibbes, Richard, 17, 52
Singer, Charles, 64
Smollett, Tobias, 84
Socratic dialogues, 84
Solomon, 50, 96
Soul, xvii, 4, 7; Aristotelian, 4, 7; Galenic, 107; "Corporeal" (Willis), 107–8
South America, 166, 182
South, Robert, 189, 222
Southerne, Thomas, 164
Spectator, The (Addison and Steele), 198
Spenser, Edmund, 86, 194
Spirits: Galenic system of, 4, 119; animal, 4, 119; vital, 4, 80; natural, 4. *See also* Soul
Spirits (angelic), sexuality of, 110–13
Spleen, 1
Sprat, Thomas, 177
Stabat Mater, 176
Steele, Richard, 196
Steele, Sir Richard, 198
Sternberg, Meir, 192–93
Sterne, Laurence, xvi, 84–85
Stoics, the, 20, 199
Stomach, 1
Stuart, House of, 182–83
Surinam, 164, 166, 168
Swift, Jonathan, 192
Sylva (Cowley), 177–79
Sylva (Evelyn), 177–78

Tallemant, Paul, 151, 152, 155
"Tell-Tale Heart" (Poe), 13
Terence, 74
Testicles, 12; male and female, 81–82
Theory and Regulation of Love, The (Norris), 185, 198
Tillotson, John, 189, 196
Timaeus (Plato), 1, 100, 199
"To Lysander at the Musick Meeting" (Behn), 149, 156, 180

Todd, Janet, 177
Tom Jones (Fielding), 87
Tongue, 1
Tristram Shandy (Sterne), 87
Trumbach, Randolph, xiii

Udall, Nicholas, 123
Urania, 93, 95–96
Uterus, 1, 52; Galenic, 3, 13–14; biblical, 30–35, 40, 56–60

Venette, Nicholas, 80
Venice Preserved (Otway), 211
Venus, 148–50, 153, 155
Vesalius, 71
Virgil, 69, 182, 211

Warner, William B., 222
Watson, Thomas, 11, 13, 16, 38, 41, 46–47, 53, 189, 193, 195, 220, 224
Way of the World, The (Congreve), 156, 198
William III and Mary II, 176
Willis, Robert, 63
Willis, Thomas, xvii, 207; on the corporeal soul, 13, 107–8; on the intellect, 108; on the sacred affections, 144–45
Wilmot, John, second earl of Rochester, xvi, 76, 100–101, 139, 149, 155–56, 200–201, 214
Wisdom, in Bible, 96, 129
Witchcraft, 61–63
Wither, George, xiv
Woman, definition of, 162
Womb. *See* Uterus
Wordsworth, William, 61
Writing, xiii, xv, xvi; early forms of, 41; act of, xvii, xviii, 24, 69–70, 83, 93–94; biblical male act of, 35–56; female act of, 151–54, 172–84, 185–228 *passim*. *See also* Heart
Wycherley, William, 155–56, 161

Yeats, William Butler, 185
Yedaiah, Isaac ben, 37
Young, Edward, 189

Zacharias, in Bible, 34, 56–57